Evidence-Based Clinical Practice: Concepts and Approaches

Evidence-Based Clinical Practice: Concepts and Approaches

Edited by

John P. Geyman, M.D.

Professor Emeritus of Family Medicine, University of Washington School
of Medicine, Seattle

Richard A. Deyo, M.D, M.P.H.

Professor of Medicine and of Health Services, University of Washington School
of Medicine and School of Public Health and Community Medicine, Seattle;
Head, Section of General Internal Medicine, University of Washington Medical
Center, Seattle

Scott D. Ramsey, M.D., Ph.D.

Assistant Professor of Internal Medicine, University of Washington School of Medicine, Seattle; Staff Physician, University of Washington Medical Center, Seattle

With 20 Contributing Authors

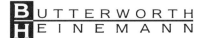

BUTTERWORTH
HEINEMANN

Boston   Oxford   Auckland   Johannesburg   Melbourne   New Delhi

Every effort has been made to ensure that the drug dosage schedules within this text are accurate and conform to standards accepted at time of publication. However, as treatment recommendations vary in the light of continuing research and clinical experience, the reader is advised to verify drug dosage schedules herein with information found on product information sheets. This is especially true in cases of new or infrequently used drugs.

Recognizing the importance of preserving what has been written, Butterworth–Heinemann prints its books on acid-free paper whenever possible.

AMERICAN FORESTS
GLOBAL ReLEAF 2000   Butterworth–Heinemann supports the efforts of American Forests and the Global ReLeaf program in its campaign for the betterment of trees, forests, and our environment.

Library of Congress Cataloging-in-Publication Data

Evidence-based clinical practice : concepts and approaches / [edited
  by] John P. Geyman, Richard A. Deyo, Scott D. Ramsey.
        p.   cm.
    Includes bibliographical references and index.
    ISBN 0-7506-7097-5 (alk. paper)
    1. Evidence-based medicine.   2. Clinical medicine--Decision
making.   I. Geyman, John P., 1931–   .   II. Deyo, Richard A.
III. Ramsey, Scott D.
    [DNLM: 1. Evidence-Based Medicine.   2. Clinical Medicine.
3. Primary Health Care.   WB 102 E927 2000]
RC48.E94   2000
616--dc21
DNLM/DLC
for Library of Congress   99-27097
                                                              CIP

British Library Cataloguing-in-Publication Data
A catalogue record for this book is available from the British Library.

The publisher offers special discounts on bulk orders of this book.
For information, please contact:

Manager of Special Sales
Butterworth–Heinemann
225 Wildwood Avenue
Woburn, MA 01801-2041
Tel: 781-904-2500
Fax: 781-904-2620

For information on all Butterworth–Heinemann publications available,
contact our World Wide Web home page at: http://www.bh.com

10 9 8 7 6 5 4 3 2 1

Printed in the United States of America

Contents

Contributing Authors

Alfred O. Berg, M.D., M.P.H.
Professor and Acting Chair of Family Medicine, University of Washington School of Medicine, Seattle

Edward J. Boyko, M.D., M.P.H.
Professor of Medicine, University of Washington School of Medicine, Seattle; Chief, General Internal Medicine Section, VA Puget Sound Health Care System, Seattle; Director, Epidemiologic Research and Information Center, Seattle

Mick Braddick, M.B., Ch.B.
Clinical Epidemiologist, Department of Provider Education and Guidelines, Group Health Cooperative of Puget Sound, Seattle

Richard A. Deyo, M.D., M.P.H.
Professor of Medicine and of Health Services, University of Washington School of Medicine and School of Public Health and Community Medicine, Seattle; Head, Section of General Internal Medicine, University of Washington Medical Center, Seattle

Sherry Dodson, M.L.S.
Clinical Medical Librarian, Health Sciences Library, University of Washington, Seattle

Mark Ebell, M.D., M.S.
Associate Professor of Family Practice, Michigan State University College of Human Medicine, East Lansing

Joann G. Elmore, M.D., M.P.H.
Associate Professor of Medicine and Adjunct Associate Professor of Epidemiology, University of Washington School of Medicine, Seattle

John P. Geyman, M.D.
Professor Emeritus of Family Medicine, University of Washington School of Medicine, Seattle

Jennifer Hrachovec, R.Ph., M.P.H.
Clinical Epidemiology Fellow, Department of Provider Education and Guidelines, Group Health Cooperative of Puget Sound, Seattle

William F. Miser, M.D., M.A.
Associate Professor of Family Medicine, Ohio State University College of Medicine, Columbus

Douglas S. Paauw, M.D., F.A.C.P.
Associate Professor of Medicine, Division of General Internal Medicine, University of Washington School of Medicine, Seattle; Attending Physician, Department of Medicine, University of Washington Medical Center and Harborview Medical Center, Seattle

Thomas H. Payne, M.D.
Clinical Assistant Professor of Medicine and Health Services, University of Washington School of Medicine, Seattle; Associate Chief Medical Officer for Clinical Information Management and Attending Physician, VA Puget Sound Health Care System, Seattle

Linda E. Pinsky, M.D.
Assistant Professor of Medicine and Adjunct Assistant Professor of Medical Education, University of Washington School of Medicine, Seattle

Scott D. Ramsey, M.D., Ph.D.
Assistant Professor of Internal Medicine, University of Washington School of Medicine, Seattle; Staff Physician, University of Washington Medical Center, Seattle

Sarah Safranek, M.L.I.S.
Information Management Librarian, Health Sciences Library and Information Center, University of Washington, Seattle

Michael E. Stuart, M.D.
Clinical Assistant Professor of Family Medicine, University of Washington School of Medicine, Seattle; Director, Department of Provider Education and Guidelines, Group Health Cooperative of Puget Sound, Seattle

Sean D. Sullivan, Ph.D.
Associate Professor, Department of Pharmacy and Health Services, School of Pharmacy, University of Washington, Seattle

Thomas R. Taylor, M.D., Ph.D., F.R.C.P.
Associate Professor of Family Medicine, University of Washington School of Medicine, Seattle; Attending Physician, Multi-Disciplinary Pain Center, University of Washington Medical Center, Seattle

Joyce E. Wipf, M.D.
Associate Professor of Medicine and Associate Director of Medicine Residency
Program, University of Washington School of Medicine, Seattle; Staff Physician,
University of Washington Medical Center and VA Puget Sound Health Care Sys-
tem, Seattle

Fredric M. Wolf, Ph.D.
Professor and Chair of Medical Education, University of Washington School of
Medicine, Seattle

Preface

The development of evidence-based medicine since the late 1980s has challenged the traditional paradigm of medical education that most practicing physicians experienced during their training. The field has been hailed by some as a fundamental intellectual advance in the process of medical education and practice, while at the same time provoking controversy and resistance by many physicians who dispute the need for this new paradigm. Regardless of the debate around the term, the emergence of evidence-based medicine has been facilitated by the increased emphasis on outcomes research and the availability of electronic databases. It continues to gather increasing interest and applications within the medical community in the United States and abroad. To the extent that this approach has called into question long-held tenets of medical education, this new paradigm has developed debate between its strong proponents and critics, which has led to confusion among many physicians pondering its real value and relevance to their everyday practice.

Although the potential value of evidence-based medicine has yet to be fully demonstrated in practice, the need for such an approach is supported by many lines of logic. Three important examples are: (1) the wide discrepancy from one part of the country to another in treatment modalities for similar problems (e.g., 20-fold differences in utilization rates for carotid endarterectomy); (2) the necessary and unavoidable emphasis on cost containment in medical care; and (3) redefinition of outcomes of care, from physician-oriented to patient-oriented concepts.

This book is derived in large part from an interdisciplinary educational initiative at the University of Washington designed to explore the strengths and limitations of evidence-based medicine in future clinical decision making. We developed six major goals for our monthly Evidence-Based Clinical Practice Rounds, which also serve as the goals for this book:

- Introduce primary care physicians, residents, and medical students to evidence-based medicine as part of clinical decision making
- Enable primary care physicians to more critically read the literature and develop new skills of self-learning
- Prepare primary care physicians and other decision makers in primary care to better evaluate clinical guidelines
- Elucidate complementary roles of clinical judgment and evidence-based approaches in individual practice settings

- Acquaint readers with techniques and limitations of cost and outcomes assessment
- Where appropriate, extend evidence-based approaches beyond care of individual patients to populations being served

The audience for this book includes primary care physicians, residents, fellows, medical students, and others involved in primary care delivery or evaluation of health care services. We have asked contributing authors to provide practical discussions of the concepts of evidence-based medicine and to illustrate them with patient vignettes wherever possible. Our aim is to expand the clinician's understanding of developments in this field, to facilitate the use of evidence-based approaches in education and practice, and to better integrate its applications with the continued importance of clinical experience and judgment.

J.P.G.
R.A.D.
S.D.R.

Chapter 1

Evidence-Based Medicine in Primary Care: An Overview*

John P. Geyman

Case 1

A 2-month-old infant was brought into a rural island clinic at 11:00 PM with a rectal temperature of 104°F. The child was in good health from birth at full term until 2 days previously, when the onset of intermittent fever to 104°F occurred. No vomiting or lethargy was present. Heart rate, blood pressure, and respiratory rate were within normal limits. No rash was present, and the neck was supple. The parents were observant and commented intelligently about the infant's condition. The family did not have health insurance. The last ferry to the mainland left 1 hour earlier. The weather conditions were conducive to flying, but emergency transportation to a hospital cost approximately $2,000.

　　The physician doubted that the child had a life-threatening illness but could not be absolutely sure. He knew that the regional children's hospital 100 miles away had emergency hospital admission protocols for a sepsis workup for infants younger than 3 months. He also knew that acute viral infection was the usual cause of illness, and that most workups had negative findings for serious illnesses. Although his reference books were current, the physician could not determine the risks or benefits of re-examining the child 8 hours later in the office versus having the child flown to the hospital for a sepsis workup. The conscientious parents had the child flown to the mainland for care after talking to a pediatrician there who recommended hospital admission (also without any estimates of risks or benefits). The workup was negative, the family acquired a sizable hospital bill, and the child was doing well without treatment 2 days later.

Case 1 describes a common problem faced almost daily by primary care physicians: how to determine risks and benefits and counsel patients and families about patient care options when needed evidence is either unavailable or unknown. The prevailing system of medical education and the practice of continued learning are not based on rigorous periodic reassessment of evidence for or against particular management options. Journals and textbooks, even those that can be rapidly accessed in the short time required for clinical decision making, are usu-

ally not helpful in determining risks and benefits. The clinician usually relies on his or her clinical experience and judgment, perhaps buttressed by the advice of colleagues or consultants who practice the same way as the clinician.

　　The rise of evidence-based medicine represents a major, but still untested, intellectual advance in clinical decision making and patient care. Evidence-based medicine generates varied reactions among physicians in community and academic settings, ranging from skepticism or outright dismissal to enthusiastic acceptance.

　　Sackett and colleagues[1] defined evidence-based medicine as the "conscientious, explicit and judicious use of current best evidence in making decisions about the care of individual patients." Evidence-based practice requires

*Reprinted with permission from JP Geyman. Evidence-based medicine in primary care: an overview. J Am Board Fam Pract 1998;11:46–56.

Table 1-1. Process of Evidence-Based Medicine

1. Select specific clinical questions from patient's problem(s)
2. Search the literature or databases for relevant clinical information
3. Appraise the evidence for validity and usefulness to the patient and practice
4. Implement useful findings in everyday practice

Source: Adapted from W Rosenberg, A Donald. Evidence-based medicine: an approach to clinical problem-solving. BMJ 1995;310:1122–1126.

the integration of the physician's clinical expertise and judgment with the best available, relevant, external evidence on a patient-by-patient basis. The process of evidence-based medicine is summarized in Table 1-1.

Evidence-based approaches could have clarified the risks and benefits of hospital admission for a sepsis workup in Case 1 and enabled better-informed partnership decision making between the physician and the parents. The physician later undertook a brief literature search that showed that the risks of bacterial meningitis and serious bacterial infection are approximately 0.5% (1 in 200) and 1.5% (3 in 200), respectively.[2,3] A practice guideline, based on meta-analysis, has been formulated for the management of infants with fever without source. The meta-analysis provides solid evidence that supports close ambulatory follow-up of low-risk infants (white blood cell count of 5,000–15,000/μl, band cell count fewer than 1,500/μl, normal urinalysis findings, and fewer than five white blood cells per high-power field in stool when diarrhea is present).[3]

A later study evaluated parent preferences for the care of febrile infants without apparent source. Parents were given a case similar to Case 1 and advised of the risks, outcomes, and costs of close ambulatory follow-up versus hospitalization for lumbar puncture and sepsis workup. Approximately 80% of the parents chose the ambulatory option, which involved less testing and treatment. Many of the parents based this choice on the fact that fewer painful tests and procedures were involved with ambulatory follow-up, the lesser likelihood of their infant receiving unnecessary antibiotics, and the assurance that re-evaluation was available if their child showed no improvement.[4]

The purpose of this book is to explore the dimensions and clinical relevance of evidence-based medicine in everyday primary care practice. More specifically, this book does the following:

1. Introduces readers to the varied problems in the prevailing clinical decision-making system that led to evidence-based medicine as a new paradigm.
2. Enables clinicians in primary care to read the literature more critically and develop new learning skills.
3. Sets forth some basic principles of evidence-based medicine, including introductory consideration of the relative quality of cost and outcome evidence.
4. Summarizes the current status of evidence-based clinical practice in primary care.
5. Provides readers with concrete and practical approaches to integrate the process of evidence-based medicine into their clinical work.

Dimensions of the Problem

Rapid Access to Relevant Information

Case 2 presents only two dimensions of a multifaceted problem facing primary care physicians during their

---

Case 2

A 50-year-old man came to a rural island clinic on a weekend with a finger injury sustained the previous evening while mooring a boat. He was in good health and was enrolled in a large health maintenance organization (HMO) in a metropolitan area 100 miles away. At examination, he had a mallet-finger injury involving the long finger of his right (dominant) hand, with loss of extension of the tip. Radiographs showed no associated fracture.

The physician was aware of the controversy surrounding conservative treatment of this injury using a splint compared with surgical repair but had no accessible evidence to assess critically the merits of both approaches. A telephone conversation with the orthopedic surgeon on call at the urban hospital associated with the patient's HMO resulted in an unequivocal recommendation for conservative treatment ("They usually do fine, and a few patients may need later surgery"). The patient was not entirely happy with this advice and requested a second opinion. Another telephone call was made to the orthopedic surgeon on call at the nearest mainland hospital. His recommendation was equally unequivocal: "Almost all of my patients showed no improvement with splinting treatment and needed surgery." The patient opted for surgery at a considerably higher expense.

encounters with patients who have common medical problems. The biggest problem is obtaining relevant evidence to assist in clinical decision making at the time of the patient's visit. Sometimes this information is available but not readily accessible. A rapid computer search could have been useful, but the physician lacked the time and expertise to perform such a search. The percentage of physicians in active practice who use computers for clinical data retrieval, although increasing, is still relatively low; for example, the American Academy of Family Physicians found that only 26% of U.S. family physicians who have office computers use them for MEDLINE searches.[5]

Without convenient access to appropriate electronic databases, retrieval of relevant and useful information in a timely manner is almost impossible. Most textbooks are dated soon after they are published, and few are grounded in evidence-based practice. Approximately 25,000 medical journals are in print at the time of this publication, and the doubling time of biomedical knowledge, which is currently 19 years, results in a fourfold increase of information within a clinician's career.[6] A physician is fortunate to find one or two useful articles in a journal issue.

Rapidly accessing electronic databases requires new skills and expertise. Given the time constraints in a physician's schedule, the physician is often frustrated by the time required to conduct a literature search. The database of the National Library of Medicine, MEDLINE, has approximately 6 million references from 4,000 journals, with about 400,000 new entries added each year.[7] When rigorous evidence-based criteria are used to screen for clinically credible and useful information in the six most important medical journals, fewer than one article per issue has been judged to be of immediate clinical value.[8] For example, one study of MEDLINE search patterns showed a low yield of useful information after an average search time of more than 20 minutes,[9] whereas another study showed that fewer than 1% of retrieved citations resulted in a new or changed clinical decision.[10]

Global Judgment by Experts

A pervasive problem for primary care physicians attempting to appraise clinical information is the conflicting recommendations by experts. Conflicting recommendations sometimes come from experts within the same specialty, but often they come from experts across specialty lines or who represent various agencies. Many, if not most, of the clinical guidelines are based on global, subjective judgments by experts rather than rigorous criteria for analysis of evidence. Berg[11] has elucidated this lack of rigor after considerable experience evaluating clinical guidelines. Slawson and colleagues[12] have observed the dilemma of "specialist ping-pong" in circumstances of conflicting data and recommendations by specialists; resolution of this problem requires an evidence-based search

for outcome-related data. Part of this problem is caused by the different patient populations seen by specialists and primary care physicians. A classic example was reported in 1980 by Ellenberg and Nelson,[13] who found widely disparate results in studies of nonfebrile seizures among children with previous febrile seizures; rates ranged from 1.5% to 4.6% in population-based studies to 2.6% to 76.9% in seizure clinic studies.

Gap between Evidence and Clinical Practice

Another complex dimension is the translation of solid scientific evidence into clinical practice. Clinicians should be aware of new evidence and be able to appraise the quality of that evidence. This discernment might result in acceptance, skepticism, or rejection of the evidence. If the evidence is accepted, many sequential barriers in the process of patient care can block its implementation. Even with evidence-based clinical guidelines, mismatches frequently occur between the circumstances of clinical trials on which the guidelines are based and actual clinical situations in which physicians encounter patients with a given problem.

Geographic Variations

Since the 1980s, studies have reflected the extreme variations in practice that exist from one part of the country to another and even within a given state. Wennberg[14] found, for example, 20-fold differences in carotid endarterectomy rates in 16 large communities in four states. Within states, he found odds of undergoing tonsillectomy during childhood ranging from 8% in one Vermont community to 70% in another, whereas in Maine, the prevalence of hysterectomy ranged from 20% to more than 70%.[14,15] A study of procedure rates for Medicare patients in 13 large metropolitan areas of the country showed variations of more than 300% for more than one-half of the procedures.[16] The results of another study showed a fourfold variation in adjusted odds ratios for the likelihood of warfarin use for patients with atrial fibrillation in the South compared with patients in the Midwest.[17] All of these examples stretch the boundaries of clinical credibility beyond reasonable variations that are expected based on clinical, demographic, or other geographic differences. These large practice variations call into question scientific truth in each instance; shifting to a more evidence-based style of practice would narrow these variations.

Cost Containment in an Era of Limits

National spending for health care services in the United States continues to rise at a rate higher than the index of inflation. Despite concerted efforts to control health care costs, the proportion of the gross domestic product expended for health care has grown from 5% in 1960 to

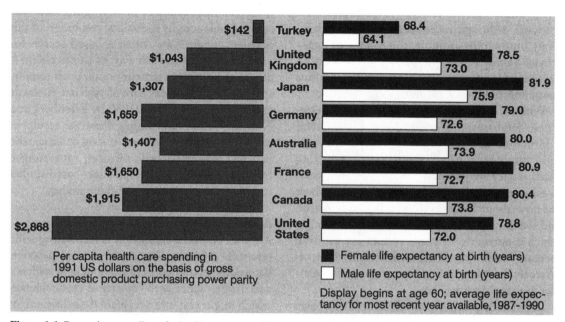

Figure 1-1. Per capita expenditure for health care versus life expectancy by country. (Reprinted with permission from MB Mengel, WL Holleman. Fundamentals of clinical practice: a textbook on the patient, doctor, and society. New York: Plenum, 1997;301. Adapted by Mengel and Holleman from GJ Scheiber, JP Poullier, LM Greenwald. Health spending, delivery, and outcomes in OECD countries. Health Aff [Millwood] 1993;12:122. Reprinted with permission. Copyright © 1993, the People-to-People Health Foundation, Inc. All Rights Reserved. Sources: OECH Health Systems: Facts and Trends. Paris: Organization for Economic Cooperation and Development, 1993; and S Letsch, et al. National health expenditures 1991. Health Care Financing Rev, Winter 1992.)

12% in 1990 to approximately 15% today.[18] This amount of spending represents one-seventh of the national economy.[19] For a family of four with an annual income of $30,000, health care spending has grown to approximately one-third of that income, or $2,500 per person.[15]

Cost containment, now a driving force in health care reform, has ignited a vigorous national debate about alternative ways of structuring and financing health care services and about managed care, value received (i.e., outcomes), and comparative benefits to the individual patient versus the population served. It makes logical and political sense to take an evidence-based approach to evaluating the need for various health care services and procedures based on analysis of costs and outcomes.

Genesis of Evidence-Based Medicine

Many forces are driving the wide application of evidence-based medicine: the need for cost containment felt by the payers of health care services (principally the government and insurance industry); advances in medical informatics that provide increased access to electronic databases, as well as the capacity to monitor practice patterns and outcomes; and continued pressure by patients and industry

to apply the latest therapies. In addition to cost, access to and quality of health care add further momentum to health care system reform efforts. As costs escalate, so does the number of uninsured, now totaling approximately 40 million people.[20] Although the U.S. health care system is touted by many to offer the highest quality of care in the world, outcome statistics, for many reasons, do not demonstrate the best outcomes. Figure 1-1 compares life expectancy and per capita health care spending in eight countries; although U.S. health care spending is nearly three times that of the United Kingdom, longevity is not better in the United States.[21,22]

The term *evidence-based medicine* has elicited confusion and misconceptions among many physicians. Sackett and colleagues[23] observed the following common misconceptions held by physicians in their work with evidence-based medicine:

1. *It's what we've always done.* Because much of medical practice is based on traditional medical education and global subjective judgment without broad access to electronic databases, this view is not well founded.
2. *It will replace clinical judgment.* Even if good external evidence is available, it might not be relevant to the care of an individual patient. More often, external evidence is either insufficient or lacking. Clinical exper-

tise and judgment are essential in everyday clinical decision making.

3. *I don't have time for it.* Lack of time is a major barrier, but continued advances in medical informatics may decrease this problem in the future. Additionally, the physician can now readily access predigested evidence-based analyses of common clinical problems through more efficient reading patterns.
4. *It will lead to "cookbook medicine."* The process of evidence-based medicine requires that physicians assess the quality and relevance of whatever current evidence can be found. In an individual clinical situation, the physician should apply the evidence only as it is appropriate to the patient's needs and preferences.

In their excellent book, *Evidence-Based Medicine: How to Practice and Teach EBM*, Sackett and coauthors[23] propose the following rationale for applying evidence-based medicine to medical education and clinical practice:

1. Increasingly available new evidence can and should lead to major changes in patient care.
2. Practicing physicians often do not obtain available relevant evidence.
3. Medical knowledge and clinical performance deteriorate with time.
4. Traditional continuing medical education (CME) is inefficient and generally does not improve clinical performance.
5. Evidence-based medicine can keep the physician up-to-date.

Conceptual Components and Outcomes of Evidence-Based Medicine

Owing to the growth of clinical research since the 1960s, the increased use of randomized clinical trials and meta-analyses, and the new emphasis on cost and outcome assessment, evidence-based medicine is being hailed as a new paradigm of medical education and practice.[24] Rooted in clinical epidemiology, evidence-based medicine can potentially inform and guide clinical decision making not only for the care of individual patients but also for cost-effectiveness analyses and for health policy for patient populations. The application of evidence-based medicine can thereby help to formulate clinical practice guidelines as summaries of rigorously appraised evidence, pathways of care, and both process- and outcomes-based performance measures of clinical practice. Table 1-2 illustrates the conceptual framework that underpins this and later chapters in this book. Figure 1-2 shows the essential components for making evidence-based clinical decisions in partnership with the patient or family within the context of everyday patient care.[25] Meta-analysis

Table 1-2. Components and Products of Evidence-Based Medicine

Components	Products
Clinical epidemiologic studies	Practice guidelines
Meta-analysis	Pathways of care
Clinical trials	Performance measures
Cost-effectiveness analysis	Process-based
Decision analysis	Outcomes-based

is a powerful tool with both strengths and limitations.[26] Properly applied, it can sort out what we know, what we do not know, and what we need to know.

Practice guidelines have proliferated since the early 1990s, as promulgated by specialty organizations, governmental agencies, and other groups. They have been of variable quality and value, depending largely on the scientific rigor of the process by which they were developed. Many, especially earlier, practice guidelines were produced without an explicit review process through global subjective judgment of an appointed panel of so-called experts. These guidelines are often flawed and not widely accepted. Increasingly, however, more guidelines are available that are evidence-based. The most desirable evidence, if and when available, includes evidence of outcomes and patient preferences, as summarized in Table 1-3.[15]

Eddy[15] proposed the following 11 principles of resource allocation in health care based on the underlying premise that resources for population-based health care are limited financially:

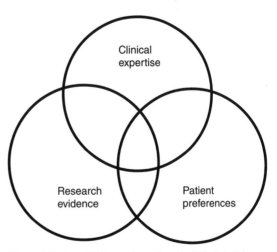

Figure 1-2. A model for evidence-based clinical decisions. (Reprinted with permission from RB Haynes, DL Sackett, JM Gray, et al. Transferring evidence from research into practice: 1. The role of clinical care research evidence in clinical decisions. ACP J Club 1996;125:A14–A16.)

Table 1-3. Hierarchy of Practice Guideline Development

1. Global subjective judgment
2. Evidence-based
3. Outcomes-based
4. Patient preference–based

Source: Adapted with permission from DM Eddy. Clinical Decision Making. From Theory to Practice: A Collection of Essays from JAMA. Boston: Jones & Bartlett Publishers, 1996;30–33.

1. Financial resources to provide health care to a population are limited.
2. It is valid and important to consider financial costs of interventions.
3. Because of financial constraints, priorities must be set.
4. It is not possible to cover from shared resources every treatment that might have some benefit.
5. The objective of health care is to maximize the health of the population served without exceeding available resources.
6. Priority of a treatment should not depend on whether the particular individuals are our personal patients.
7. Priority setting requires estimates of benefits, harms, and costs.
8. Empiric evidence should take priority in assessing benefits, harms, and costs.
9. A treatment must meet three criteria before being promoted for use:
   a. Compared with no treatment, treatment is effective in improving health outcomes.
   b. Compared with no treatment, benefits outweigh harms of outcomes.
   c. Compared with the next best alternative treatment, treatment is a good use of resources for the population served (principle 5).
10. Patient preferences should be sought as much as possible in making judgments of benefits, harms, and costs of a treatment.
11. In determining whether a treatment satisfies principle 9, the burden of proof is on those promoting its use.

These principles may seem obvious and unassailable, but many examples exist to prove that they have not been followed. Electronic fetal monitoring, for example, is widely applied with major impacts on perinatal care without meeting any of the criteria in principle 9.

Present Status of Evidence-Based Practice

Sources for Evidence-Based Medicine

A steadily advancing wave of interest in evidence-based medicine is influencing medical education and clinical practice. Some books and journals are taking an evidence-based approach, as are some CME programs. An increasing number of clinical practice guidelines are being developed through rigorous analysis and appraisal methods. The Agency for Health Care Policy and Research, which has created 19 practice guidelines, is establishing a group of evidence-based practice centers around the country to develop guidelines on a contractual basis.[27] It has also created a national guideline clearinghouse on the Internet, which is now operational.[28] A study of the use of practice guidelines by HMOs showed that 80% used guidelines developed by the HMO, whereas an equal number adapted them from external sources[29]; in many instances, these guidelines were increasingly evidence-based.

Two major types of electronic databases exist. One is bibliographic, such as MEDLINE, which selects relevant citations. The other provides direct access to publications of relevant clinical evidence. Examples of the second type include the *ACP Journal Club*, (a bimonthly supplement of the *Annals of Internal Medicine*), InfoPOEMs (formerly the *Journal of Family Practice* Journal Club), and the Cochrane Database of Systematic Reviews.[30] All are available on the Internet.

In only a few studies was the potential availability of evidence relevant to the wide spectrum of clinical problems in primary care examined. Two such early reports, however, suggest a surprisingly high degree of relevance. In a retrospective study in a suburban training general practice in Leeds, England, 81% of interventions were based on randomized controlled trial evidence or convincing nonexperimental evidence.[31] In another study that examined the treatments provided to 109 consecutive inpatients on a general medical ward in Oxford, England, 82% of treatments were evidence-based (53% with randomized, controlled trial support and 29% with convincing, nonexperimental evidence).[32]

Application of Evidence-Based Medicine in Clinical Practice

Slawson and colleagues[12] have suggested a useful approach that can be used by physicians to gather evidence and appraise its clinical importance. They acknowledged that, given the clinician's shortage of time and overload of information from various sources, clinically useful information must be accessible within the constraints of limited time and be both relevant and valid for the clinician's practice. They combined these variables in a "usefulness equation" (Figure 1-3).

Whatever effort a clinician is making to increase his or her medical knowledge about clinical questions, an initial relevance test concerning the prevalence of clinical problems in practice can help to guide decisions and make reading, attendance at CME conferences, or other CME approaches more efficient. Further critical appraisal of new information is aided by evaluating the usefulness of such

$$\text{Usefulness} = \frac{\text{relevance x validity}}{\text{work}}$$

Figure 1-3. Usefulness equation. (Reprinted with permission from DC Slawson, AF Shaughnessy, JH Bennett. Becoming a medical information master: feeling good about not knowing everything. J Fam Pract 1994;38:505–513.)

information. Slawson and colleagues[12] observed that patient-oriented evidence that matters, in terms of demonstrated positive outcomes important to patients, is far more useful than disease-oriented evidence that represents intermediate outcomes without demonstrable positive outcomes to patients. Table 1-4 displays four clinical illustrations of this important distinction. For example, the knowledge of whether a new therapy decreases mortality, morbidity, or major complications of diabetes mellitus is more useful to the clinician than the knowledge of whether the new therapy merely leads to better control as measured by hemoglobin A_{1c} tests, an intermediate outcome.

Validity assessment can be approached individually or by using validity appraisals established by others. In either event, a clinical study being appraised must be evaluated for internal validity (Are the results valid for patients in the study? Was the study randomized?) and external validity (Can the findings of the study be generalized to one's patient and practice?). Haynes and colleagues[33] developed a "bare-bones users' guide" for appraisal of the validity of clinical studies (Table 1-5).

The process used by the U.S. Preventive Services Task Force[34] serves as an excellent example of an explicitly rigorous application of an evidence-based appraisal of evidence for or against screening and preventive procedures (Table 1-6).

The major problem in practicing evidence-based medicine is finding relevant evidence in a timely way so that it can be integrated into clinical decision making in everyday practice. As electronic databases become more complete and user friendly, this problem should be alleviated. At the time of this publication, the Cochrane Library, for example, has nearly 600 completed systematic reviews on file, with 5,000–10,000 reviews projected by 2002. In addition, this library also has a Database of Abstracts of Reviews of Effectiveness (DARE).[35]

Toward an Evidence-Based Practice

A clinician can take a number of practical, concrete steps toward establishing an evidence-based approach to practice. The following steps are recommended for this initial effort:

1. Subscribe to *Evidence-Based Medicine*, bimonthly structured abstracts with evidence-based commentaries published by the American College of Physicians, Philadelphia (800-523-1546).
2. Increase reading of predigested information relevant to your practice from sources listed in Table 1-7.
3. Refocus reading habits to include sources in the Further Reading list.
4. Join or establish an evidence-based journal club in your area, with hospital staff or in a group practice.

Table 1-4. Examples of Hypothetical Disease-Oriented Evidence (DOE) and Patient-Oriented Evidence That Matters (POEM) Studies

DOE ──► POEM		
Number of Assumptions Required to Assume Patients Will Benefit		
High ──► Low		
Drug A lowers cholesterol	Drug A decreases cardiovascular mortality/morbidity	Decreases overall mortality
PSA screening detects prostate cancer most of the time and at an early stage	PSA screening decreases mortality	PSA screening improves quality of life
Corticosteroid use decreases neutrophil chemotaxis in patients with asthma	Corticosteroid use decreases admissions, length of hospital stay, and symptoms of acute asthma	Corticosteroid use decreases asthma-related mortality
Tight control of type 1 diabetes mellitus can keep fasting blood glucose <140 mg/dl	Tight control of type 1 diabetes can decrease microvascular complications	Tight control of type 1 diabetes can decrease mortality and improve quality of life

PSA = prostate-specific antigen.
Note: Not all POEM trials have been performed.
Source: Adapted from DC Slawson, AF Shaughnessy, JH Bennett. Becoming a medical information master: feeling good about not knowing everything. J Fam Pract 1994;38:505–513.

Table 1-5. Bare-Bones Users' Guides for Appraisal of the Validity of Medical Studies

Purpose of Study	Guides		
Therapy	Concealed, random allocation of patients to comparison groups	Outcome measure of known or probable clinical importance	Few lost to follow-up compared with number of bad outcomes
Diagnosis	Patients to whom you would want to apply the test in practice	Objective or reproducible diagnostic standard applied to all participants	Blinded assessment of test and diagnostic standards
Prognosis	Inception cohort early in the course of the disorder and initially free of the outcome of interest	Objective or reproducible assessment of clinically important outcomes	Few lost to follow-up compared with number of bad outcomes
Cause	Clearly defined comparison group or those at risk for, or having, the outcome of interest	Blinding of observers of outcome to exposure; blinding of observers of exposure to outcome	
Reviews	Explicit criteria for selecting articles and rating validity	Comprehensive search for all relevant articles	

Source: Reprinted with permission from RB Haynes, DL Sackett, JA Gray, et al. Transferring evidence from research into practice: 2. Getting the evidence straight. ACP J Club 1997;126:A14–A16.

Table 1-6. An Evidence-Based Approach to Guideline Development by the U.S. Preventive Services Task Force: Rating the Quality of Evidence and Strength of Recommendations

Quality of evidence
A. Evidence obtained from at least one properly designed randomized controlled trial.
B1. Evidence obtained from well-designed controlled trials without randomization.
B2. Evidence obtained from well-designed cohort or case-control analytic studies, preferably from more than one center or research group.
B3. Evidence obtained from multiple time series with or without the intervention. Dramatic results in uncontrolled experiments (e.g., the results of the introduction of penicillin treatment in the 1940s) could also be regarded as this type of evidence.
C. Opinions of respected authorities, based on clinical experience; descriptive studies or reports of expert committees.

Strength of recommendations
A. Good evidence supports the recommendation that the condition be specifically considered in a periodic health examination.
B. Fair evidence supports the recommendation that the condition be specifically considered in a periodic health examination.
C. Poor evidence exists regarding the inclusion of the condition in the periodic health examination, but recommendations may be made on other grounds.
D. Fair evidence supports the recommendation that the condition be excluded from consideration in a periodic health examination.
E. Good evidence supports the recommendation that the condition be excluded from consideration in a periodic health examination.

Source: Adapted from U.S. Preventive Services Task Force Staff. The Guide to Clinical Preventive Services: Report of the United States Preventive Services Task Force (2nd ed). Philadelphia: Williams & Wilkins, 1996;861–862.

5. Meet with a librarian at your nearest health sciences library to arrange a tutorial or workshop on current search tools, such as MEDLINE.
6. Establish access through an office or home computer to the Internet and the Web sites listed in Table 1-7.
7. Reorient your CME to evidence-based courses as they become more available.

Time is the major limitation faced by the busy primary care physician in the trenches of everyday practice. Targeted reading of predigested evidence-based references, however, can make already allocated reading time more efficient and productive. In addition, as electronic aids to practice become widely available in primary care settings, barriers to evidence-based practice should diminish. As

Table 1-7. Sources of High-Quality Evidence

Source	Description and/or Web Address
Primary (undigested) sources	
MEDLINE	National Library of Medicine database with citations from approximately 4,000 journals dating back to 1966
EMBASE	Derived from *Excerpta Medica*, with some citations in pharmaceutical literature not available in MEDLINE; since 1974
Secondary (predigested sources)	
American College of Physicians, *ACP Journal Club*	*ACP Journal Club* on CD-ROM; http://www.acponline.org
InfoPOEMs (formerly *Journal of Family Practice* Journal Club)	http://www.infopoems.com
Best Evidence	CD-ROM started in 1997 with all first years of *ACP Journal Club* and all of *Evidence-Based Medicine*
Centre for Evidence-Based Medicine	http://cebm.jr2.ox.ac.uk
Cochrane Collaboration	http://hiru.mcmaster.ca/COCHRANE
Bandolier (full text)	http://www.jr2.ox.ac.uk:80/Bandolier
National Guideline Clearinghouse (Agency for Health Care Policy and Research)	http://www.ngc.gov
Physicians' Online	Free MEDLINE access; inexpensive Internet access if signed up; http://www.po.com

Becker[36] observed, the availability of a palmtop computer with comprehensive, current clinical information is already on the immediate horizon.

References

1. Sackett DL, Rosenberg WM, Gray JA, et al. Evidence based medicine: what it is and what it isn't. BMJ 1996;312:71–72.
2. Baraff LJ, Oslund SA, Schriger DL, Stephen ML. Probability of bacterial infections in febrile infants less than three months of age: a meta-analysis. Pediatr Infect Dis J 1992;11:257–264.
3. Baraff LJ, Bass JW, Fleisher GR, et al. Practice guideline for the management of infants and children 0 to 36 months of age with fever without source. Agency for Health Care Policy and Research. Ann Emerg Med 1993;22:1198–1210.
4. Oppenheim PI, Sotiropoulos G, Baraff LJ. Incorporating patient preferences into practice guidelines: management of children with fever without source. Ann Emerg Med 1994;24:836–841.
5. Is anyone using computerized records? Fam Pract Manage 1997;4:96.
6. Wyatt J. Use and sources of medical knowledge. Lancet 1991;338:1368–1373.
7. Arndt KA. Information excess in medicine. Overview, relevance to dermatology, and strategies for coping. Arch Dermatol 1992;128:1249–1256.
8. Haynes RB. Where's the meat in clinical journals? Ann Intern Med 1993;19(Suppl):A22.
9. Haynes RB, McKibbon KA, Walker CJ, et al. Online access to MEDLINE in clinical settings. A study of use and usefulness. Ann Intern Med 1990;112:78–84.
10. Haynes RB, Johnston ME, McKibbon KA, Walker CJ. A randomized controlled trial of a program to enhance clinical use of MEDLINE. Online J Curr Clin Trials 1993;May 11:Doc No. 56.
11. Berg AO. Clinical practice policies: believe only some of what you read. Fam Pract Manage 1996;3:58–70.
12. Slawson DC, Shaughnessy AF, Bennett JH. Becoming a medical information master: feeling good about not knowing everything. J Fam Pract 1994;38:505–513.
13. Ellenberg JH, Nelson KB. Sample selection and the natural history of disease. Studies of febrile seizures. JAMA 1980;243:1337–1340.
14. Wennberg J. Dealing with medical practice variations: a proposal for action. Health Aff (Millwood) 1984;3:6–32.
15. Eddy DM. Clinical Decision Making. From Theory to Practice: A Collection of Essays from JAMA. Boston: Jones & Bartlett Publishers, 1996;5.
16. Chassin MR, Brook RH, Park RE, et al. Variations in the use of medical and surgical services by the Medicare population. N Engl J Med 1986;314:285–290.
17. Stafford RS, Singer DE. National patterns of warfarin use in atrial fibrillation. Arch Intern Med 1996;156:2537–2541.
18. Letsch S, Lazenby HC, Levit KR, Cowan CA. National health expenditures: 1991. Health Care Financ Rev 1991;14:1–30.
19. Burner S, Waldo D. National health expenditure projection, 1994–2005. Health Care Financ Rev 1995;16 (Summer):221–242.
20. U.S. Bureau of the Census. Health insurance coverage:

1995. Current population reports. Washington, DC: Government Printing Office, 1996;60–195.

21. Mengel MB, Holleman WL (eds). Fundamentals of Clinical Practice: A Textbook on the Patient, Doctor, and Society. New York: Plenum Medical Book, 1997;301.

22. Schieber GJ, Poullier JP, Greenwald LM. Health spending, delivery, and outcomes in OECD countries. Health Aff (Millwood) 1993;12:120–129.

23. Sackett DL, Richardson WS, Rosenberg W, Haynes RB. Evidence-Based Medicine: How to Practice and Teach EBM. New York: Churchill Livingstone, 1997;2–16.

24. Evidence-Based Medicine Working Group. Evidence-based medicine. A new approach to teaching the practice of medicine. JAMA 1992;268:2420–2425.

25. Haynes RB, Sackett DL, Gray JA, et al. Transferring evidence from research into practice: 1. The role of clinical care research evidence in clinical decisions. ACP J Club 1996;125:A14–16.

26. Bailar JC III. The promise and problems of meta-analysis. N Engl J Med 1997;337:559–560.

27. Practice Trends. AHCPR moves on. Fam Pract News April 15, 1997;70.

28. Practice beat—practice parameters. Coming soon, a most logical idea: the clearinghouse. Med Economics July 28, 1997;29–33.

29. Rosenberg W, Donald A. Evidence-based medicine: an approach to clinical problem-solving. BMJ 1995;310:1122–1126.

30. Frieden J. Plans push use of evidence-based guidelines. Fam Pract News April 15, 1997;70.

31. Gill P, Dowell AC, Neal RD, et al. Evidence-based general practice: a retrospective study of interventions in one training practice. BMJ 1996;312:819–821.

32. Ellis J, Mulligan I, Rowe J, Sackett DL. Inpatient general medicine is evidence based. Lancet 1995;346:407–410.

33. Haynes RB, Sackett DL, Gray JA, et al. Transferring evidence from research into practice: 2. Getting the evidence straight. ACP J Club 1997;126:A14–A16.

34. U.S. Preventive Services Task Force Staff. The guide to clinical preventive services: report of the United States Preventive Services Task Force (2nd ed). Philadelphia: Williams & Wilkins, 1996;861–862.

35. Bennett JW, Glazious P. Evidence-based practice. What does it really mean? Dis Manage Health Outcomes 1997;1:277–285.

36. Becker LA. Computers for clinical practice—not yet, but soon. J Fam Pract 1997;45:127–128.

Further Reading

Articles

Information Mastery

Shaughnessy AF, Slawson DC, Bennett JH. Becoming an information master: a guidebook to the medical information jungle. J Fam Pract 1994;39:489–499.

Critical Appraisal of Literature

Drummond MF, Richardson WS, O'Brien BJ, et al. Users' guides to the medical literature. XIII: How to use an article on economic analysis of clinical practice. A. Are the results of the study valid? Evidence-Based Medicine Working Group. JAMA 1997;277:1552–1557.

Fletcher RH, Fletcher SW. Evidence-based approach to the medical literature. J Gen Intern Med 1997;12(Suppl 2):S5–S14.

Greenhalgh J. How to read a paper. The MEDLINE database. BMJ 1997;315:180–183.

Guyatt GH, Naylor CD, Juniper E, et al. Users' guides to the medical literature. XII: How to use articles about health-related quality of life. Evidence-Based Medicine Working Group. JAMA 1997;277:1232–1237.

Guyatt GH, Sackett DL, Cook DJ. Users' guides to the medical literature. II: How to use an article about therapy or prevention. A. Are the results of the study valid? Evidence-Based Medicine Working Group. JAMA 1993;270:2598–2601.

Guyatt GH, Sackett DL, Sinclair JC, et al. Users' guides to the medical literature. IX: A method for grading health care recommendations. Evidence-Based Medicine Working Group. JAMA 1995;274:1800–1804.

Haynes RB, Wilczynski N, McKibbon KA, et al. Developing optimal search strategies for detecting clinically sound studies in MEDLINE. J Am Med Inform Assoc 1994;1:447–458.

Jaeschke R, Guyatt G, Sackett DL. Users' guides to the medical literature. III: How to use an article about a diagnostic test. A. Are the results of the study valid? Evidence-Based Medicine Working Group. JAMA 1994;271:389–391.

Jaeschke R, Guyatt GH, Sackett DL. Users' guides to the medical literature. III. How to use an article about a diagnostic test. B. What are the results and will they help me in caring for my patients? Evidence-Based Medicine Working Group. JAMA 1994;271:703–707.

Laupacis A, Wells G, Richardson WS, Tugwell P. Users' guides to the medical literature. V: How to use an article about prognosis. Evidence-Based Medicine Working Group. JAMA 1994;272:234–237.

Levine M, Walter S, Lee H, et al. Users' guides to the medical literature. IV: How to use an article about harm. Evidence-Based Medicine Working Group. JAMA 1994;271:1615–1619.

Naylor CD, Guyatt GH. Users' guides to the medical literature. X: How to use an article reporting variations in the outcomes of health services. Evidence-Based Medicine Working Group. JAMA 1996;275:554–558.

Naylor CD, Guyatt GH. Users' guides to the medical literature. XI: How to use an article about a clinical utilization review. Evidence-Based Medicine Working Group. JAMA 1996;275:1435–1439.

O'Brien BJ, Heyland D, Richardson WS, et al. Users' guides to the medical literature. XIII: How to use an article on economic analysis of clinical practice. B. What are the results and will they help me in caring for my patients?

Evidence-Based Medicine Working Group. JAMA 1997;277:1802–1806.

Oxman AD, Cook DJ, Guyatt GH. Users' guides to the medical literature. VI: How to use an overview. Evidence-Based Medicine Working Group. JAMA 1994;272:1367–1371.

Oxman AD, Sackett DL, Guyatt GH. Users' guides to the medical literature. I: How to get started. Evidence-Based Medicine Working Group. JAMA 1993;270:2093–2095.

Richardson WS, Detsky AS. Users' guides to the medical literature. VII: How to use a clinical decision analysis. A. Are the results of the study valid? Evidence-Based Medicine Working Group. JAMA 1995;273:1292–1295.

Shaughnessy AF, Slawson DC. Getting the most from review articles: a guide for readers and writers. Am Fam Physician 1997;55:2155–2160.

Wilson MC, Hayward RS, Tunis SR, et al. Users' guides to the medical literature. VIII: How to use clinical practice guidelines. B. What are the recommendations and will they help you in caring for your patients? Evidence-Based Medicine Working Group. JAMA 1995;274:1630–1632.

Internet Resources

Anthes DL, Berry RE, Lanning A. Internet resources for family physicians. Can Fam Physician 1997;43:1104–1113.

Gagne J. Netview. Med Software Rev 1997;May:9–10.

Books

Goroll AH, May LA, Mulley AG Jr (eds). Primary Care Medicine: Office Evaluation and Management of the Adult Patient (3rd ed). Philadelphia: JB Lippincott, 1995.

Panzer RJ, Black ER, Griner PF (eds). Diagnostic Strategies for Common Medical Problems. Philadelphia: American College of Physicians, 1991.

Pareras LG. Medicine and the Internet: Reference Guide. Philadelphia: Lippincott–Raven, 1996.

Sackett DL, Haynes RB, Tugwell P. Clinical Epidemiology: A Basic Science for Clinical Medicine (2nd ed). Philadelphia: Lippincott–Raven, 1991.

Chapter 2

Did We Learn Evidence-Based Medicine in Medical School? Some Common Medical Mythology*

Douglas S. Paauw

Despite the advances in medicine occurring daily, physicians are slow to change their practices. Many interventions have been studied, including continuing medical education courses, computerized reminder systems, printed monographs, and continuing medical education home reading materials.[1,2] The most common forms of updating information, continuing medical education courses and home reading materials, have little impact on changing professional practices.[1,2] Physicians rely on a core knowledge base acquired in medical school and through subsequent experiential learning. Much of what is practiced and taught in medicine is based on plausible theory, but in some cases, no direct evidence supports it. Some practices are "grandfathered" in without anyone questioning the validity of what is being taught or practiced.

The purpose of this chapter is to look at several medical myths and explore available literature to counter or offer alternatives to long-held beliefs.

Methods

A MEDLINE search for relevant English-language articles published between January 1976 and July 1998 was conducted using a search for the following terms or combination of terms: myths, oral vitamin B_{12} replacement, eye patch and corneal abrasion, adverse effects of beta blockers, beta blockers and hypoglycemia, beta blockers and depression, insulin sliding scale, and narcotics and abdominal pain. Relevant articles and bibliographies were reviewed to identify articles published before 1976 as well as to identify other articles not included in the original search.

*Reprinted with permission from DS Paauw. Did we learn evidence-based medicine in medical school? Some common medical mythology. J Am Board Fam Pract 1999;12:143–149.

Some Common Medical Myths

Myth 1: Replacement of Vitamin B_{12} Deficiency Owing to Pernicious Anemia Must Not Be Done Orally

The classic teaching in medical school is that vitamin B_{12} deficiency in patients with pernicious anemia is due to poor vitamin B_{12} absorption, owing to a lack of intrinsic factor, and that replacement must be given intramuscularly. This belief was presented in the following statement of the *United States Pharmacopeia* Anti-Anemia Preparations Advisory Board: "In the management of a disease for which parenteral therapy with vitamin B_{12} is a completely adequate and wholly reliable form of therapy, it is unwise to use a type of treatment which is, at best, unpredictably effective."[3] Studies in the 1950s showed that vitamin B_{12} can be absorbed orally in patients with pernicious anemia and that two mechanisms of absorption of vitamin B_{12} exist: one that involves intrinsic factor and one that does not.[4] Several studies showed that oral replacement with vitamin B_{12} can lead to resolution of the anemia.[5–8] When the doses of oral B_{12} were less than 300 mcg daily, serum levels were usually not in the normal range.[5,7] Normalization of serum levels was readily achievable when patients received 300–1,000 mcg of vitamin B_{12} daily.[5,6] In one study, 64 patients receiving 500 or 1,000 mg of vitamin B_{12} orally daily for pernicious anemia all had normal serum vitamin B_{12} levels, normalization of hemoglobins, and no neurologic complications at follow-up after 5 years.[6] Oral replacement of vitamin B_{12} with 1,000 mg daily keeps bodily stores of vitamin B_{12} as adequately filled as intramuscular delivery.[9] In another study, 33 patients were randomized to receive oral cobalamin, 2,000 µg daily or 1,000 µg intramuscularly on days 1, 3, 7, 10, 14, 21, 30, 60, and 90.[10] The oral

---

Case 1

An 84-year-old woman was seen in a clinic for weakness and fatigue. Physical examination revealed a normal mental status and evidence of bilateral lower extremity neuropathy. Her hematocrit was 23, with a hemoglobin of 7.3 g/liter and a mean corpuscular volume of 117. Serum cobalamin level was 80 (Nl >200), and urinary methylmalonic acid level was high. A Schilling test was abnormal and corrected with addition of intrinsic factor, indicating pernicious anemia. She was given loading doses of hydroxocobalamin intramuscularly and told she needed a monthly injection of hydroxocobalamin to manage her disease.

---

treatment group had higher serum vitamin B_{12} levels, lower serum methylmalonic acid levels, and correction of all hematologic and neurologic abnormalities.

The cost of oral and parenteral vitamin B_{12} replacement is comparable. The cost of 100 tablets of 1,000 mcg of vitamin B_{12} is less than $10. Thirty doses of vitamin B_{12} for injection is also less than $10, but charges for administration either by clinic personnel or a visiting nurse dramatically increase the monthly cost. If the patient is able to give himself or herself the vitamin B_{12} injection, the additional cost is the cost of the monthly syringe, needle, and alcohol wipes.

Why is oral vitamin B_{12} not widely used for replacement? Most physicians do not believe that vitamin B_{12} can be replaced orally. In a 1991 survey of internists, 94% were not aware of an available, effective oral therapy for vitamin B_{12} replacement.[11] In the same survey, 88% of the internists stated that an oral replacement form of vitamin B_{12} would be useful in their practice. This same study was repeated in 1996, with 73% of internists surveyed not aware of an effective oral therapy for vitamin B_{12} replacement.[12]

This myth combines several features seen in medical myths. It makes some sense from a pathophysiologic standpoint: Vitamin B_{12} requires intrinsic factor; if one does not have intrinsic factor, how does one absorb vitamin B_{12}? The studies that refuted the myth were published at a time (1960s) when oral vitamin B_{12} was not available in the United States, so oral replacement was not standard practice. Finally, the earliest studies on oral vitamin B_{12} replacement using low doses of vitamin B_{12} were failures.

Myth 2: Patching the Eye Improves Comfort and Healing in Patients with Corneal Abrasions

The traditional treatment for corneal abrasions is to apply a firm eye patch for several days.[13] This standard approach is not based on any evidence of benefit of healing or decreased pain. A study in 1960 evaluated differences in healing of corneal abrasions in patients with an eye pad compared with patients without an eye pad.[14] No differences were seen in healing, and the author concluded that simple corneal abrasions should be treated without an eye pad.[14] Several more recent studies have supported the recommendation to avoid patching the eye in patients with simple corneal abrasions.[15–17] The largest of these studies involved 201 patients with corneal abrasions.[16] The patients who did not receive an eye patch had less pain and faster healing of the corneal abrasions.

No human studies were done to support the initial use of eye patches for the treatment of corneal abrasions. The first study questioning this practice, published in 1960, showed no benefit of eye patching. Despite evidence to the contrary, eye patching continued to be the standard of care for treatment of corneal abrasions and still is a common treatment offered for patients with corneal abrasion.[18]

Myth 3: Patients with Diabetes Are at Increased Risk for Hypoglycemic Unawareness if on a Beta Blocker

This patient with diabetes meets treatment guidelines for pharmacologic therapy for his hypertension. A beta blocker would offer both antihypertensive treatment and a cardio-

---

Case 2

A 26-year-old man was evaluated for right eye pain. He was poked in the eye while playing basketball. He described considerable right eye discomfort but no visual changes. On examination with sodium fluorescein, he had evidence of a corneal abrasion. He was instructed to wear an eye patch over the right eye for the next 48 hours.

Case 3

A 48-year-old man with Type 1 diabetes presented for primary care. He had a history of gout, hypertension, and coronary artery disease, and he experienced a myocardial infarction 9 months ago. He was treated with lisinopril for his hypertension, but this was stopped 2 months later because of the development of angioedema. On examination, he had a blood pressure of 160/95 and pulse of 80; on eye examination he had nonproliferative retinopathy in both eyes and bilateral neuropathy in both lower extremities. He was started on diltiazem hydrochloride for his hypertension.

---

protective benefit after a myocardial infarction. Concern about the side effects of beta blockers limits their use despite clear evidence of benefit. In the Cardiac Arrhythmia Suppression Trial study,[19] 50% of the patients received a calcium channel blocker after a myocardial infarction compared with approximately 30% receiving a beta blocker. The cardiovascular benefit of beta blockers in patients with diabetes who have had a myocardial infarction is striking. The mortality benefit in individuals with diabetes treated with a beta blocker after a myocardial infarction is 48%, with a 78% decrease in reinfarction.[20]

In patients with insulin-treated diabetes, a concern exists that the use of beta blockers reduces or eliminates the warning symptoms of hypoglycemia. This concern was addressed by Barnett and colleagues in a prospective study of 150 insulin-treated diabetics.[21] Fifty insulin-treated patients taking beta blockers were compared with 100 insulin-treated diabetics not on beta blockers. The patients kept a diary recording all episodes of hypoglycemia and all warning symptoms. The incidence of loss of consciousness from hypoglycemia was the same in both groups and was not related to the dose of beta blocker given. All symptoms of hypoglycemia were similar in both groups, with the exception of diaphoresis, which was more common in the beta blocker group. In another study, patients with diabetes on beta blockers were given insulin infusions to decrease blood sugar, and symptoms were recorded. The patients on beta blockers did not have hypoglycemic unawareness. They did have adrenergic symptoms at lower blood glucose levels than

the diabetic controls not on beta blockers, but their overall symptom scores were higher because of an increased perception of diaphoresis in the beta blocker–treated patients.[22] In one retrospective cohort study, more than 13,000 patients with diabetes treated with either oral hypoglycemics or insulin were studied to determine whether antihypertensive agents predisposed patients to serious hypoglycemic events. No class of antihypotensive medication (including beta blockers) was found to predispose treated patients with diabetes to serious hypoglycemic events.[23]

Myth 4: Beta Blockers Are an Important Cause of Depression

Early reports of possible beta blocker–induced depression surfaced soon after the beta blocker propranolol became available in the 1960s. A frequently cited reference is a letter to the *British Medical Journal* in which Waal reported that 20 of 89 patients on propranolol volunteered or exhibited depressive symptoms.[24] Forty percent of these patients were classified as having grade I depression symptoms of irritability, insomnia, nightmares, and fatigue. No control group of patients was evaluated to ascertain the prevalence of these symptoms in patients treated with other antihypertensives or in nonhypertensive patients. Pollack and colleagues reported on a series of three patients who developed symptoms of depression after starting propranolol and concluded that depression after the administration of propranolol was a real phenomenon.[25]

Case 4

A 67-year-old man was admitted to a clinic with severe chest pain, and a diagnosis of an acute inferior myocardial infarction was made. He underwent coronary artery catheterization and had significant atherosclerotic disease in his left anterior descending and right coronary arteries. He was started on atenolol, simvastatin, aspirin, and nitroglycerin (as needed). Three months after the infarct, he returned for a clinic visit with symptoms of insomnia, difficulty concentrating, feelings of worthlessness, and fatigue. He had no history of depression. He was tapered off atenolol and started on sertraline hydrochloride.

Case 5

A 33-year-old man presented to the emergency department with acute abdominal pain. He had the sudden onset of pain in the middle of his abdomen approximately 2 hours earlier. The pain was worse with movement, particularly during the car ride to the hospital. He recently injured his leg snowboarding and was taking a large amount of aspirin to relieve the pain. On examination, the patient had a rigid abdomen with tenderness on palpation. He asked for pain medication but was told he needed to be evaluated by the surgeon before medication would be considered.

A number of studies have concluded that the prevalence of depression in patients on beta blockers is not increased.[26–31] Schleifer and colleagues evaluated 190 patients who sustained a myocardial infarction for evidence of depression. The patients were interviewed 8–10 days after the infarct and again at 3 months. No antianginal or antihypertensive medications, including beta blockers, were associated with an increase in depression.[26] Carney et al.[27] evaluated 75 patients undergoing elective cardiac catheterization using psychiatric interview and psychological assessments. One-half of the patients in the study were receiving beta blockers. Thirty-three percent of the patients who were not receiving beta blockers met the *Diagnostic and Statistical Manual of Mental Disorders*, Third Edition, criteria for depression, and 21% of the beta blocker–treated patients met criteria for depression. In a study of depression in new users of antihypertensive medications using the Harvard Community Health Plan medication registry, the rates of depression were no higher in beta blocker users than in users of other antihypertensives.[29] Thiessen and colleagues studied the rates of antidepressant prescriptions after beta blocker prescriptions using the records of the Saskatchewan prescription drug plan.[30] Their study found that 6.4% of beta blocker users received a prescription for an antidepressant within 30 days of receiving a beta blocker prescription compared with 2.8% of the reference group. A similar study design by Hallas et al.[32] showed no increase in antidepressant prescribing after patients received a beta blocker.

Much concern about the possibility that beta blockers could cause depression was generated by early case reports and subsequent case series, none of which evaluated the prevalence of depression in a control group. Confounding the issue is the side effect of fatigue, which is frequently reported in patients on beta blockers.[33] Patients may be incorrectly diagnosed with depression if fatigue is the only depressive symptom present. Depression after major medical illness, such as a myocardial infarction, is common. As several studies have shown,[26,27] depression is common in patients with coronary artery disease regardless of the medications they are taking. No large, controlled prospective trials have addressed the issue of depression in beta blocker users. The beneficial effects of beta blockers should not be overlooked in patients with a history of depression, as the small possibility of a depressive effect due to the beta blocker may be outweighed by the beneficial effect of the beta blocker.

Myth 5: Giving Narcotics to a Patient with a Possible Acute Abdomen May Mask the Signs and Make It Difficult to Make a Diagnosis

Standard teaching in medical school is to withhold narcotics from patients with possible acute abdomen syndromes because the narcotic may mask important signs and delay or prevent an accurate diagnosis. *Cope's Early Diagnosis of the Acute Abdomen*, a book read by most medical students, has endorsed this position. This quote appeared in the fifteenth edition: "If morphine be given, it is possible for a patient to die happy in the belief that he is on the road to recovery, and in some cases the medical attendant may for a time be induced to share the elusive hope."[34] An even stronger position was taken in the next edition of *Cope's* text: "The patient cried out for relief, the relatives are insistent that something should be done, and the humane disciple of Aesculapius may think it is his first duty to diminish or banish the too obvious agony by administering a narcotic. Such a policy is a mistake. Though it may appear cruel, it is really kind to withhold morphine until a reasonable diagnosis has been made."[35]

No controlled trials ever questioned this long-held belief until a study done by Attard et al., which was published in 1992.[36] In this study, 100 patients were evaluated by the admitting officers at one hospital and given either a narcotic intramuscularly or saline intramuscularly. Surgeons who subsequently followed the patients felt equally confident in diagnosis and management of both groups. The decision to operate or observe was incorrect in two patients in the narcotic group and nine in the saline group. Another study,[37] which used intravenous morphine or placebo in 71 patients for the treatment of acute abdominal pain, found no difference in the accuracy of diagnosis between groups. Three diagnostic or management errors were made in each group. Myth 5 has been spread both through the use of a well-respected text

---

Case 6

A 58-year-old woman with Type 2 diabetes was admitted to the hospital for treatment of a diabetic foot ulcer. She noticed increasing blood sugars over the past week as her ulcer worsened. Her other medical problems included coronary artery disease with a history of a myocardial infarction 2 years ago and a history of hypertension. Her medications included isosorbide dinitrate, 20 mg orally three times daily; enalapril, 10 mg orally every morning; enteric coated aspirin, 325 mg daily; and glyburide, 10 mg orally twice daily. Laboratory workups on admission provided the following results: Na, 130 mEq/liter; K, 3.8 mmol/liter; Cl, 98 mmol/liter; HCO_3, 24 mEq/liter; and glucose, 440 mmol/liter. She was treated with intravenous ampicillin sulbactam for her foot ulcer and started on a sliding-scale insulin regimen for management of her diabetes.

---

and by surgical dogma. The hypothesis made some sense, so it was not tested for many years. Now, with two placebo-controlled trials showing no harm with pain control, practices may start to change, although such change will be slow for a belief held for several generations.

Myth 6: Sliding-Scale Insulin Therapy Is Effective and Appropriate Therapy for Managing Diabetes in Hospitalized Patients

Most training in the management of diabetes mellitus in the United States takes place during medical school and residency in the inpatient setting. The use of sliding-scale insulin injections is a commonly used management strategy for hospitalized inpatients.[38,39] In a study of medical inpatients, physicians prescribed a sliding scale for 61% of 218 patients with a history of diabetes who were admitted to the hospital for reasons other than metabolic control.[40] It is not clear how this practice began; no studies show benefit of the sliding-scale approach to diabetes management. It is firmly entrenched as a popular method of "cookbook medicine," usually learned during residency training.[38] Initial sliding scales gave insulin based on urine glucose levels, whereas current sliding scales give insulin based on regularly obtained fingerstick glucose values, usually obtained at 4- to 6-hour intervals. Problems with this approach include giving insulin retrospectively for high blood glucose levels and not giving insulin when the patient achieves euglycemia, regardless of caloric intake. Insulin is not given in anticipation of rising blood glucose levels with meals. Patients frequently receive blood glucose monitoring at bedtime or even during the night when no food intake occurs. Treating elevated evening blood glucose levels with regular insulin increases the risk of hypoglycemic episodes while the patient is asleep and less likely to be able to call for assistance.

Several studies have evaluated the efficacy of sliding-scale insulin therapy. Gearheart and colleagues evaluated outcomes of patients admitted for treatment of diabetic ketoacidosis.[41] Insulin therapy was categorized as sliding scale, proactive (prospective regimen of insulin in anticipation of glucose levels), or combination (routine insulin ordered with an additional sliding scale). Patients treated with sliding-scale insulin had higher median glucose values than the other two regimens. The patients who received the proactive regimen were hospitalized for fewer than the combination and sliding-scale groups (4.4 vs. 6.3 vs. 6.3 days, respectively). MacMillan found similar problems with sliding-scale insulin.[42] In a retrospective study of children admitted to a hospital with diabetic ketoacidosis, the group that received sliding-scale insulin had a longer duration of ketosis and worse glucose control than children who received long-acting insulin. In one study, Queale et al. reviewed the diabetes management of 171 hospitalized patients with diabetes.[43] One hundred thirty of the patients were placed on sliding-scale insulin regimens. When used alone (i.e., without long-acting insulin), the sliding-scale insulin regimens were associated with a threefold higher risk of hyperglycemic episodes compared with patients who received no pharmacologic regimen. This study also touches on other problems with sliding-scale insulin regimens, namely, that they are rarely modified and that one size fits all. Patients at highest risk in this study for hypoglycemia were men with low body weight and individuals with low serum albumin levels. The sliding-scale regimen written on admission to the hospital was rarely modified during the hospitalization.[43]

Alternatives to sliding-scale insulin for management of the hospitalized patient with diabetes include intravenous insulin drips in the patient who is not able to eat or long-acting daily insulin with pre-meal adjustments in regular insulin dosing based on an insulin algorithm.[44] Algorithms differ from sliding scales in that they are connected to meal times, taking into account calorie load and activity level.[44,45] A key factor in safely giving insulin in the hospital setting is checking blood glucose levels around meal time and making any adjustment to short-acting insulin doses based on both premeal glucose level and anticipated caloric intake.

Why did sliding-scale insulin use become such a wide-spread practice? It simplifies diabetes management into a simple, easy-to-remember formula. This is probably the reason it has endured despite a lack of evidence in the literature to support its use. It allows preordered insulin doses to be given automatically, based on serum glucose monitoring, without interrupting the physician for intermittent insulin orders. The few studies published suggest that it is an inferior management choice compared with longer-acting insulin or intravenous insulin infusions.

Summary

Medical myths occur for many different reasons. A common thread is that they all make some pathophysiologic sense. A good example of this is the concern for use of oral cobalamin in the treatment of pernicious anemia. The difficulty in absorbing vitamin B_{12} when intrinsic factor is not available does not make oral replacement impossible; the dose should be higher. Pathophysiologic concerns have also been a key reason for avoidance of beta blocker use in patients with diabetes. The fear is that beta blockers will block adrenergic symptoms and patients will not know when they are hypoglycemic. Studies addressing this issue found no problems with increased severe episodes of hypoglycemia in patients on beta blockers or increased hypoglycemic unawareness. Several researchers commented on the unanticipated symptom of increased sweating associated with hypoglycemia in patients with diabetes on beta blockers. Another important concept behind some medical myths is the over-reliance on case reports or authoritative text. The concern for depression associated with beta blocker use grew out of one widely referenced case report.[24] Subsequent studies have not provided convincing evidence for a strong association with beta blocker use and depression. The strong position taken against narcotic use in *Cope's Early Diagnosis of the Acute Abdomen* is probably the reason for the perpetuation of the practice of avoiding narcotics for pain relief in patients with undiagnosed acute abdominal conditions. The only two studies addressing this issue showed no problems with diagnosis caused by providing narcotic pain relief.[31,32]

Newer therapies usually undergo closer scrutiny before being accepted. This often includes placebo-controlled trials to show the efficacy of a medication. This may not be the case with newer technologies. It is harder to evaluate the benefit of a technology against noncomparable, older technologies. Right heart catheterization (Swan-Ganz catheter) was a technology that was widely used before any outcome studies became available. Multiple reports since the late 1980s have shown increased mortality and increased use of resources in patients who received right heart catheterization.[46,47] Most new drug therapies require randomized data to show effects before wide-spread use and acceptance occur. Older, widely accepted therapies may not be backed by controlled-trial data, and change is difficult once practice patterns are widespread.

Physicians should ask the question "Will this help my patient live better or longer?" when prescribing a therapy. These myths underscore the importance and usefulness of outcome-based research to guide physicians in their practices.

References

1. Davis DA, Thomson MA, Oxman AD, Haynes RB. Changing physicians performance. A systemic review of the effect of continuing medical education strategies. JAMA 1995;274:700–705.
2. Evans CE, Haynes RB, Birkett NJ, et al. Does a mailed continuing medical education program improve physician performance? JAMA 1986;255:501–504.
3. Bethell FH, Castle WB, Conley CL, London IM. Present status of treatment of pernicious anemia: ninth announcement of USP Anti-Anemia Preparations Advisory Board. JAMA 1959;171:2092–2094.
4. Doscherholmen A, Hagen PS. A dual mechanism of vitamin B_{12} plasma absorption. J Clin Invest 1957;36:1551–1557.
5. Brody EA, Estren S, Wasserman LR. Treatment of pernicious anemia by oral administration of vitamin B_{12} without added intrinsic factor. N Engl J Med 1959;260:361–367.
6. Berlin H, Berlin R, Brante G. Oral treatment of pernicious anemia with high doses of vitamin B_{12} without intrinsic factor. Acta Med Scand 1968;184:247–258.
7. McIntyre PA, Hahn R, Masters JM, Krevans JR. Treatment of pernicious anemia with orally administered cyanocobalamin (vitamin B_{12}). Arch Intern Med 1960;106:280–292.
8. Waife SO, Jansen CJ, Crabtree RE, et al. Oral vitamin B_{12} without intrinsic factor in the treatment of pernicious anemia. Ann Intern Med 1963;58:810–817.
9. Berlin R, Berlin H, Brante G, Pilbrant A. Vitamin B_{12} body stores during oral and parenteral treatment of pernicious anaemia. Acta Med Scand 1978;204:81–84.
10. Kuzminsk AM, Del Giacco EJ, Allen RH, et al. Effective treatment of cobalamin deficiency with oral cobalamin. Blood 1998;92:1191–1198.
11. Lederle FA. Oral cobalamin for pernicious anemia. Medicine's best kept secret? JAMA 1991;265:94–95.
12. Lederle FA. Oral cobalamin for pernicious anemia: back from the verge of extinction. J Am Geriatr Soc 1998;46:1125–1127.
13. Pousada L. Emergency Medicine. Baltimore: Williams & Wilkins, 1989.
14. Jackson H. Effect of eye pads in healing of simple corneal abrasions. BMJ 1960;2:713.
15. Hurlbert MF. Efficacy of eyepad in corneal healing after corneal foreign body removal. Lancet 1991;337:643.

16. Kaiser PK. A comparison of pressure patching versus no patching for corneal abrasions due to trauma of foreign body removal. Ophthalmology 1995;102:1936–1942.

17. Kirkpatrick JN, Hoh HB, Cook SD. No eye pad for corneal abrasions. Eye 1993;7:468–471.

18. Hardwood Nuss AC. Eye Trauma in the Clinical Practice of Emergency Medicine. Philadelphia: Lippincott–Raven, 1996.

19. The Cardiac Arrhythmia Suppression Trial (CAST) Investigators. Preliminary report: effect of encainide and flecainide on mortality in a randomized trial of arrhythmia suppression after myocardial infarction. N Engl J Med 1989;321:406–412.

20. Kendall MJ, Lynch KP, Hjalmarson A, Kjekshus J. Beta-blockers and sudden cardiac death. Ann Intern Med 1995;123:358–367.

21. Barnett AH, Leslie D, Watkins PJ. Can insulin-treated diabetics be given beta-adrenergic blocking drugs? BMJ 1980;280:976–978.

22. Hirsch IB, Boyle PJ, Craft S, Cryer PE. Higher glycemic thresholds for symptoms during beta-adrenergic blockade in IDDM. Diabetes 1991;40:1177–1186.

23. Shorr RI, Ray WA, Daugherty JR, Griffin MR. Antihypertensives and the risk of serious hypoglycemia in older persons using insulin or sulfonylureas. JAMA 1997;278:40–43.

24. Waal HJ. Propranolol induced depression. BMJ 1967;2:50.

25. Pollack MH, Rosenbaum JF, Cassem NH. Propranolol and depression revisited: three cases and a review. J Nerv Ment Dis 1985;173:118–119.

26. Schleifer SJ, State WR, Macari Hindson MM, et al. Digitalis and beta-blocking agents: effects on depression following myocardial infarction. Am Heart J 1991;121:1397–1402.

27. Carney R, Rich M, teVelde A, et al. Prevalence of major depressive disorder in patients receiving beta-blocker therapy versus other medications. Am J Med 1987;83:223–226.

28. Sorgi P, Ratey J, Knoedler D, et al. Depression during treatment with beta-blockers: results from a double-blind placebo-controlled study. J Neuropsychiatry Clin Neurosci 1992;4:187–188.

29. Gerstman BB, Jolson HM, Baver M, et al. The incidence of depression in new users of beta-blockers and selected antihypertensives. J Clin Epidemiol 1996;49:809–815.

30. Thiessen BQ, Wallace SM, Blackburn JL, Wilson TW. Increased prescribing of antidepressants subsequent to beta-blocker therapy. Arch Intern Med 1990;150:2286–2290.

31. Palac DM, Cornish RD, McDonald WJ, et al. Cognitive function in hypertensives treated with atenolol or propranolol. J Gen Intern Med 1990;5:310–318.

32. Hallas J. Evidence of depression provoked by cardiovascular medication: a prescription sequence symmetry analysis. Epidemiology 1996;7:478–484.

33. Medical research council working party on mild to moderate hypertension. Adverse reactions to bendrofluazide and propranolol for the treatment of mild hypertension. Lancet 1981;2:539–543.

34. Silen W (ed). Cope's Early Diagnosis of the Acute Abdomen (15th ed). New York: Oxford University Press, 1979.

35. Silen W (ed). Cope's Early Diagnosis of the Acute Abdomen (16th ed). New York: Oxford University Press, 1983.

36. Attard AR, Corlett MJ, Kidner NJ. Safety of early pain relief for acute abdominal pain. BMJ 1992;305:554–556.

37. Pace S, Burke TF. Intravenous morphine for early pain relief in patients with acute abdominal pain. Acad Emerg Med 1996;3:1086–1092.

38. Katz CM. How efficient is sliding-scale insulin therapy? Problems with a "cookbook" approach in hospitalized patients. Postgrad Med 1991;89:46–48, 51–54, 57.

39. MacMillan DR. Insulin adjustment by the sliding scale method—a straw man who won't stay down? J Ky Med Assoc 1991;89:211–212.

40. Queale WS, Sadler AJ, Bancati FL. The use of sliding scales in medical inpatients with diabetes mellitus. J Gen Intern Med 1995;10(Suppl):47.

41. Gearhart JG, Duncan JL III, Replogle WH, et al. Efficacy of sliding-scale insulin therapy: a comparison with prospective regimens. Fam Pract Res J 1994;14:313–322.

42. MacMillan DR. The fallacy of insulin adjustment by the sliding scale. J Ky Med Assoc 1970;68:577–579.

43. Queale WS, Seidler AJ, Brancati FL. Glycemic control and sliding scale insulin use in medical inpatients with diabetes mellitus. Arch Intern Med 1997;157:545–552.

44. Hirsch IB, Paauw DS, Brunzell J. Inpatient management of adults with diabetes. Diabetes Care 1995;18:870–878.

45. Hirsch IB, Farkas-Hirsch R, Skyler JS. Intensive insulin therapy for treatment of type 1 diabetes. Diabetes Care 1990;13:1265–1283.

46. Connors AF, Speroff T, Dawson NV, et al. The effectiveness of right heart catheterization in the initial care of critically ill patients. JAMA 1996;276:889–897.

47. Gore JM, Goldberg RJ, Spodick DH, et al. A community-wide assessment of the use of pulmonary artery catheters in patients with acute myocardial infarction. Chest 1987;92:721–731.

Chapter 3
Dimensions of Evidence*

Alfred O. Berg

In the January/February 1998 issue of the *Journal of the American Board of Family Practice*, John Geyman introduced the subject of evidence-based medicine by presenting an overview of the gap between evidence and practice and by describing the challenges that will arise as we attempt to fill the gap.[1]

A number of concerns are driving the evidence-based approach. First, the usual sources of clinical advice, namely, expert opinions, have proved to be variable and unreliable. When one asks a group of experts a straightforward clinical question, one is likely to get a range of answers rather than a single answer that is based on evidence. The American Medical Association Diagnosis and Treatment Therapeutic Assessment, in which experts are polled, always elicits diverse responses, with convergences of opinion being uncommon. An evidence-based approach indicates which of the treatment options is best supported by scientific data. Also, tremendous geographic variation exists in the use of some diagnostic and therapeutic modalities, without a basis for the variation in the prevalence or incidence of the disease. An evidence-based approach limits variation to only those options with the best evidence, regardless of geographic location. Another concern is the gap that exists between practice and evidence. The gap arises when clinicians do not have evidence, and when clinicians have evidence but do not apply it. An evidence-based approach identifies which of these problems should be addressed. Also, costs of medical care in the United States are higher, absolutely and proportionally, than in any other industrialized country. An evidence-based approach can potentially constrain costs, because standards to accept (and pay for) a new intervention are high (an evidence-based approach could also prove an expensive intervention to be worthwhile, of course, but

more examples of the former exist). Last is the growing concern about quality. Is it possible that all processes lead to similar good outcomes? Likely not, and one of the goals of an evidence-based approach is to recognize which strategies predictably lead to the best outcomes.

This chapter discusses dimensions of evidence as a historical and philosophic preamble to later chapters in the book that refine concepts of evidence, outcomes, quality, and cost. Using brief clinical scenarios in which one physician asks another a question about a patient, I explore some of the ways in which physicians define and use evidence in clinical practice. I use the question "Does it work?" about a clinical intervention because the "it" can be a fact about etiology or prognosis, a diagnostic test, or a therapeutic or preventive intervention. The underlying question is whether the advice is "true," forcing us to consider the quality of evidence that supports it. I conclude with a summary of one of the popular methods used to answer some of the shortcomings illustrated in the scenarios—constructing clinical practice guidelines.

Illustrative Clinical Scenarios

Trust Me

Dr. Smith: So, which statin would you recommend?
Dr. Jones: Atorvastatin is the drug of choice.
(Translation: Does it work? It does if I say so.)

In a busy clinical setting, Dr. Smith asks a straightforward question, and Dr. Jones provides a straightforward answer. Dr. Smith is likely to implement the advice (at least for now) without questioning it. This model dates to the prescientific era when trainees were apprenticed to an experienced physician and simply emulated their practice without questioning it. This model is also very common today and is probably the dominant form of

*Reprinted with permission from AO Berg. Dimensions of evidence. J Am Board Fam Pract 1998;11:216–223.

teaching in the clinical setting.[2] The problem from an evidence-based perspective is that the inputs and processes are not explicit—the questioner does not know what factors went into making the recommendation and how they were processed before giving the advice. The advice may or may not be based on evidence, and it may or may not be true.

Deferral to Authority

Dr. Smith: So, which statin would you recommend?

Dr. Jones: I prefer atorvastatin, and the last time I sent someone over to the lipid clinic, that was Dr. Doe's recommendation as well.

(Translation: Does it work? It does if Dr. Expert says so.)

This scenario is a variant of the first, often heard when Dr. Jones is reasonably certain of an answer but wants to bolster her position by referring to an expert's opinion. Expertise and specialized knowledge are highly valued in our society. Rarely do physicians question authorities in specialized areas. The relationship between referring physicians and their consultants is complex, but usually the expert claims to have the answer and the referring physician accepts it. The problem from an evidence-based perspective is similar to that in the first scenario: The inputs and processes are not explicit. The advice may or may not be based on evidence. The advice may or may not be correct. An evidence-based approach directly confronts the expertise of the expert, in some cases uncomfortably so, by questioning the scientific basis for the recommendation. An evidence-based consultation provides both a recommendation and the supporting data rather than the recommendation alone.

In My Experience

Dr. Smith: So, which statin would you recommend?

Dr. Jones: I don't really like any of them. I have had good experience with diet and cholestyramine, and I never prescribe 3-hydroxy-3-methylglutaryl coenzyme A reductase inhibitors.

(Translation: Does it work? It does if it seems to.)

This response usually is not stated quite this way; rather, it comes out as "in my clinical experience . . ." Physicians develop strong opinions about what does and does not work based on their own clinical experience. Thus, physicians for many years have used numerous treatments for multiple sclerosis and have convinced themselves that the treatments work based on their own clinical experience. Most treatments have not withstood the test of a properly conducted clinical trial, yet many are still in use by physicians because their experiences are limited to a small number of patients, the course of the disease is unpredictable, and most patients seem to improve.

In this scenario, a physician is using an outdated drug as first-line therapy. It was probably the drug of choice when the physician left residency, but progress has surpassed him. Clinical knowledge decreases with time.[3] Year of graduation from residency is an important predictor of the drug formulary used by the average physician.[4]

Clinical experience is the source for many therapies that have proved efficacious, of course, but it is also the source for interventions of disproved or unknown efficacy. Much of the controversy surrounding alternative medicine can be viewed from this perspective. Because so many human ailments are self-limited, practitioners of aromatherapy, reflexology, and Rolfing are able to persuade themselves that their interventions work when no scientific evidence exists to prove that they do.

The Pathophysiologic Model

Resident (at 2 AM): This low-risk woman is at term and in labor. Is there anything else I should be doing right now?

Attending: No, get some rest. The external fetal monitor will collect all the information we need to monitor labor.

(Translation: Does it work? It does if it makes sense that it would.)

This interaction illustrates the major focus of clinical practice and scientific work since the mid-1800s. Many clinical interventions are used because the basic pathophysiology makes sense, even though they are lacking true outcome data to show a positive effect. Electronic fetal monitoring makes sense based on what is known about maternal and fetal physiology, the natural history of labor, and how physicians make decisions, but the evidence supporting the clinical usefulness of routine electronic fetal monitoring is very thin, with the best-quality studies showing the least benefit.[5]

In the past, it was sufficient to understand the pathophysiologic process underlying a condition and prescribe treatments that interrupted the process. It is now known that this logical linkage is potentially dangerous because it has not worked or has caused harm in some cases. The arrhythmia suppression trials are an example: Promising drugs were found to suppress arrhythmias but sometimes at the expense of a patient's life.[6]

Everyone Else Is Doing It

Dr. Smith: I have a 55-year-old man in for a complete physical, and he's asking about screening for prostate cancer.

Dr. Jones (medical director): Make sure you do a digital rectal examination and get a prostate-specific antigen. We'll get sued if you don't do the screening and he develops prostate cancer, because screening is the standard in our community.

(Translation: Does it work? It does if everyone agrees that it does.)

This answer is common and potentially dangerous. The problem is that if everyone assumes the answer to be X, but X has never been subjected to properly conducted clinical studies, everyone could be blissfully unaware that they are wrong. It is not known whether the medical director's advice is right, because no solid evidence exists to prove that screening for prostate cancer with prostate-specific antigen is beneficial, although it is practically the standard of care in this country. The unquestioned use of radical mastectomy for breast cancer is a sobering example of a case in which the presumption of benefit was so strong for so many decades that the first physicians who questioned it were professionally isolated.

The U.S. Preventive Services Task Force was surprised to discover the poor quality of evidence supporting preventive interventions already in wide practice.[7] To suggest that placebo-controlled randomized trials are needed to assess quality and quantity of life is a radical notion for many clinical conditions. I have learned to be guarded when the consensus on what to do appears to be the strongest.

A Reference Standard?

Dr. Smith: I have a 26-year-old man with his first episode of low back pain. What can I recommend?

Dr. Jones: (silent)

(Translation: Does it work? What should Dr. Jones recommend?)

Much of what physicians do in clinical medicine has not been subjected to well-designed scientific studies. Randomized controlled trials (RCTs) are the reference standard for interventions, but RCTs are not perfect and do not apply to studies of cause, diagnosis, or prognosis. RCTs are not often conducted on patients similar to those encountered in practice, and the selection process and follow-up of patients in an RCT are usually quite different from what one might achieve in a typical practice setting. Some clinical interventions will never be subjected to an RCT.

Nevertheless, evidence from RCTs are, at least for now, the most scientific point of entry into a discussion with a patient about what his or her options are for a therapeutic or preventive intervention. If no data are available, the discussion has a different end point than if data are available, and the main issue is determining whether the data apply to the patient in the examining room.

It is incredibly rare, however, that a single RCT, even if well designed, answers the question for all patients in all settings. Medical research almost never provides silver bullets. If physicians want their clinical practice to be

based on high-quality evidence, they should ask the questions: Which evidence? What defines high quality? How much do we need?

Clinical Practice Guidelines

One approach to answering these questions is to develop a systematic way of defining, collecting, analyzing, and summarizing the evidence into a clinical practice guideline. The process of constructing an evidence-based clinical practice guideline is described by many authors, but all have in common the following steps:

1. Define the question.
2. Find the evidence.
3. Analyze the evidence.
4. Summarize the evidence.

Define the Question

Defining the question sounds easy, but it can be challenging. A panel of experts constructing a clinical guideline can spend many hours, even days, focusing and refining the question. David Sackett proposed the following list of the central tasks of clinical work[8]:

Clinical findings: how to gather and interpret findings properly from the history and physical examination

Etiology: how to recognize causes for diseases, including iatrogenesis

Differential diagnosis: how to discriminate and rank the alternatives by likelihood, seriousness, and treatability

Diagnostic tests: how to select and interpret diagnostic tests, taking into account their precision, accuracy, acceptability, cost, and safety

Prognosis: how to estimate the patient's course with time and anticipate complications

Therapy: how to select treatments that do more good than harm and that are worth the efforts and costs of using them

Prevention: how to reduce the chance of disease by detecting and modifying risk factors and how to diagnose early disease by screening

For each of these clinical tasks, there are four elements of a well-formulated question:

1. Who is the patient or what is the problem being addressed?
2. What is the intervention?
3. What are the alternatives?
4. What are the outcomes?

For example, if one were looking for a therapy for heart failure, the intervention might be an angiotensin-

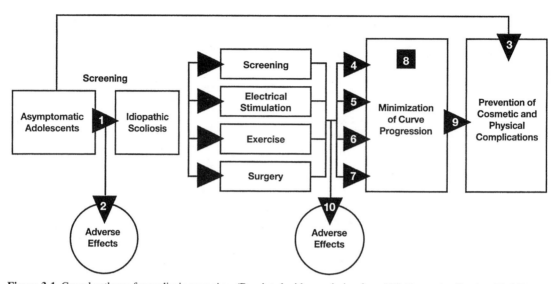

Figure 3-1. Causal pathway for scoliosis screening. (Reprinted with permission from U.S. Preventive Services Task Force. Screening for adolescent idiopathic scoliosis. JAMA 1993;269:2664–2666.)

converting enzyme inhibitor, an alternative might be diuretics alone, and the outcomes might be the correction of the heart failure or mortality.

In defining clinical questions, rigorous evidence-based reviews often include evidence maps or causal pathways, laying out in advance how a clinical problem is thought to work. This map then directs the literature review. Figure 3-1 presents a causal pathway for a secondary prevention intervention—screening for adolescent idiopathic scoliosis—used by the U.S. Preventive Services Task Force in conducting an evidence-based review to determine whether screening worked.[9] In the causal pathway, each numbered link defines a clinical question for which an evidence search was conducted (the results of the search also appear in the figure).

Find the Evidence

Once the clinical questions are clear, one is ready to gather and summarize the evidence. To give some accountability to the process, the methods must be systematic, thorough, and explicit. MEDLINE is the best-known database; however, it targets a minority of the biomedical journals worldwide (although, arguably, it indexes nearly all the important ones), and not all MEDLINE-based search products work in the same way. More than 30 proprietary versions are available, and the same search strategy yields slightly different results for each. Furthermore, relevant evidence may be unpublished, indexed incorrectly so that a search does not capture it, or published before 1966 (thus predating MEDLINE).

For these reasons, truly comprehensive searches use databases and strategies that go beyond MEDLINE. For

the physician, however, the problem is the reverse: MEDLINE searches produce too much information, not too little. As a result, interest has arisen in constructing physician-friendly databases that are more likely to be clinically on target. The *ACP Journal Club* and a similar product put out by the *Journal of Family Practice* Journal Club are attempts in this direction, but others exist, such as the new journal *Evidence-Based Medicine* and the Cochrane database. The Agency for Health Care Policy and Research has constructed a national guideline clearinghouse with a Web page that catalogues and indexes clinical guidelines, including evaluative and comparative information for topics that are addressed by more than one guideline. In the future, every practicing physician should be adept at using electronic databases and determining which databases fit which clinical needs best.

Analyze the Evidence

Once assembled, the evidence should be reviewed for applicability and quality. Reviewing the quality of evidence has been the subject of countless journal clubs and seminars for many years. In this review process, everything physicians learn about evaluating published research comes into practice. The standards for judging the quality of research on diagnostic tests, prognosis, treatment, and adverse events are very high indeed and getting higher every year. As these standards are applied, fewer articles pass muster. Those working in evidence-based medicine are nearly unanimous in demanding high-quality, randomized trials for interventions. However, case studies, case series, observational studies, and uncontrolled trials on interventions still dominate the medical literature.

Table 3-1. Quality of Evidence

I. Evidence obtained from at least one properly ran-
    domized controlled trial.
II.1. Evidence obtained from well-designed controlled
    trials without randomization.
II.2. Evidence obtained from well-designed cohort or
    case-controlled analytic studies, preferably from
    more than one center or research group.
II.3. Evidence obtained from multiple time series with or
    without the intervention. Dramatic results in uncon-
    trolled experiments (e.g., the results of the introduc-
    tion of penicillin treatment in the 1940s) could also
    be regarded as this type of evidence.
III. Opinions of respected authorities based on clinical
    experience, descriptive studies and case reports, or
    reports of expert committees.

For the foreseeable future, high-quality evidence will not be available for many important clinical questions. In these circumstances, an evidence-based approach at minimum requires explicit criteria for categorizing the design (e.g., case-control study, randomized controlled trial) and judging the quality of a study. Many resources are available to help make these judgments. The grading of evidence used by the U.S. Preventive Services Task Force is a typical example of categorizing studies (Table 3-1).[7] Category-specific criteria for judging the quality of a study are also available from the many sources that address critical reading skills.[10]

Summarize the Evidence

The last step in conducting an evidence review is to summarize collected evidence in some useful way. Two products are discussed here: evidence tables and outcomes tables (also referred to as *balance sheets*).

An evidence table is simply a systematic way of displaying information from multiple studies so that they can be compared. For example, the table would have a row for each study included in the database, with the columns containing study characteristics, such as patient population studied, duration, specific interventions, outcomes, and actual data for groups and subgroups. Evidence tables allow a user to scan quickly those study characteristics that are relevant to the question at hand. A sample evidence table summarizing some of the principal breast cancer screening trials is presented in Table 3-2.[10]

An outcomes table takes the materials from the evidence tables and summarizes them even more concisely. In general, an outcomes table displays the alternative interventions and outcomes in a way that users can understand. A classic outcomes table covering breast cancer screening in women ages 55 to 65 years is presented in Table 3-3.[10] The natural history and benefits and harms from the interventions are the rows, and the alternative interventions are the columns. A complete outcomes table presents harms as well as benefits, using data collected and summarized with the same care and rigor for both.

It is important to point out that the numbers in an outcomes table are not directive—that is, reasonable physicians and patients might make different decisions based on the individual values they place on the risks and outcomes. The patient's informed preferences are extremely important as well.

Conclusion

Practicing evidence-based medicine requires a shift in the clinical thought processes that most physicians were trained to use. In the past, clinical decisions and clinical advice relied on clinical experience, expert opinions, collegial relationships, pathophysiology, common sense, community standards, published materials, and other sources. The practice of evidence-based medicine uses the same sources for clinical advice but passes all of them through the filter of the following question: "On what evidence is the advice based?" A properly constructed clinical practice guideline has the potential to serve as a lens for the evidence that does exist (i.e., that has passed through the filtering question), focusing it on specific clinical issues in an explicit and accountable way.

Not all evidence is of the same quality. Evidence from a properly conducted randomized clinical trial is more likely to be true than evidence based on one physician's clinical experience or personal opinion; but in giving and receiving advice, one rarely pauses to consider what the quality of the underlying evidence might be. I recommend pausing more often.

Table 3-2. Evidence of the Effectiveness of Breast Cancer Screening for Women 50 Years and Older[a]

Study	Age (yrs)	Design	Size (Number)	Length of Follow-Up (yrs)	BPE	MGY	Scheduled Frequency (yrs)	Approximate Dilution	Reported Results
Sweden, 1977[b]	50–74	RCT	Control patients: 41,104 Screened patients: 58,148	7.0	No	1 view	2	0.20	RR: 0.61 CL = 0.44, 0.84
Nijmegen, 1975[c]	50–64	MCCS	Cases: 27 Controls: 135	7.0	No	1 view	2		OR: 0.26 CL = 0.1, 0.67
Health Insurance Plan Project, 1963[d]	50–65	RCT	Control patients: 16,089 Screened patients: 16,151	9.0	Yes	2 views	1	0.40	Control patients: 80 of 16,089 Screened patients: 52 of 16,151
DOM, 1975[e]	50–64	MCCS	Cases: 54 Controls: 162	7.0	Yes	2 views	1–2		OR: 0.31 CL = 0.15, 0.65
Florence, 1979[f]	40–70	MCCS	Cases: 57 Controls: 186	7.0	No	2 views	2.5		OR: 0.24 CL = 0.13, 0.42
Malmok, 1976[g]	55–74	RCT	Control patients: 8,490 Screened patients: 8,507	8.8	No	2 views	18–24 mos	0.28	RR: 0.79 CL = 0.51, 1.24
United Kingdom, 1979[h]	45–64	CT	Control patients: 127,117 Screened patients: 45,841	6.5	Yes	Mixed	BPE: 1 MGY: 2	0.34	RR: 0.8 CL = 0.64, 1.01

BPE = breast physician examination; CL = confidence limit; CT = controlled trial; MCCS = matched case-control study; MGY = mammography; OR = odds ratio; RCT = randomized controlled trial; RR = relative risk.

[a]To permit comparisons, results are reported for 6–10 years of follow-up. Longer follow-up results are available from some studies. Reported results incorporate any adjustments performed by the investigator.

[b]Tabar L, Faberberg G, Day NE, Holmberg L. What is the optimum interval between mammographic screening examinations? An analysis based on the latest results of the Swedish two-county breast cancer screening trial. Br J Cancer 1987;55:547–551.

[c]Verbeek AL, Hendriks JH, Holland R, et al. Reduction of breast cancer mortality through mass screening with modern mammography. First results of the Nijmegen project, 1975–1981. Lancet 1984;1:1222–1224; Verbeek AL, Hendriks JH, Holland R, et al. Mammographic screening and breast cancer mortality: age-specific effects in Nijmegen Project, 1975–82 [letter]. Lancet 1985;1:865–866.

[d]Shapiro S, Venet W, Strax P, et al. Ten- to fourteen-year effect of screening on breast cancer mortality. J Natl Cancer Inst 1982;69:349–355; Shapiro S, Venet W, Strax P, et al. Selection, follow-up, and analysis in the Health Insurance Plan Study: a randomized trial with breast cancer screening. Natl Cancer Inst Monogr 1985;67:65–74; Shapiro S, Venet W, Strax P. Periodic Screening for Breast Cancer: The Health Insurance Plan Project and Its Sequelae, 1963–1986. Baltimore: Johns Hopkins University Press, 1988.

[e]Collette HJ, Day NE, Romback JJ, deWaard F. Evaluation of screening for breast cancer in a non-randomised study (the DOM project) by means of a case-control study. Lancet 1984;1:1224–1226.

[f]Palli D, Del Turco MR, Buiatti E, et al. A case-control study of the efficacy of a non-randomized breast cancer screening program in Florence (Italy). Int J Cancer 1986;38:501–504.

[g]Andersson I, Aspergren K, Janson L, et al. Mammographic screening and mortality from breast cancer: the Malmo mammographic screening trial. BMJ 1988;297:943–948.

[h]First results on mortality reduction in the UK trial of early detection of breast cancer. UK Trial of Early Detection of Breast Cancer Group. Lancet 1988;2:411–416.

Source: Adapted from DM Eddy. A Manual for Assessing Health Practices and Designing Practice Policies: The Explicit Approach. Philadelphia: American College of Physicians, 1992;45. With permission from the American College of Physicians.

Table 3-3. A Balance Sheet for Outcomes of 10 Years of Annual Breast Cancer Screening with Breast Physical Examination and Mammography in Women 55–65 Years Old

		Probability or Magnitude		
	Event	**Without Screening**	**With Screening**	**Differences Caused by Screening**
Background	Develop breast cancer in 10-yr period (probability)	2.33% (233/10,000)	2.33% (233/10,000)	0% (0/10,000)
Benefits	Die (ever) from a breast cancer that develops in a 10-yr period (probability)	1.23% (123/10,000)	0.73% (95% CL, 0.41–0.93%) (73/10,000)	0.50% (95% CL, 0.30–0.82%) (50/10,000)
	Reassurance[a] from knowledge that probability of cancer is decreased by 1.7% (probability)	0% (0/10,000)	78.61%[b] (7,861/10,000)	78.61% (7,861/10,000)
Harms	Number of physical and mammographic examinations (inconvenience, anxiety, discomfort)	0	10	10
	False-positive result during 10 yrs (probability)	0% (0/10,000)	20% (2,000/10,000)	20% (2,000/10,000)
	New breast cancer caused by 10 yrs of radiation (probability)	0% (0/10,000)	0.0004% (1/250,000)	0.0004% (1/250,000)

CL = confidence limit.
[a]Without screening, the probability that a woman will have breast cancer during the 10 years is approximately 2.33%. If the screening test results are negative, the probability that she will have breast cancer during the 10 years is decreased to approximately 0.60%. Thus, if a woman has 10 examinations with negative results, her probability of developing breast cancer in the 10 years is decreased by 1.73% (2.33% – 0.60% = 1.73%). The probability that all 10 tests will have negative results is 78.61%.
[b]The probability that all 10 test results will be negative.
Source: Reprinted with permission from DM Eddy. A Manual for Assessing Health Practices and Designing Practice Policies: The Explicit Approach. Philadelphia: American College of Physicians, 1992;56. With permission from the American College of Physicians.

References

1. Geyman JP. Evidence-based medicine in primary care: an overview. J Am Board Fam Pract 1998;11:46–56.
2. Covell DG, Uman GC, Manning PR. Information needs in office practice: are they being met? Ann Intern Med 1985;103:596–599.
3. Ramsey PG, Carline JD, Inui TS, et al. Changes over time in the knowledge base of practicing internists. JAMA 1991;266:1103–1107.
4. Sackett DL, Haynes RB, Taylor DW, et al. Clinical determinants of the decision to treat primary hypertension. Clin Res 1977;24:648.
5. Vintzileos AM, Nochimson DJ, Guzman ER, et al. Intrapartum electronic fetal heart rate monitoring versus intermittent auscultation: a meta-analysis. Obstet Gynecol 1995;85:149–155.
6. Echt DS, Liebson PR, Mitchell LB, et al. Mortality and morbidity in patients receiving encainide, flecainide, or placebo. The Cardiac Arrhythmia Suppression Trial. N Engl J Med 1991;324:781–788.
7. U.S. Preventive Services Task Force. Guide to Clinical Preventive Services (2nd ed). Baltimore: Williams & Wilkins, 1996.
8. Sackett DL, Richardson WS, Rosenberg W, Haynes RB. Evidence-based medicine: how to practice and teach EBM. New York: Churchill Livingstone, 1997.
9. U.S. Preventive Services Task Force. Screening for adolescent idiopathic scoliosis. JAMA 1993;269:2664–2666.
10. Eddy DM. A Manual for Assessing Health Practices and Designing Practice Policies: The Explicit Approach. Philadelphia: American College of Physicians, 1992.

Chapter 4
Strategies for Finding Evidence

Sarah Safranek and Sherry Dodson

The exponential growth of medical literature has made it virtually impossible for practicing physicians to stay abreast of new treatment and diagnostic options. In 1992, the Evidence-Based Medicine Working Group recommended that physicians rely on medical literature to keep their clinical practices current with the most recent advances in medical science.[1–3] However, several studies have indicated that physicians in practice make little use of the medical literature. Studies by both Covell et al.[4] and Gorman and Helfand[5] involved observations and interviews with practicing physicians during office hours. They noted that, although questions about patient care arise frequently while physicians see patients, most of these questions go unanswered and are never pursued. Gorman and Helfand found that as many as 70% of patient care questions are not pursued at all, and that the other 25–30% of questions are investigated with resources other than journal literature—that is, textbooks, colleagues, and consultants. MEDLINE and the resulting journal literature were only consulted 2% of the time in Gorman and Helfand's study. The main resources that were used by the primary care physicians in the study (textbooks and drug resources such as the *Physicians' Desk Reference*) are, by nature, out of date and may contain erroneous information.

Although huge investments, most notably by the National Library of Medicine (NLM), have been made to make search systems less expensive, easier to use, and more accessible, many barriers remain before the use of search systems is commonplace in a physician's practice. Fortunately for primary care physicians, helpful new tools continue to appear. In this chapter we discuss connecting to the Internet, and we explore some of the newer tools and online services that provide more immediate access to relevant literature for patient care decision making. We also look at search strategies to help the practicing physician find the best evidence in journal literature.

Connecting to the Internet

Universities, government offices, associations, societies, businesses, and individuals are bringing an increasing volume of biomedical information online. Connecting to the Internet is the first important step to help health care professionals quickly identify needed clinical information. The 1997 American Interactive Healthcare Professionals Survey was completed in July 1997 and involved focus groups and telephone interviews with health care executives nationwide. According to the survey findings, the percentage of physicians actively using the Internet is in the range of 25–30%, and an additional 16% say they are interested in going online but require instruction.[6] For those not yet connected, we briefly discuss the necessary requirements and various options.

Hooking up to the Internet requires four basic components: a computer, a modem, Internet software, and an Internet Service Provider (ISP).

Computer

Computer technology is changing so rapidly that it is not realistic to recommend a particular configuration. Either a Macintosh or a Windows machine is capable of connecting to the Internet. A few strategies to help guide computer purchase decisions are to ask the library staff at the hospital where you admit patients, to consult with colleagues who already have computers, or to call the regional National Network of Libraries of Medicine to discuss options in your area (800-338-7657).

Modem

The modem is the device that connects the computer via a telephone line to an ISP. Modems may be housed inside your computer or linked externally by a cable. Internal modems are generally less expensive than external modems; however, external modems may be a bit easier for the novice to set up and program. Modems have different data transmission speeds as measured by kilobits per second of data, and a faster modem allows you to download and work much more efficiently. It is always important to buy the fastest modem that you can afford because it saves time and aggravation on the Internet.

Internet Software

The software instructs the computer and the modem how to access the Internet through the ISP. Typically, Internet software is provided by the ISP and may include a communications package to connect the computer to the Internet by telephone, a World Wide Web browser, an electronic mail program, and a newsgroup reader.

Internet Service Provider

Many avenues exist for securing an ISP, including signing up with one of the national commercial online services, selecting a local ISP, or exploring government or educational affiliations. Each has advantages and disadvantages (Table 4-1).

National online services include America Online,[7] CompuServe,[8] Microsoft Network,[9] and Prodigy.[10] In addition to Internet access, these companies provide a number of proprietary services exclusive to subscribers, such as discussion forums, news, and entertainment. For a novice user, these services have the advantage of being easy to set up and use. They also benefit people who travel frequently because their broad geographic coverage allows members to sign on from virtually any North American location without dialing long distance. One disadvantage is that these national online services tend to be more costly than a local ISP. Another potential problem

of national online services is that they have more control over what members can see on the Internet, so that members cannot necessarily view whichever sites they choose. Most of the large online services offer free trials with no risk or obligation. It may be worthwhile to try a service for a month and then look at commercial trade magazines for articles that evaluate national online services.[11]

Local ISPs may be another good option for connecting to the Internet. The number of local ISPs is increasing at an astonishing rate as a result of fierce competition for a share of the Internet market. Typically, local ISPs provide free connectivity software either contained on a CD-ROM or downloadable from the provider's server. The major advantages of using a local ISP are that they are generally less expensive than national online services and they provide access to all of the Internet. The major disadvantage of a local ISP in today's competitive market is that they may not have the resources to support their subscribers, resulting in busy phone lines and difficulties in establishing and maintaining connections.

Institutional affiliations with government or educational agencies may provide individuals with Internet connections through their institution's computer networks. The advantages of connecting to the Internet via institutional affiliations are that the software is often free or available for a small fee (there may be free access or small fees for connect time), and that governmental or educational institutions are more likely to remain stable. Academic or educational affiliates may also benefit from access to the array of clinical tools and databases provided by their institution. Accessing the Internet through institutional affiliations carries the disadvantages of lack of privacy and institutional restrictions on personal use. For the computer novice, configuring the computer and software may be a formidable task.

Once connected to the Internet, the next step for the primary care professional is efficient access and use of MEDLINE and the other specialized evidence-based medicine tools, such as the Cochrane database, *ACP Journal Club*, InfoPOEMs (formerly *Journal of Family Practice* Journal Club), and *Best Evidence*. Primary care practitioners confront many questions in an average workday concerning a wide variety of patient management issues. Although tools such as Cochrane are beginning to address many of these primary care issues with the goal of evaluating interventions in all areas of health care, MEDLINE is the fundamental source of evidence-based literature.

Table 4-1. Internet Service Provider Options

Internet Service Provider	Advantages	Disadvantages
National	Full range of bundled software	Generally more expensive
	Ease of making connection	May restrict access to some resources
	Widespread availability	
Local	Generally less expensive	Less stable
	Unrestricted access	
Institutional affiliations	Stability	Difficulties setting up
	Often free or available for small fee	Lack of privacy

Accessing MEDLINE

MEDLINE, an electronic database produced by the NLM, indexes approximately 3,900 biomedical journals. Decisions on journal inclusion in the MEDLINE database are made by a scholarly committee on the basis of scope, quality, and

---

Case 1

Mr. and Mrs. Jones present to your office with their 6-year-old son, Taylor, who has the chief complaint of 2 weeks of hay fever symptoms. They have tried over-the-counter antihistamines, but Taylor has fallen asleep in his first grade class. Mr. Jones asks, "Are there medications that Taylor can take that won't make him drowsy? My wife takes Claritin [loratadine] for her hay fever. Is that safe for children?" You decide to do a MEDLINE search for more information.

---

type of content; quality of editorial work and production; and journal audience. MEDLINE is available from multiple commercial vendors who buy the data from the NLM to repackage and sell to subscribers, and in the past few years, Internet Web sites, such as HealthGate,[12] Medscape,[13] and numerous others, have offered free search interfaces to MEDLINE sponsored by advertisers. In the spring of 1997, however, MEDLINE became accessible on the Internet free of charge via the NLM's PubMed search system.

PubMed consists of the full MEDLINE file (*Index Medicus* 1966 to the present, *International Nursing Index*, and *Index to Dental Literature*), PREMEDLINE (new records in the process of being indexed that have not yet been added to MEDLINE), and all citations from participating journals that are only selectively indexed in standard MEDLINE. Many hospitals and medical libraries subscribe to MEDLINE from SilverPlatter, Ovid, or other companies. However, the currentness of PubMed (weekly updates of MEDLINE and daily additions to PREMEDLINE), free access, and special evidence-based medicine search enhancements make it the most attractive MEDLINE option.

Once you have located citations in MEDLINE, the next step is to obtain the full text of the articles. PubMed contains a small number of links to journal publishers' Web pages that provide full-text articles for a fee and to a few publishers who provide the full text for free. These links are expected to increase as more publishers establish online services. An additional option is Loansome Doc, an online document ordering system that allows you to send your article requests electronically from PubMed to a medical library. Information about Loansome Doc and a phone number for assistance in identifying libraries in your region can be found in the Help sections of PubMed.

The challenge facing the evidence-based medicine searcher is how to extract from MEDLINE's 9 million citations those relevant research articles that have used appropriate evidence-based study methodologies. PubMed offers several approaches to searching: a basic mode in which simple one-sentence queries can be entered, as well as advanced features such as Boolean searching, a medical subject heading (MeSH) browser, and an evidence-filtered search tool, Clinical Queries.

Because of its currentness, wide availability, and special search features, we focus our discussion of search techniques on PubMed. However, most of the techniques we discuss can be adapted easily to other MEDLINE search interfaces.

Optimal Search Strategies in MEDLINE for Evidence-Based Materials

Learning to search MEDLINE efficiently and comprehensively for current evidence is challenging even for experienced searchers. The following techniques will help maximize relevant retrieval, and we also recommend taking a class to develop searching skills. The Further Reading section at the end of this chapter lists a series of very helpful case-based MEDLINE search tip articles. PubMed's online help also can serve as a training tool, and training workbooks are available from the NLM Web site.[14]

Questions you might wish to answer for Mr. and Mrs. Jones and their son include: Are there antihistamines for children that do not cause drowsiness? Is Claritin appropriate for pediatric usage? Are any side effects associated with Claritin in children? What is the dosage for 6-year-olds?

Basic Search

Enter some key terms at the PubMed basic search screen (Figure 4-1) for quick results, for example, "hay fever child Claritin."

Scanning through the first few titles, you see that at least one study exists that is controlled and double-blinded. At this point, you could click on the See Related Articles link next to the citation to retrieve a set of citations that closely relate to the selected article. This feature can be helpful in augmenting search results when the initial retrieval is small.

Clinical Queries

Alternatively, enter the key terms in the PubMed Clinical Queries search mode. Clinical Queries allows you to focus your search on one of four study areas—therapy, diagnosis, etiology, or prognosis—and retrieve only articles that report research conducted using specific methodologies. You may choose a *sensitive* search (i.e., retrieving most relevant articles and probably some less relevant

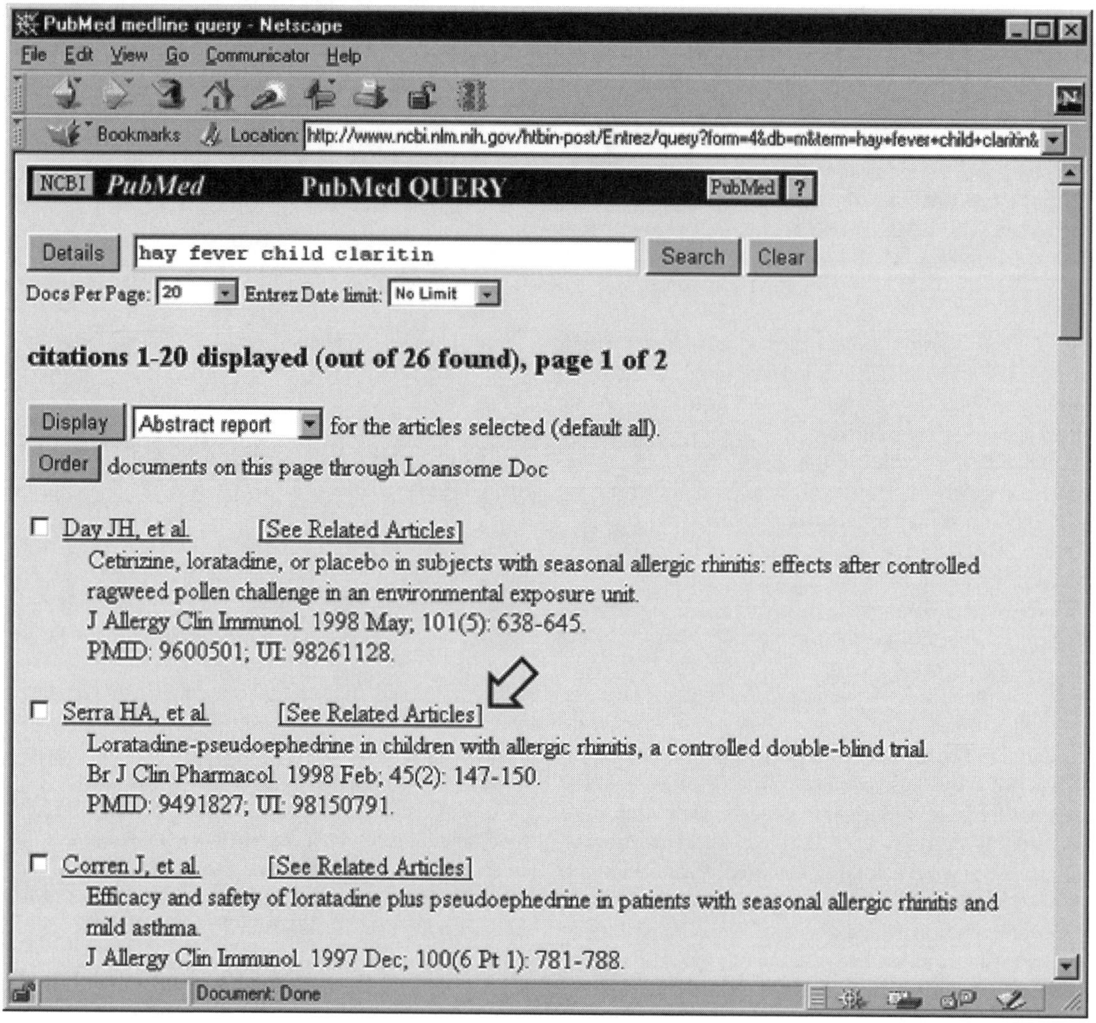

Figure 4-1. Search for *hay fever* and *child* and *claritin* on the basic search screen.

ones) or a more *specific* search (i.e., retrieving mostly relevant articles but probably omitting a few) (Figure 4-2). Search words are combined with collections of search terms or filters that restrict retrieval to particular types of research. The filters are drawn from a study by Haynes and colleagues at McMaster University identifying optimum MEDLINE strategies.[15] For example, if you selected the therapy category and chose the specificity focus, the results would be restricted to articles that included the words *double-blinded* or *placebo*. The filtering terms used to search for each of the study categories are listed in a table linked to the Clinical Queries screen.

Advanced Searching

The basic and Clinical Queries modes work well for the questions in Case 1. However, thought and strategy are often required to convert clinical questions into useful search results. Palmer, Lusher, and Snowball[16] suggest formulating the clinical problem in terms of the patient or condition, the intervention being considered, and the clinical outcome.

> Patient/Condition: 6-year-old with hay fever
> Intervention: treatment, no treatment, Claritin
> Outcome: pediatric toxicity, cost, off-label use, unknown long-term risks, controls symptoms without drowsiness, improved daytime function

Now that your information need is broken down into parts, identify the most important concepts in your question and their relationship to one another. The process of converting your question can be divided into these additional steps: (1) identifying synonyms for each concept, (2) prioritizing the concepts, and (3) constructing logical relationships between concepts.[17]

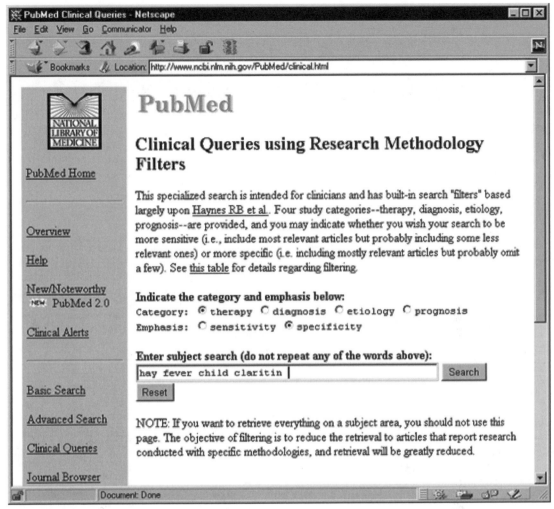

Figure 4-2. Search for *hay fever* and *child* and *claritin* on the Clinical Queries search screen.

List synonyms for the key concepts you have identified:

Child OR children OR pediatric* OR paediatric*
Hay fever OR allergic rhinitis
Claritin OR loratadine

Choose words that might be used by authors in abstracts or titles. For instance, in this example we included both hay fever and allergic rhinitis. Consider singular and plural forms of words and British and American spelling variations. The Boolean operator OR allows you to broaden a concept and include synonyms. The truncation symbol (*) is used to pick up variant endings.

Truncation

Most search systems designate truncation symbols that can be used to collect variations, plurals, and various forms of words. For example, pediatric* in PubMed would retrieve pediatric, pediatrics, or pediatrician. Because each search system may designate different truncation symbols, check the Help file for examples in the system you are using.

Select the concept that is most important to the question, and use the others to modify or narrow the search results.

1. Hay fever
2. Child OR children
3. Loratadine OR Claritin

Combining these concepts using the Boolean operator AND retrieves citations that discuss all three concepts in one article.

Hay fever AND (child OR children) AND (loratadine OR Claritin)

Concepts are generally processed from left to right, but that order can be overcome by using parentheses. Terms nested in parentheses will be processed first.

The third Boolean operator NOT allows you to remove records containing a particular word or concept from your search results. For example, you could exclude studies on loratadine in adults from your strategy:

> Hay fever AND (child OR children) AND (loratadine OR Claritin) NOT adult

It is important to make judicious use of the Boolean operator NOT because you risk eliminating relevant results. The above search would eliminate articles on the topic that discussed the use of loratadine in adults, but would also exclude those about the use of loratadine in both children and adults. All citations discussing adults are eliminated.

Medical Subject Headings

MeSHs are controlled indexing terms assigned to each MEDLINE citation that describe the content of the article. Searchers can use the subject headings to search a topic without considering the variety of ways individual authors may have referred to that topic. For example, using the MeSH term *lung neoplasms* locates articles in which the authors discuss lung cancer, tumors of the lung, lung carcinoma, and other related conditions. MEDLINE indexers choose subject headings from a thesaurus or list of terms (the MeSH Annotated Alphabetic List published annually by the NLM). Usually, six to 12 headings are assigned to each article, with several designated as major headings to represent the most significant topics covered in the article.

PubMed Medical Subject Heading Browser

Many MEDLINE vendors provide electronic access to MeSH vocabulary. In PubMed, the MeSH browser offers cross-referencing to preferred terms: typing in the word *allergy* (not an official MeSH term) provides a pointer to the MeSH term *hypersensitivity*. The browser allows you to view and select terms from the MeSH tree, or hierarchy of terms. Another way to identify subject headings is to search using natural language (key words), look for a relevant article, and view its subject headings in the MEDLINE record.

Figure 4-3 shows the MeSH browser view for the term *hypersensitivity*. It falls under the broader term *immunologic diseases* in the MeSH tree, and includes narrower terms beneath it, such as *respiratory hypersensitivity*.

Each article is indexed under the most specific MeSH terms available. For example, an article on allergy to alder trees is indexed under *hay fever*, not under the broader heading *respiratory hypersensitivity*.

Exploding

Exploding is a MEDLINE search function that allows you to include in your search the more specific terms that fall beneath a given term in the hierarchy of MeSH terms. For example, if you exploded the MeSH term *respiratory hypersensitivity*, you would retrieve articles indexed to all of the MeSH terms falling beneath it in the hierarchy, including *asthma*, *hay fever*, and *perennial allergic rhinitis*. Exploding is useful if you wish to expand your search to include related terms without identifying and typing them in individually. Terms are automatically exploded in PubMed by default.

Subheadings

Subheadings are terms that can be used to search frequently discussed aspects of a topic, such as therapy, surgery, epidemiology, etiology, and the like. Subheadings are added to MeSH terms to further describe the focus of the article. For example:

> Hay fever/drug therapy
> Loratadine/adverse effects

You can view a complete list of subheadings in the Help section of PubMed.

Publication Types

Another effective way to search quickly for studies that use the best evidence-based methodologies is to limit your search by type of research study. For example, you can restrict your search to meta-analyses, randomized controlled trials, clinical trials, reviews, or one of the other available publication types used in MEDLINE records. View the list of MEDLINE Publication Types in PubMed Help.

> Hay fever AND (child OR children) AND (loratadine OR Claritin) AND randomized controlled trial

The above strategies are summarized in Table 4-2 as approaches that enable you to narrow or broaden your search.

Strategies for Increasing or Decreasing Your Search Retrieval

Planned enhancements to PubMed, which include a limits menu for human versus animal studies, age groups, and articles in English, and a search filter option that restricts retrieval to 121 major clinical journal titles, will make searching more efficient.

MEDLINE is an important source of current evidence. PubMed Clinical Queries filtering and other search features

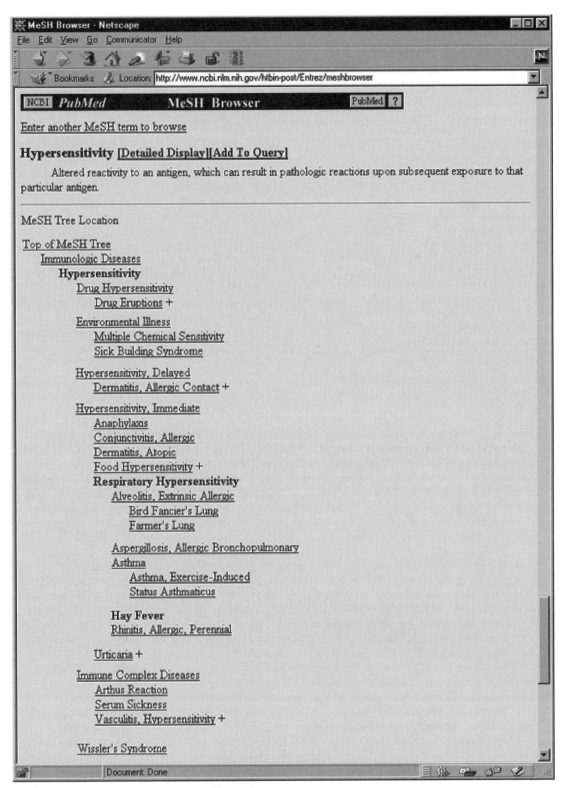

Figure 4-3. Medical Subject Headings browser (MeSH) showing tree structure hierarchy for the term *hypersensitivity*.

Table 4-2. Search Strategies

Strategies to narrow or refine a search
Use major subject headings:
   Hay fever[majr]
Use subheadings with MeSH headings:
   Hay fever/drug therapy
Limit to particular publication types:
   Hay fever AND randomized controlled trial
Limit to English language:
   Hay fever AND eng[la]
Limit to particular years or even days using the Entry Date:
   Limit feature
Limit to words in the title:
   Hay fever[ti]
Use the Boolean operators AND or NOT
Strategies to broaden a search
Use truncation symbol (*) to pick up variant endings
   Pediatric*
Decrease the number of concepts searched
Use the Boolean operator OR with additional synonyms
Explode subject headings to include more specific terms
Include all subheadings
Include all publication types

MeSH = medical subject headings.

increase the likelihood of useful results. However, searching and evaluating all relevant, evidence-based research on a topic in MEDLINE can be extremely time consuming owing to inconsistencies in indexing, the complexity of language, and the large volume of literature. In the following case, we focus on some of the tools that provide clinicians ready access to systematic reviews and structured abstracts.

A full-text, quality-filtered review, such as the one found by Dr. Davis in the Cochrane Library, originates from the results of exhaustive searches in MEDLINE and other databases that are then rigorously analyzed by subject research groups.

Although the PubMed system response time is fast (recently implemented system enhancements have increased the speed so that a search that previously took 18 seconds now runs in fewer than 2 seconds), considerable time and skill are often necessary to create a search strategy that locates a manageable number of relevant citations in MEDLINE. Additional time is required to obtain the complete articles and appraise their content, making MEDLINE somewhat impractical for use at the point of care.

A sound strategy for finding patient care information is to first check the Cochrane Library or some of the other

Case 2

Dr. Davis, a first-year medicine resident doing an ambulatory rotation, saw a 71-year-old male patient whose chief complaint was memory disturbances due to early Alzheimer's disease symptoms. At a noon conference, one of the young faculty members had reported on the use of tacrine in a patient very similar to Dr. Davis' patient. Dr. Davis decided to search for more information regarding the use of tacrine for memory loss. She wanted to look at research on the effectiveness and side effects of tacrine to help decide whether it would be a suitable drug for her clinic patient. Dr. Davis had chosen to present this patient the following Tuesday at a clinical problem-solving meeting in which her task was to defend the literature on which she based her choice of therapy.

First, Dr. Davis searched the Web version of the Cochrane Library. Produced by the Cochrane Collaboration, the library provides a fast way to identify systematic reviews. The Cochrane Collaboration is an international organization that aims to prepare, maintain, and promote the accessibility of systematic reviews on health care interventions.[18,19] The Cochrane Library, 1998 Issue 4, currently has 576 completed systematic reviews that involve extensive searches of electronic databases, including MEDLINE, and hand searches of journal issues on a wide variety of topics. Jadad and colleagues compared Cochrane reviews with reviews published in paper journals and found that Cochrane reviews were updated more frequently and included elements that made them less prone to bias.[20]

Dr. Davis's search of the Cochrane Library using the MeSH term *tacrine* yielded a systematic review on the use of tacrine in Alzheimer's disease dated March 1997 (Figure 4-4). It examined evidence of beneficial effects of tacrine in Alzheimer's disease and assessed the safety profile for serious adverse effects.[21]

Through a search of the *ACP Journal Club* Web site,[22] Dr. Davis located a review of a 1997 position paper considering tacrine therapy for Alzheimer's disease in the March/April 1998 issue of *ACP Journal Club*.[23]

She turned to PubMed MEDLINE to check for more recent materials and first tried the Clinical Queries therapy filter with the MeSH headings *tacrine* AND *Alzheimer disease*. The search resulted in more than 90 citations, so to further narrow the focus, she used both *Alzheimer disease/drug therapy* and *tacrine/therapeutic use* as major subject headings, specified the randomized controlled trial publication type, and limited the retrieval to English language. This strategy resulted in approximately 40 citations, including an article published in 1998 that she had not located in Cochrane or the *ACP Journal Club*.

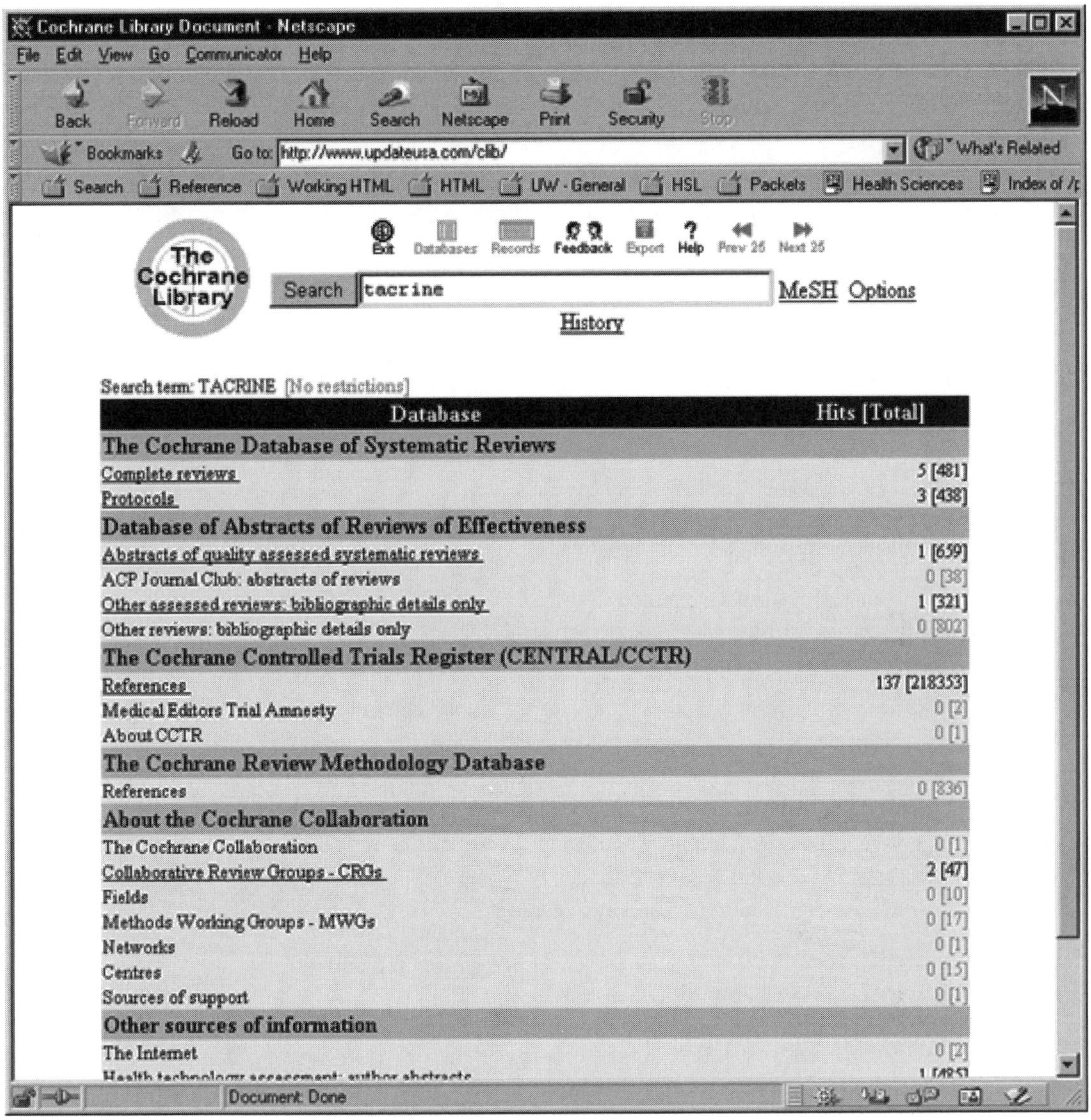

Figure 4-4. Search for systematic reviews of *tacrine* in the Cochrane Library.

sources of relevant clinical evidence, such as *ACP Journal Club* and InfoPOEMs. Next turn to MEDLINE to look for primary research, more recent studies, or topics not addressed in the specialized evidence-based medicine resources. Perhaps the best strategy for the busy health care professional is to develop a working relationship with the librarian in your hospital or institution. The librarian will often be your most helpful colleague in these efforts, whether that assistance is locating the information for you, aiding you with search strategies, or pointing out the latest evidence-based resources.

An annotated list of useful electronic and Web evidence-based medicine resources is presented in Evidence-Based Electronic Resources. Development of integrated ways of

searching MEDLINE, Cochrane, and other disparate resources would be very useful, an idea that is not lost on search interface developers. The future will likely bring one-stop search products providing a single interface to various resources, making locating useful evidence-based information quicker and more straightforward.

References

1. Huth EJ. The underused medical literature. Ann Intern Med 1989;110:99–100.
2. Kassirer J. Learning medicine: too many books, too few journals. N Engl J Med 1992;326:1427–1428.

3. Evidence-Based Medicine Working Group. Evidence-based medicine: a new approach to teaching the practice of medicine. JAMA 1992;268:2420–2425.
4. Covell DJ, Uman GC, Manning PR. Information needs in office practice: are they being met? Ann Intern Med 1985;103:596–599.
5. Gorman PN, Helfand M. Information seeking in primary care: how physicians choose which clinical questions to pursue and which to leave unanswered. Med Decis Making 1995;15:113–119.
6. Brown MS. Physicians on the Internet: ambivalence and resistance about to give way to acceptance. Medicine on the Net 1998;4:19–21.
7. America Online. Available at: http://www.aol.com. Accessed June 25, 1998.
8. CompuServe. Available at: http://www.compuserve.com. Accessed June 25, 1998.
9. Microsoft Network. Available at: http://www.msn.com. Accessed June 25, 1998.
10. Prodigy. Available at: http://www.prodigy.com. Accessed June 25, 1998.
11. Pompili T, et al. Online services. (America Online, CompuServe Interactive, the Microsoft Network, and Prodigy Internet). PC Magazine 1997;16:200–206.
12. HealthGate. Available at: http://www.healthgate.com. Accessed June 25, 1998.
13. Medscape. Available at: http://www.medscape.com. Accessed June 25, 1998.
14. National Library of Medicine MEDLINE training manuals. Available at: http://www.nlm.nih.gov/pubs/web_based.html. Accessed June 25, 1998.
15. Hanes RB, Wilczynski N, McKibbon KA, et al. Developing optimal search strategies for detecting clinically sound studies in MEDLINE. J Am Med Inform Assoc 1994;1:447–458.
16. Palmer J, Lusher A, Snowball R. Searching for the evidence. Genitourin Med 1997;73:70-72.
17. Duffel P. Constructing a search strategy. CINAHLnews 1995;14:1–2.
18. Bero L, Rennie D. The Cochrane Collaboration: preparing, maintaining, and disseminating reviews of the effects of health care. JAMA 1995;274:1935–1938.
19. Jadad AR, Haynes RB. The Cochrane Collaboration: advances and challenges in improving evidence-based decision making. Med Decis Making 1998;279:611–614.
20. Jadad AR, Cook DJ, Jones A, et al. Methodology and reports of systematic reviews and meta-analysis: a comparison of Cochrane Reviews with articles published in paper-based journals. JAMA 1998;280:278–280.
21. Qizilbash N, Birks J, Lopez Arrieta J, et al. The efficacy of tacrine in Alzheimer's disease (03/01/97). Cochrane Database of Systematic Reviews, Issue 2, 1998. Edmonton: Synapse Publishing.
22. *ACP Journal Club* [serial online]. Available at: http://www.acponline.org/journals/acpjc/jcmenu.htm. Accessed June 25, 1998.
23. Hirsh CH. Commentary on "Tacrine has limited efficacy for Alzheimer disease." ACP J Club 1998; 128:46. Comment on Glennie J, for the Canadian Coordinating Office for Health Technology Assessment (CCOHTA). The efficacy of tacrine and the measurement of outcomes in Alzheimer's disease. CCOHTA Technology Overview: Pharmaceuticals 1997 July; Issue 5.

Further Reading

Cochrane Collaboration

Dickersin K, Manheimer E. The Cochrane Collaboration: evaluation of health care and services using systematic reviews of the results of randomized controlled trials. Clin Obstet Gynecol 1998;41:315–331.
Hunt DL, McKibbon KA. Locating and appraising systematic reviews. Ann Intern Med 1997;126:532–538.
Jadad AR, Haynes RB. The Cochrane Collaboration—advances and challenges in improving evidence-based decision making. Med Decis Making 1998;18:2–9.

Connecting to the Internet

Chi-Lum BI, Glowniak JV, Gosbee J, et al. The physician's guide to the Internet. Patient Care 1997;31:26–53.
Ho K, Grunfeld A. An Internet primer for emergency physicians: part 1. J Emerg Med 1996;14:771–776.
Klemenz B, McSherry D. Obtaining medical information from the Internet. J R Coll Physicians Lond 1997;31: 410–413.
Wang KK, Wong Kee Song LM. The physician and the Internet. Mayo Clin Proc 1997;72:66–71.

Searching MEDLINE

Dorsch J. Evidence Based Medicine: Finding the Best Clinical Literature. Library of the Health Sciences, University of Illinois at Chicago. Available at: http://www.uic.edu/~jod/ebm.html. Accessed June 25, 1998.
Dwyer C. Pointers for making the most of your MEDLINE searches. October 1997. ACP Observer. Available at: http://www.acponline.org/journals/news/oct97/medline.html. Accessed June 25, 1998.
Greenhalgh T. How to read a paper. The MEDLINE database. BMJ 1997;315:180–183.
Hunt DL, McKibbon KA. Locating and appraising systematic reviews. Ann Intern Med 1997;126:532–538.
Lowe HJ, Barnett GO. Understanding and using the medical subject headings (MeSH) vocabulary to perform literature searches. JAMA 1994;271:1103–1108.
McKibbon KA, Walker-Dilks CJ. Beyond *ACP Journal Club*: how to harness MEDLINE to solve clinical problems. ACP J Club 1994;120(Suppl 2):A10–A12.
McKibbon KA, Walker-Dilks CJ. Beyond *ACP Journal Club*: how to harness MEDLINE for therapy problems. ACP J Club 1994;121(Suppl 1):A10–A12.
McKibbon KA, Walker-Dilks CJ. Beyond *ACP Journal*

Club: how to harness MEDLINE for diagnostic problems. ACP J Club 1994;121(Suppl 2):A10–A12.

McKibbon KA, Walker-Dilks CJ, Haynes RB, Wilczynski N. Beyond *ACP Journal Club*: how to harness MEDLINE for prognosis problems. ACP J Club 1995;123:A12–A14.

McKibbon KA, Walker-Dilks CJ, Wilczynski NL, Haynes RB. Beyond *ACP Journal Club*: how to harness MEDLINE for review articles. ACP J Club 1996;124:A12–A13.

Walker-Dilks CJ, McKibbon KA, Haynes RB. Beyond *ACP Journal Club*: how to harness MEDLINE for etiology problems. ACP J Club 1994;121:A10–A11.

Physicians' Information-Seeking Behavior

Chamblis ML, Conley J. Answering clinical questions. J Fam Pract 1996;43:140–144.

Ely JW, Burch RJ, Vinson DC. The information needs of family physicians: case specific clinical questions. J Fam Pract 1992;35:265–269.

Forsythe DE, Buchanan BG. Expanding the concept of medical information: an observational study of physicians' information needs. Comput Biomed Res 1992;25: 181–200.

Gorman PN, Ash J, Wykoff L. Can primary care physicians' questions be answered using the medical literature? Bull Med Libr Assoc 1994;82:140–146.

Haynes RB, McKibbon A, Walker CJ, et al. Online access to MEDLINE in clinical settings. Ann Intern Med 1990;112:78–84.

Lindberg DAB, Siegel ER, Rapp BA, et al. Use of MEDLINE by physicians for clinical problem solving. JAMA 1993;269:3124–3129.

Osheroff JA , Bankowitz RA. Physician's use of computer software in answering clinical questions. Bull Med Libr Assoc 1993;81:11–19.

Osheroff JA, Forsythe DE, Buchanan BG, et al. Physicians' information needs: an analysis of questions posed during clinical teaching. Ann Intern Med 1991;114: 576–581.

Timpka T, Ekstrom M, Bjurulf P. Information needs and information seeking behavior in primary health care. Scand J Prim Health Care 1989;7:105–109.

Thompson ML. Characteristics of information resources preferred by primary care providers. Bull Med Libr Assoc 1997;85:187–192.

Evidence-Based Electronic Resources

ACP Journal Club, six issues per year. $59 per year for individuals, $80 per year for institutions. American College of Physicians (Philadelphia, PA). Available at: http://www.acponline.org/journals/acpjc/jcmenu.htm. Provides structured abstracts and expert commentary on scientifically strong, clinically relevant articles selected by criteria outlined in each issue. Articles are chosen from more than 35 internal medicine journals.

Bandolier, free access on the Internet. National Health Service Research and Development Directorate (Oxford, England). Available at: http://www.jr2.ox.ac.uk/Bandolier/index.html. *Bandolier* is a literature review source published monthly at Oxford University containing evidence-supported information. Topics range from the humorous to the technical, but the majority of information is concise and useful.

Best Evidence, annual CD-ROM. $75 for individuals. American College of Physicians (Philadelphia, PA). Available at: http://www.acponline.org/catalog/cbi/best_evidence.htm. Cumulates both *ACP Journal Club* (1991–1997) and *Evidence-Based Medicine* (December 1995–1997) so that they both can be searched on a single CD-ROM.

Cochrane Library, quarterly updates. $225 per year for individuals. Update Software Ltd. (Oxford, England). Available at: http://www.update-software.com. In the United States, Update Software Inc. Available at: http://www.updateusa.com. Composed of four sections: the Cochrane Database of Systematic Reviews, the Database of Abstracts of Reviews of Effectiveness, the Cochrane Controlled Trials Registry, and the Cochrane Review Methodology Database.

Evidence-Based Medicine, six issues per year. $85 per year for individuals, $136 per year for institutions. American College of Physicians (Philadelphia, PA) and BMJ Publishing Group (London). Available at: http://www.acponline.org/journals/ebm/ebmmenu.htm. Similar in format to *ACP Journal Club* and also includes articles from more than 50 journals in the subject areas of family medicine, internal medicine (with key selections from *ACP Journal Club*), general surgery, pediatrics, obstetrics, gynecology, psychiatry, and anesthesiology.

Evidence-Based Practice, monthly newsletter. $90 per year for physicians, $80 per year for nurse practitioners or physician assistants. Dowden Publishing Co. More than 85 journals reviewed monthly by the editors, with 25–30 synopses each month of POEMs (patient-oriented evidence that matters).

Health Services/Technology Assessment Text (*HSTAT*). Available at: http://text.nlm.nih.gov. *HSTAT* is a free electronic resource developed at the NLM that provides access to the full text of documents useful in health care decision making. Included are clinical practice guidelines, quick-reference guides for clinicians, consumer brochures, evidence reports from the Agency for Health Care Policy and Research, National Institutes of Health clinical studies, and additional federal resources. *HSTAT* also provides a link to the Centers for Disease Control and Prevention's Prevention Guidelines Database.

InfoPOEMs (formerly *Journal of Family Practice* Journal Club). Available at: http://www.infopoems.com. InfoPOEMs is designed to support the evidence-based practice of medicine. Each month, more than 80 journals are reviewed to identify the eight articles with patient-oriented outcomes that have the greatest potential to change the way primary care clinicians practice. These articles are then critically appraised by expert family physicians, educators, and/or pharmacologists.

National Guideline Clearinghouse. Available at: http://www.

ngc.gov. A public resource for evidence-based clinical practice guidelines sponsored by the Agency for Health Care Policy and Research in partnership with the American Medical Association and the American Association of Health Plans.

PubMed. Available at: http://www.ncbi.nlm.nih.gov/PubMed. The NLM's free Web interface to the MEDLINE database.

Turning Research into Practice (TRIP). Primary Care Clinical Effectiveness Team, Gwent Health Authority. Available at: http://www.gwent.nhs.gov.uk/trip/test-search.html. Provides a single searchable index to 23 evidence-based medicine resources ranging from the Cochrane Database of Systematic Reviews to the *ACP Journal Club*, *MD Digest*, *Bandolier*, Scottish Intercollegiate Guidelines Network (SIGN), *Journal of Family Practice*, Development and Evaluation Committee Reports (DEC), and various sets of practice guidelines. The 3,463 entries are searchable by title.

Chapter 5
Critical Appraisal of the Literature: How to Assess an Article and Still Enjoy Life*

William F. Miser

Case 1

A 47-year-old perimenopausal woman, in your office for a well-woman examination, has a newspaper clipping given to her by a friend. The clipping reviews a recent article published in a well-known national medical journal that warns against the use of hormonal replacement therapy (HRT) because of an increased risk of breast cancer.[1] Although she is at low risk for this cancer and her breast examination is normal, she resists your recommendation to begin HRT. When you discuss with her the results of an article that demonstrated that postmenopausal use of estrogen reduces the risk of severe coronary heart disease,[2] she counters with another article from the same issue that concludes that cardiovascular mortality is increased in estrogen users.[3] As you review these studies, you do not recognize that all have serious flaws. Also, you do not have available more methodologically sound articles that demonstrate the overwhelming benefit of HRT[4–6] with no increased risk in breast cancer.[7–9] She leaves triumphantly from your office without a prescription, and you feel confused about the overall benefit of HRT.

After you make a mental note to read more about HRT, you see your next patient, a 28-year-old man with allergic rhinitis. He hands you a study he obtained from the Internet that concludes that the latest antihistamine is far superior in efficacy to all other antihistamines currently available on the market. He asks you for this new prescription, realizing that his health insurance company will not approve it unless you justify to them why he should take this particular antihistamine. You promise to review the article and call him later in the week with his prescription.

The mother of your next patient, a 12-year-old boy, requests a test with which you are unfamiliar. She hands you yet another article suggesting that physicians who do not offer this test are guilty of negligence. As you review this study, you wish that you remembered more about how to critically assess an article, and you hope that the rest of the day goes better.

This scenario is occurring more frequently as patients are increasingly gaining access to medical information and then looking to their physicians for its interpretation. Gone are the days when physicians' opinions went unchallenged by uninformed patients. Our society is inundated with medical advice and contrasting views from newspaper, radio, television, popular lay journals,

and the Internet, and physicians are faced with the task of damage control.

Physicians also encounter constantly changing recommendations for clinical practice and an "information jungle."[10,11] With 6 million medical articles published each year, the amount of information available is overwhelming.[12] If clinicians, trying to keep up with all of the literature, were to read two articles per day, in just 1 year they would fall 82 centuries behind in their reading!

Despite the gargantuan volume of medical literature, less than 15% of all articles published on a particular

*Reprinted with permission from WF Miser. Critical appraisal of the literature. J Am Board Fam Pract 1999;12:(in press).

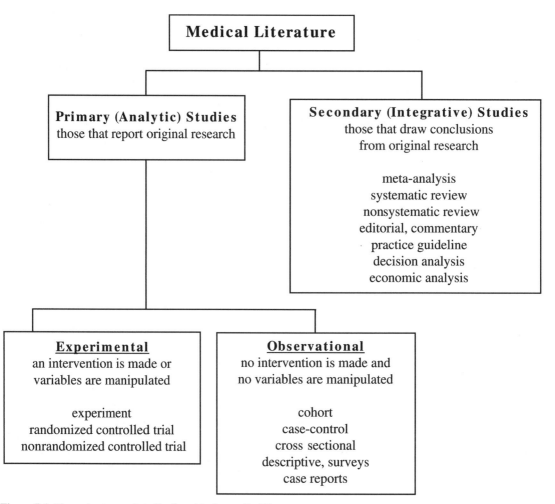

Figure 5-1. The major types of studies found in the medical literature.

topic are useful.[13] Most articles are not peer-reviewed, are sponsored by those with commercial interests, or arrive free in the mail. Even articles published in the most prestigious journals are far from perfect. Analyses of clinical trials published in a wide variety of journals have identified large deficiencies in design, analysis, and reporting; although improving, the average quality score of clinical trials since the 1970s is less than 50%.[14–16] As a result, many diagnostic tests and therapies are not rigorously evaluated before being established as a routine part of practice; this leads to the widespread use of tests with unproved efficacy and treatments that are either ineffective or that may do more harm than good.[17] As such, readers must take personal responsibility for judging the validity and clinical importance of the medical literature.

The challenge to physicians is to provide up-to-date medical care incorporating valid new information. Our

ultimate goal as clinicians should be to help patients live long, functional, satisfying, and pain- and symptom-free lives. To do this requires us to balance compassion with competence. One of the essential skills needed to maintain competence, to provide patients with the best possible care, and to do more good than harm is the ability to critically appraise the literature. We must be able to find potentially relevant information, to filter out the best quality information from the much larger volume of less credible information, and then to judge whether to believe the information that remains.[12]

The two major types of studies (Figure 5-1) reported in the medical literature are those that (1) report original research (i.e., analytic, primary studies) and (2) summarize or draw conclusions from original research (i.e., integrative, secondary studies). Primary studies can be either experimental (an intervention is made) or observational (no intervention is made). The purpose of this chapter is

---

Case 2

Croup season is approaching, and you have a rather large pediatric population in your practice. Since you finished your residency, you have been treating croup with mist therapy but have been dissatisfied with its results. You talk to a colleague about this problem, and she hands you an article published in 1998 in the *Journal of the American Medical Association* (*JAMA*), "Nebulized budesonide and oral dexamethasone for treatment of croup: a randomized controlled trial."[44] You were taught that the use of corticosteroids for croup is controversial and should be reserved for patients in the hospital. You have a few minutes before seeing your next patient but are unsure whether you have the time to read this article.

---

to provide an overview of a systematic, efficient, and effective approach to the critical review of original research. This information is pertinent to physicians regardless of their setting, be it an academic medical center or a rural solo practice. Owing to space limitations, this chapter cannot cover everything in exhaustive detail, and the reader is encouraged to refer to the Further Reading section at the end of the chapter for more assistance.

Critical Appraisal of an Article

It is important for you as a clinician to master the skills of critical appraisal of the literature if you are to apply "evidence-based medicine" to the daily clinical problems you encounter. However, most busy clinicians do not have hours to spend critiquing an article; they need a brief, efficient screening method that allows them to determine whether the information is valid and applicable to their practice. By applying the techniques offered here, you can approach the literature confidently and base your clinical decisions on "evidence rather than hope."[18]

This approach is modified and adapted from several excellent sources. The Department of Clinical Epidemiology and Biostatistics at McMaster University published a series of useful guides in 1981 to help the busy clinician critically read clinical articles about diagnosis, prognosis, etiology, and therapy.[19–23] These guides have been updated and expanded to focus more on the practical issues of first finding pertinent articles and then validating (believing) and applying the information to patient care.[18,24–43] The recommendations from these users' guides form the foundation on which techniques developed by Slawson, Shaugnessy, and Bennett[10,11] are modified and added.

The process of appraising an article consists of three steps: (1) conducting an initial validity and relevance screen, (2) determining the intent of the article, and (3) evaluating the validity of the article based on its intent. This chapter focuses on the type of study most germane to clinical practice: a therapeutic intervention. To make the most of this exercise, it would be helpful

for you to obtain a copy of the article mentioned in Case 2 and to follow the steps outlined in the following sections. The users' guides and other resources listed at the end of this chapter are helpful in learning how to appraise other types of articles.

Step One: Conduct an Initial Validity and Relevance Screen

The first step when looking at an article is to ask yourself, "Is this article worth taking the time to review in depth?" This can be answered in a few seconds by asking six simple questions (Form 5-1). A "stop" or "pause" answer to any of these questions should prompt you to seriously consider whether you should spend the time to critically review the study. The article mentioned in Case 2 is used to illustrate these points.

1. *Is the article from a peer-reviewed journal?* Most national and specialty journals published in the United States are peer-reviewed; if in doubt, this answer can be found in the journal's Instructions for Authors section. Typically, those journals sent to clinicians unsolicited and free of charge are "throwaway" journals, so called because that is exactly what you should do with them. These journals, although attractive in appearance, are not peer-reviewed but instead are geared toward generating income from advertising.[12,18]

Articles published in the major peer-reviewed journals have already undergone an extensive process to weed out flawed studies and to improve the quality of the ones subsequently accepted for publication. Typically, when an investigator submits a manuscript to a peer-reviewed journal, the editor first establishes whether the manuscript is suitable for that journal and then, if acceptable, sends it to several reviewers for analysis. Peer reviewers are not part of the editorial staff but usually are volunteers who have expertise in both the subject matter and research design. The purpose of the peer review is to act as a sieve by detecting studies that are flawed by poor design, are trivial, or are uninterpretable. This process, along with subsequent revisions and editing, improves the quality of the

---

Form 5-1. Initial Validity and Relevance Screen*

Is this article worth taking the time to review in depth?

1. Is the article from a peer-reviewed journal? (Articles published in a peer-reviewed journal have already gone through an extensive review and editing process.) Yes (go on) No (stop)
2. Is the location of the study similar to mine, so that the results, if valid, would apply to my practice? Yes (go on) No (stop)
3. Is the study sponsored by an organization that may influence the study design or results? Yes (pause) No (go on)

Read the conclusion of the abstract to determine relevance.

4. Will this information, if true, have a direct impact on the health of my patients, and is it something they will care about? Yes (go on) No (stop)
5. Is the problem addressed one that is common to my practice, and is the intervention or test feasible and available to me? Yes (go on) No (stop)
6. Will this information, if true, require me to change my current practice? Yes (go on) No (stop)

---

*A "stop" or "pause" answer to any of the questions should prompt you to seriously question whether you should take the time to critically review the article.

Source: Questions 4–6 adapted from D Slawson, A Shaughnessy, M Ebell, H Barry. Mastering medical information and the role of POEMs: patient-oriented evidence that matters. J Fam Pract 1997;45:195–196.

---

paper and its statistical analyses.[45–48] *Annals of Internal Medicine*, for example, receives more than 1,200 original research manuscript submissions each year. The editorial staff reject half after an internal review, and the remaining half are sent to at least two peers for review. Of the original 1,200 submissions, only 15% are published.[49]

Because of these strengths, peer review is the accepted method for improving the quality of the science reported in the medical literature.[50] This mechanism is far from perfect, however, and it does not guarantee that the published article is without flaw or bias.[13] Other types of publication biases are inherent in the process despite an adequate peer review process. Studies showing statistically significant ("positive") results and having larger sample sizes are more likely to be written and submitted by authors and subsequently accepted and published than are nonsignificant ("negative") studies.[51–54] Also, the speed of publication depends on the direction and strength of the trial results; trials with negative results take twice as long to be published as do positive trials.[55] Finally, no matter how good the peer review system, fraudulent research, although rare, is extremely hard to identify.[56]

The article you are assessing is published in *JAMA*. You are almost certain that this is a peer-reviewed journal; the Instructions for Authors section confirms this ("*JAMA* is an international, peer-reviewed, general medical journal . . ."). You answer yes to this question.

2. *Is the location of the study similar to mine, so that the results, if valid, would apply to my practice?* This question can be answered by reviewing information about the authors on the first page of an article (typically at the bottom of the page). If you have a rural general practice and you are assessing a study performed in a university subspecialty clinic, you may want to pause and consider the potential biases that may be present. This is a "soft" area, and you should rarely reject an article outright at this juncture; however, large differences in location should raise caution in your mind.

In the article you are assessing, you notice at the bottom of the first page that the study was performed in two university hospitals in Canada. Although no reason exists to believe children with croup for whom you provide care are different from those seen in Canada, you begin to wonder if the study done in a tertiary care center is applicable to your practice. You decide to continue critiquing this article but make a mental note to consider this issue later.

3. *Is the study sponsored by an organization that may influence the study design or results?* This question considers the potential bias that may occur from outside funding. In most journals, investigators are required to identify sources of funding for their study. Clinicians should be wary of published symposiums sponsored by pharmaceutical companies. Although found in peer-reviewed journals, they tend to be promotional in nature, to have misleading titles, and to use brand names, and they are less likely to be peer-reviewed in the same manner as other articles in the parent journal.[57] Also, randomized clinical trials (RCTs) published in journal supplements are generally of inferior quality compared with articles published in the parent journal.[58] This is not to say that all studies sponsored by commercial interests are biased; on the contrary, numerous well-designed studies published in the literature are sponsored by the pharmaceutical industry. If a pharmaceutical company or other commercial organization funded the study, however, you should look for

Table 5-1. Major Clinical Categories of Primary Research and Their Preferred Study Designs

Clinical Category	Preferred Study Design
Therapy: tests the effectiveness of a treatment such as a drug, surgical procedure, or other intervention	Randomized, double-blinded, placebo-controlled trial
Diagnosis and screening: measures the validity (Is it dependable?) and reliability (Will the same results be obtained every time?) of a diagnostic test, or evaluates the effectiveness of a test in detecting disease at a presymptomatic stage when applied to a large population	Cross-sectional survey (comparing the new test with a "gold standard")
Causation: assesses whether a substance is related to the development of an illness or condition	Cohort or case-control
Prognosis: determines the outcome of a disease	Longitudinal cohort study

Source: Adapted from T Greenhalgh. How to read a paper: getting your bearings (deciding what the paper is about). BMJ 1997;315:243–246.

assurances from investigators that the design and results were not influenced by that association.

You again review the information about the authors and look at the end of the article for this information. You find that funding support is from several foundations, none of which has commercial interests in the drugs used in the study.

The answers to the next three questions dealing with clinical relevance to your practice can be obtained by reading the conclusion and selected portions of the abstract. Clinical relevance is important not only to physicians but also to their patients. Rarely is it worthwhile to read an article about an uncommon condition you have never encountered in your practice or about a treatment or diagnostic test that is not, and never will be, available to you. Reading these types of articles may satisfy your intellectual curiosity but will not impact your practice. Slawson and colleagues emphasized that for a busy clinician, articles concerned with patient-oriented evidence that matters are far more useful than those articles that report disease-oriented evidence.[10,59] So, given a choice between reading an article that describes the sensitivity and specificity of a screening test in detecting cancer (disease-oriented evidence) and one that shows that those who undergo this screening enjoy an improved quality and length of life (patient-oriented evidence that matters), you would probably want to choose the latter.

4. *Will this information, if true, have a direct impact on the health of my patients, and is it something they will care about?* You read this conclusion of the abstract: "Based on the similar outcomes in the 3 groups, oral dexamethasone is the preferred intervention because of its ease of administration, lower cost, and more widespread availability." You scan the rest of the abstract and find that the outcomes were a croup score, hospital admission rates, time spent in the emergency department, return visits, and ongoing symptoms at 1 week. Because these are outcomes that you and your patients care about, you answer yes to this question.

5. *Is the problem addressed one that is common to my practice, and is the intervention or test feasible and available to me?* If you are in a practice that sees very few children or rarely sees croup, you may decide the answer is no and go on to read other articles. You decide the answer to this is yes, however, because croup is a common problem seen in your practice, and oral dexamethasone is something you could easily stock in your office.

6. *Will this information, if true, require me to change my current practice?* Because you have never used oral dexamethasone in the outpatient treatment of croup, your answer to this question is yes.

In only a few seconds, you have quickly answered six pertinent questions that allow you to decide if you want to take the time to critically review this article. This "weeding" tool allows you to recycle those articles that are not relevant to your practice, thus allowing more time to examine the validity of those few articles that may have an impact on the care of your patients.

Step Two: Determine the Intent of the Article

If you decide to continue with the article after completing step one, your next task is to determine why the study was performed and what clinical question(s) the investigators were addressing.[60] The four major clinical categories found in articles of primary (original) research are: (1) therapy, (2) diagnosis and screening, (3) causation, and (4) prognosis (Table 5-1). The answer to this step often can be found by reading the abstract and, if needed, by skimming the introduction (usually found in the last paragraph) to determine the purpose of the study.

For the article mentioned in Case 2, the investigators address a therapeutic intervention (the use of oral dexamethasone in treating mild to moderate croup). Because you are seriously considering including this therapeutic intervention in your practice, you decide you

Form 5-2. Validity Screen for an Article about Therapy*

If the article passes the initial screen in Form 5-1, proceed with the following critical assessment by reading the article's Methods section.

1. Is the study a randomized controlled trial?		
How were patients selected for the trial?		
Were they properly randomized into groups using concealed assignment?	Yes (go on)	No (stop)
2. Are the subjects in the study similar to mine?	Yes (go on)	No (stop)
3. Are all participants who entered the trial properly accounted for at its conclusion?		
Was follow-up complete and were few lost to follow-up compared with the number of bad outcomes?		
Were patients analyzed in the groups to which they were initially randomized (intention-to-treat analysis)?	Yes (go on)	No (stop)
4. Was everyone involved in the study (subjects and investigators) "blind" to treatment?	Yes	No
5. Were the intervention and control groups similar at the start of the trial?		
(Check "Table 1" of article)	Yes	No
6. Were the groups treated equally (aside from the experimental intervention)?	Yes	No
7. Are the results clinically as well as statistically significant?		
Were the outcomes measured clinically important?	Yes	No
8. If a negative trial, was a power analysis done?	Yes	No
9. Were other factors present that might have affected the outcome?	Yes	No
10. Are the treatment benefits worth the potential harms and costs?	Yes	No

*A "stop" answer to any of the questions should prompt you to seriously question whether the results of the study are valid and whether you should use this therapeutic intervention.

Source: Adapted from material developed by the Department of Clinical Epidemiology and Biostatistics at McMaster University. G Guyatt, D Sackett, D Cook. Users' guides to the medical literature. II: How to use an article about therapy or prevention? A. Are the results of the study valid? Evidence-Based Medicine Working Group. JAMA 1993;270:2598–2601; the Information Mastery Working Group. D Slawson, A Shaughnessy, J Bennett. Becoming a medical information master: feeling good about not knowing everything. J Fam Pract 1994;38:505–513.

should spend the time to critically evaluate the conclusions of the study.

Step Three: Evaluate the Validity of the Article Based on Its Intent

After successfully passing the first two steps, the article should be critically assessed for its validity and applicability to your practice setting. Each of the four clinical categories found in Table 5-1 has a preferred study design and critical items to ensure its validity. The users' guides published by the Department of Clinical Epidemiology and Biostatistics at McMaster University provide a useful list of questions to help you with this assessment. Adaptations of these lists of questions are found in Forms 5-2 through 5-5.

To get started on this step, read the entire abstract; survey the boldface headings; review the tables, graphs, and illustrations; and then skim-read the first sentence of each paragraph to quickly grasp the organization of the article. You then need to focus on the methods section, answering a specific list of questions based on the intent of the article. Because the article from Case 2 deals with

a therapeutic intervention, you begin reading the methods section of the article and addressing the questions listed in Form 5-2.

1. *Is the study a randomized controlled trial?* RCTs (Figure 5-2) are considered the "gold standard" design to determine the effectiveness of treatment. The power of RCTs lies in their use of randomization. At the start of a trial, participants are randomly allocated by a process equivalent to the flip of a coin to either one intervention (e.g., a new antihypertensive) or another (e.g., an established antihypertensive or placebo). Both groups are then followed for a specified period, and defined outcomes (e.g., blood pressure, myocardial infarction, death) are measured and analyzed at the conclusion.

Randomization diminishes the potential for investigators selecting individuals in a way that would unfairly bias one treatment group over another (i.e., selection bias). It is important to determine how the investigators actually performed the randomization. Although infrequently reported in the past, most journals now require a standard format that provides this information.[15] Various techniques can be used for randomization.[61] Investigators

Form 5-3. Validity Screen for an Article about a Diagnostic Test*

If the article passes the initial screen in Form 5-1, proceed with the following critical assessment by reading the article's Methods section.

1. What is the disease being addressed and what is the diagnostic test?

   _____

2. Was the new test compared with an acceptable "gold standard" test and were both tests applied in a uniformly blind manner? — Yes (go on) No (stop)
3. Did the patient sample include an appropriate spectrum of patients to whom the diagnostic test will be applied in clinical practice? — Yes (go on) No (stop)
4. Is the new test reasonable? What are its limitations? — Yes (go on) No (stop)
   Explain: _____
5. In terms of prevalence of disease, are the study subjects similar to my patients? (Varying prevalences will affect the predictive value of the test in my practice.) — Yes No
6. Will my patients be better off as a result of this test? — Yes No
7. What are the sensitivity, specificity, and predictive values of the test?

   Sensitivity = (a) / (a + c) = _____
   Specificity = (d) / (b + d) = _____
   Positive predictive value = (a) / (a + b) = _____
   Negative predictive value = (c) / (c + d) = _____

Test Result	"Gold Standard" Result	
	Positive	Negative
Positive	a	b
Negative	c	d

*A "stop" answer to any of the questions should prompt you to seriously question whether the results of the study are valid and whether you should use this diagnostic test.

Source: Adapted from material developed by the Department of Clinical Epidemiology and Biostatistics at McMaster University. R Jaeschke, G Guyatt, D Sackett. Users' guides to the medical literature. III: How to use an article about a diagnostic test. A. Are the results of the study valid? Evidence-Based Medicine Working Group. JAMA 1994;271:389–391; the Information Mastery Working Group. D Slawson, A Shaughnessy, J Bennett. Becoming a medical information master: feeling good about not knowing everything. J Fam Pract 1994;38:505–513.

Form 5-4. Validity Screen for an Article about Causation*

If the article passes the initial screen in Form 5-1, proceed with the following critical assessment by reading the article's Methods section.

1. Was a clearly defined comparison group or those at risk for, or having, the outcome of interest included? — Yes (go on) No (stop)
2. Were the outcomes and exposures measured in the same way in the groups being compared? — Yes (go on) No (stop)
3. Were the observers blinded to the exposure of outcome and to the outcome? — Yes (go on) No (stop)
4. Was follow-up sufficiently long and complete? — Yes (go on) No (stop)
5. Is the temporal relationship correct? (Does the exposure to the agent precede the outcome?) — Yes No
6. Is there a dose-response gradient? (As the quantity or the duration of exposure to the agent increases, does the risk of outcome likewise increase?) — Yes No
7. How strong is the association between exposure and outcome? (Is the relative risk or odds ratio large?) — Yes No

*A "stop" answer to any of the questions should prompt you to seriously question whether the results of the study are valid and whether the item in question is really a causative factor.

Source: Adapted from material developed by the Department of Clinical Epidemiology and Biostatistics at McMaster University. M Levine, S Walter, H Lee, et al. Users' guides to the medical literature. IV: How to use an article about harm. Evidence-Based Medicine Working Group. JAMA 1994;271:1615–1619.

may use simple randomization, in which each participant has an equal chance of being assigned to one group or another, without regard to previous assignments of other participants. Sometimes, this type of randomization results in one treatment group being larger than another or, by chance, one group having important baseline differences that may affect the study. To avoid these problems, investigators may use blocked randomization (i.e., groups are equal in size) or stratified randomization (i.e., subjects are randomized within groups based on potential confounding factors, such as age or gender).

To determine the assignment of participants, investigators should use a table of random numbers or a computer that produces a random sequence. The final allocation of participants to the study should be concealed from both investigators and participants. If investigators responsible for assigning subjects are aware of the allocation, they may unwittingly (or otherwise) assign those with a better prognosis to the treatment group and those with a worse prognosis to the control group. RCTs that have inadequate allocation concealment yield an inflated treatment effect that is as much as 30% better than in trials with proper concealment.[62,63]

In the article you are assessing, you find in the second paragraph of the Methods section that the study design was an RCT and that subjects were randomized to one of three groups: nebulized budesonide and oral placebo, placebo nebulizer and oral dexamethasone, and nebulized budesonide and oral dexamethasone. A central pharmacy randomized the patients into these groups using computer-generated random numbers in random blocks of six or nine to ensure equal distribution among the groups and then stratified them by study site. The randomization list was kept in the central pharmacy to ensure allocation concealment. You answer yes to this question and proceed with your assessment.

2. *Are the subjects in the study similar to mine?* To be generalizable (i.e., to have external validity), the subjects in the study should be similar to the patients you care for in your practice. A common problem encountered by primary care physicians is interpreting the results of studies done on patients in subspecialty care clinics. The group of men in a university urology clinic participating in a study on early detection of prostate cancer may be different from the group of men seen in a typical primary care clinic. It is important to determine who was included and who was excluded from the study. You find that the study subjects were children, ages 3 months to 5 years, who presented with mild to moderate croup. Because you provide care for children in this age group, and after noting the exclusion criteria, you answer yes to this question.

3. *Are all participants who entered the trial properly accounted for at its conclusion?* Another strength of RCTs is that participants are followed prospectively. However, it is important that these participants be accounted for at the end of the trial to avoid a "loss of subjects bias," which can occur through the course of a prospective study as subjects drop out of the investigation for various reasons. They may have lost interest, moved out of the area, developed intolerable side effects, or died. The subjects who are lost to follow-up may be different from those who remain, and the groups studied may have different rates of drop-outs. An attrition rate of more than 10% for short-term trials and 15% for long-term trials may invalidate the results of the study.

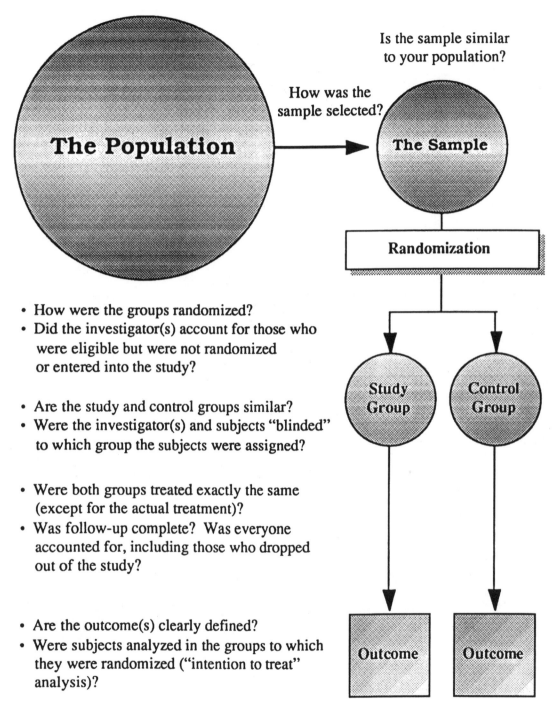

Is the sample similar
to your population?

How was the
sample selected?

The Population

The Sample

Randomization

- How were the groups randomized?
- Did the investigator(s) account for those who
  were eligible but were not randomized
  or entered into the study?

- Are the study and control groups similar?
- Were the investigator(s) and subjects "blinded"
  to which group the subjects were assigned?

- Were both groups treated exactly the same
  (except for the actual treatment)?
- Was follow-up complete? Was everyone
  accounted for, including those who dropped
  out of the study?

- Are the outcome(s) clearly defined?
- Were subjects analyzed in the groups to which
  they were randomized ("intention to treat"
  analysis)?

Study Group

Control Group

Outcome

Outcome

Figure 5-2. The randomized controlled trial, considered the "gold standard" for studies dealing with treatment or other interventions.

At the conclusion of the study, subjects should be analyzed in the group in which they were originally randomized, even if they were noncompliant or switched groups (intention-to-treat analysis). For example, researchers in a study wish to determine the best treat- ment approach to carotid stenosis, and patients are randomized to either carotid endarterectomy or medical management. Because it would be unethical to perform "sham" surgery, investigators and patients cannot be blinded to their treatment group. If, during the initial evaluation, individuals randomized to endarterectomy were found to be poor surgical candidates, they may be treated medically. At the conclusion of the study, however, their outcomes (e.g., stroke, death) should be included in the surgical group, even if they did not have surgery; to do otherwise would unfairly inflate the benefit of the surgical approach.

Most journals require a specific format for reporting RCTs, which includes a chart that allows you to easily follow the flow of subjects through the study.[15] In the article you are assessing, you notice in the chart that all but 1 of 198 participants were followed to study completion, which is an outstanding follow-up. You also notice in the methods section that the "primary analysis was based on the intention-to-treat principle." You answer yes to this question.

4. *Was everyone involved in the study (subjects and investigators) "blind" to treatment?* Investigator bias may occur when those making the observations may unintentionally "shade" the results to confirm the hypothesis or to influence the subjects. This bias can be prevented by the process of blinding, in which neither the investigators nor the subjects are aware of group assignment (double-blinded). For example, in a study comparing a new antihypertensive drug to a placebo, neither the investigators nor the subjects should be aware of what the subjects are taking. The study medication should be indistinguishable from the comparison medication or placebo; it should have the same look and taste and be taken at the same frequency. If the study medication has a certain bitter taste or other side effect and the comparison medication does not, patients may be able to guess which medicine they are taking, which may influence how they perceive their improvement.

In the article you are assessing, you find that the dexamethasone syrup and placebo syrup were identical in taste and appearance. Because budesonide was slightly opaque and the nebulized placebo was clear saline, the investigators took extra precautions by packaging the solutions in brown syringes. The investigators went further by asking the research assistants and subjects to guess which intervention the patients received; their responses were no greater than chance alone, indicating the blinding was successful. Assured that this was a properly conducted double-blinded study, you answer yes to this question.

5. *Were the intervention and control groups similar at the start of the trial?* Through the process of randomization, you expect the groups to be similar at the beginning of a trial. Because this may not always be the case, investigators should provide a group comparison. This information is usually found in the first table in the article.

In the article you are assessing, you find the groups to be similar, but not exact, in gender, age, history, croup score, and vital signs. Those in the dexamethasone-treated group had a slightly higher percentage of preceding upper respiratory tract infections than did those in the budesonide-treated group (67% vs. 54%). Although the investigators do not include an analysis on whether this is statistically significant, it is unlikely that such a small difference would be clinically significant. In areas such as these, you must use your clinical experience and judgment to determine whether small differences are likely to influence outcomes. You are satisfied that the groups are similar enough and answer yes to this question.

6. *Were the groups treated equally (aside from the experimental intervention)?* To ensure both that the study was properly blinded and that other unknown determinants are not a factor in the results, the groups should be treated equally except for the therapeutic intervention. In the study you are assessing, you find that every subject was treated in the same manner—everyone received an oral syrup (dexamethasone or placebo) and a nebulized solution (budesonide or placebo) and were assessed and followed equally. Had the investigators not given the subjects randomized to the oral dexamethasone a nebulized solution, both the investigators and subjects would know the therapeutic group in which the subjects were placed, thereby introducing a bias. Also, the possibility cannot be excluded that the actual treatment benefit was due to the process of nebulization itself and not to the budesonide. Because the investigators took these precautions, you answer yes to this question.

7. *Are the results clinically as well as statistically significant?* Statistics are mathematic techniques of gathering, organizing, describing, analyzing, and interpreting numeric data.[64] Through their use, investigators try to convince readers that the results of their study are valid. Internal validity addresses how well the study was done and determines whether the results reflect truth instead of occurring by chance alone. External validity considers whether the results are generalizable to patients outside of the study. Both types of validity are important.

The choice of statistical test depends on the study design, the types of data analyzed, and whether the groups are independent or paired. The three main types of data are categorical (i.e., nominal), ordinal, and continuous (i.e., interval). An observation made on more than one individual or group is independent (e.g., measuring serum cholesterol in two groups of subjects), whereas making more than one observation on an individual is paired (e.g., measuring serum cholesterol in an individual before and after treatment). Based on this information, one can then select an appropriate statistical test (Table 5-2). Be suspicious of a study that has a standard set of data collected in a standard way but are analyzed by a test that has an unpronounceable name and is not listed in a standard statistical textbook; the investigators may be attempting to prove that something is statistically significant when it truly is not.[65]

Two types of errors can occur when comparing the results of a study with "reality" (Figure 5-3). A type I

Table 5-2. A Practical Guide to Commonly Used Tests*

Categorical, 2 Samples	Categorical, >2 Samples	Ordinal	Continuous
	Tests for association between two independent variables		
Chi-square	—	—	—
Fisher exact			
Chi-square ($r \times r$)	Chi-square ($r \times r$)	—	—
Mann-Whitney U	Kruskal-Wallis one-way	Spearman's r	—
Wilcoxon rank sum	analysis of variance (ANOVA)	Kendall tau	
Student t	ANOVA	Kendall tau	Pearson correlation
		Spearman's r	Linear regression
		ANOVA	Multiple regression
	Tests for association between paired observations		
McNemar	Cochran Q	Wilcoxon signed rank	Paired t
		Friedman two-way ANOVA	

*The test chosen depends on study design, types of variables analyzed, and whether observations are independent or paired. Categorical (nominal) data can be grouped but not ordered (e.g., eye color, gender, race, religion). Ordinal data can be grouped and ordered (e.g., sense of well-being: excellent, very good, fair, poor). Continuous data have order and magnitude (e.g., age, blood pressure, cholesterol, weight).

error occurs when the study finds a difference between groups when no difference actually exists. This type of error is similar to a jury finding an innocent person guilty of committing a crime. The investigators usually indicate the maximum acceptable risk (i.e., alpha level) they are willing to tolerate in reaching this false-positive conclusion. Usually, the alpha level is arbitrarily set at 0.05 (or lower), which means that the investigators are willing to take a 5% risk that any differences found in the study were due to chance. At the completion of the study, the investigators then calculate the probability, known as the *P value*, that a type I error occurred. When the *P* value is lower than the alpha value (e.g., *P* <.05), the investigators conclude that the results are "statistically significant."

Statistical significance does not always correlate with *clinical* significance (Table 5-3). In a large study, very small differences can be statistically significant. For example, a study comparing two antihypertensives in more than 1,000 subjects may find a statistically significant difference in mean blood pressures of only 3 mm Hg, which is trivial in the clinical realm. A *P* value of less than .0001 is no more clinically significant than a value of

less than .05. The smaller *P* value only means that the risk of drawing a false-positive conclusion is less (fewer than 1 in 1,000 vs. fewer than 50 in 1,000). When analyzing an article, beware of being seduced by statistical significance and accepting it in lieu of clinical significance; both must be considered.

Instead of using *P* values, investigators are increasingly using confidence intervals (CIs) to determine the significance of a difference. The problem with *P* values is that they convey no information about the size of differences or associations found in the study.[66] Also, *P* values provide a dichotomous answer—the results are either significant or not significant. In contrast, the CI provides a range that will, with a high degree of probability, contain the true value, and provides more information than *P* values alone.[67–69] The larger the sample size, the narrower and more precise the CI. A standard method used is the 95% CI, which provides the boundaries in which a 95% chance exists that the true value falls within that range. For example, a randomized clinical trial demonstrates that 50% of patients treated with Drug A are cured compared with 45% of those treated with Drug B. Statistical analy-

Figure 5-3. Potential outcomes of statistical decisions. If the study concludes that a difference exists when, in reality, no difference in the population exists, a type I error has occurred. A type II error occurs if the study concludes that no difference exists when, in reality, a difference exists in the population.

In Reality . . .

Study Conclusion . . .		A difference exists	No difference exists
	A difference exists	Correct	Type I error (alpha)
	No difference exists	Type II error (beta)	Correct

Table 5.3 Four Questions to Ask
when Assessing Significance

---

1. Are the differences noted between groups likely due to chance (type I error)?
2. If differences were not due to chance, were they due to flaws or biases of the study?
3. If differences are statistically significant, are they also clinically significant?
4. If differences are not statistically significant, did a type II error occur?

---

sis of this 5% difference produces a *P* value of less than .001 and a 95% CI of 0–10%. The investigators conclude that this is a statistically significant improvement based on the *P* value. As a reader, however, you decide on the basis of the 95% CI range of 0–10% that a difference of 5% is not clinically significant.

In the article you are assessing, no statistical difference was found among the groups in terms of the change in croup score from baseline to final study assessment, time in the emergency department, hospitalization, and use of supplemental glucocorticoids. This study is considered a "negative" trial (no differences found). As such, you go on to the next question, which addresses these types of studies.

8. *If a negative trial, was a power analysis done?* A type II error (see Figure 5-3) occurs when the study finds no difference between groups when a difference actually exists in the population.[70] This type of error is similar to a jury finding a criminal innocent of committing a crime. The odds of reaching a false-negative conclusion, known as *beta*, is typically set at 0.20 (20% chance). The power of a test (1 − beta) is the ability to find a difference when one actually exists and depends on (1) the number of subjects in the study (i.e., the more subjects, the greater the power), and (2) the size of the difference (known as *effect size*) between groups (i.e., the larger the difference, the greater the power). Typically, the effect size investigators choose depends on ethical, economic, and pragmatic issues and can be categorized into small (10–25%), medium

(26–50%), and large (greater than 50%).[71] When looking at the effect size chosen by the investigators, ask whether you consider this difference to be clinically meaningful.

Before the start of a study, the investigators should do a power analysis to determine how many subjects should be included in the study. However, this is often not done. Only 32% of the RCTs with negative results published between 1975 and 1990 in *JAMA*, *Lancet*, and *New England Journal of Medicine* reported sample size calculations; on review, the majority of these trials had too few patients, which led to insufficient statistical power to detect a 25% or 50% difference.[72] Other studies have shown similar deficiencies in other journals and disciplines.[14,48,73,74] Whenever you read an article reporting a negative result, ask whether the sample size was large enough to permit investigators to draw such a conclusion. If a power analysis was done, check to see if the study had the required number of subjects. If a power analysis was not done, view the conclusions with skepticism—it may be that the sample size was not large enough to detect a difference.

In the article you are assessing, you find that the investigators did perform a power analysis that, using the criteria established above, required a minimum sample size of 62 participants per group. You notice that, in the final analysis, each group had more than this number. You are assured that this study had adequate power to detect a type II error and answer yes to this question.

9. *Were other factors present that might have affected the outcome?* At times, an outcome may be due to factors other than the intervention. For example, the simple act of observing subjects can affect an outcome (Hawthorne effect). This effect occurs when subjects change their normal behavior because they are aware of being observed. To minimize this effect, the study groups should be observed equally. Also, randomization and sufficiently large sample size assure that both known and unknown determinants of an outcome are evenly distributed between groups. As you read through an article, think about potential influences that could impact one group more than another and thus affect the outcome.

In the article you are assessing, the investigators treated each of the groups equally (except for the inter-

---

Conclusion of Case 2

After a thorough assessment of this article, you conclude that it is well designed with valid results. You feel confident that oral dexamethasone should be stocked in your office during croup season and that you will institute this as a standard within your practice. As you apply this therapy, you also make a commitment to monitor its benefits and risks to your patients and to scan the literature for future articles that may offer additional information about croup therapy. Consistency of the results in your practice, as well as across multiple published studies, is one characteristic of the scientific process that leads to acceptance and implementation.

vention drugs). They also looked at factors such as prior upper respiratory tract infections and episodes of croup, which could have had a potential impact. Because you can think of no factors, you answer no to this question.

10. *Are the treatment benefits worth the potential harms and costs?* This final question forces us to weigh the cost of the treatment against the potential benefit and to consider potential harm of the therapy. One common method used to weigh the benefits of treatment is the number needed to treat (NNT). The NNT takes into consideration the likelihood of an outcome or side effect.[26] Generally, the less common a potential outcome (e.g., death), the greater the number of patients that would require treatment to prevent one outcome. For example, a calculation may show that 30 people with severe stenosis must be treated with an anticoagulant to prevent one stroke. If sudden death is a risk of a medication used to treat a benign condition, one must question the actual benefit of that drug.

The investigators addressed this issue in the results section. Because the therapeutic interventions were equal, oral dexamethasone was recommended as the preferred therapy because it is less expensive and easier to administer.

A Final Word

With some practice and the use of the worksheets, one can quickly (within a few minutes) perform a critical assessment of an article. While performing this appraisal, it is important to keep in mind that few articles are perfect. A critical assessment is rarely black and white but often comes in shades of gray.[24] Only you can answer for yourself the exact shade of gray that you are willing to accept when deciding to apply the results of the study to your practice. By applying the knowledge, principles, and techniques presented in this chapter, however, you can more confidently recognize the various shades of gray and reject those articles that are seriously flawed.

References

1. Colditz G, Hankinson S, Hunter D, et al. The use of estrogens and progestins and the risk of breast cancer in postmenopausal women. N Engl J Med 1995; 332:1589–1593.
2. Stampfer M, Willett W, Colditz G, et al. A prospective study of postmenopausal estrogen therapy and coronary heart disease. N Engl J Med 1985; 313:1044–1049.
3. Wilson P, Garrison R, Castelli W. Postmenopausal estrogen use, cigarette smoking, and cardiovascular morbidity in women over 50. The Framingham Study. N Engl J Med 1985;313:1038–1043.
4. Stampfer M, Colditz G, Willett W, et al. Postmenopausal estrogen therapy and cardiovascular disease. Ten-year follow-up from the Nurses' Health Study. N Engl J Med 1991;325:756–762.
5. American College of Physicians. Guidelines for counseling postmenopausal women about preventive hormone therapy. Ann Intern Med 1992;117:1038–1041.
6. Gorsky R, Koplan J, Peterson H, Thacker S. Relative risks and benefits of long-term estrogen replacement therapy: a decision analysis. Obstet Gynecol 1994;83:161–166.
7. Dupont W, Page D. Menopausal estrogen replacement therapy and breast cancer. Arch Intern Med 1991;15: 66–79.
8. The Writing Group for the PEPI Trial. Effects of estrogen or estrogen/progestin regimens on heart disease risk factors in postmenopausal women: The Postmenopausal Estrogen/Progestin Interventions (PEPI) Trial. JAMA 1995;273:199–208.
9. Stanford J, Weiss N, Voigt L, et al. Combined estrogen and progestin hormone replacement therapy in relation to risk of breast cancer in middle-aged women. JAMA 1995;274:137–142.
10. Slawson D, Shaughnessy A, Bennett J. Becoming a medical information master: feeling good about not knowing everything. J Fam Pract 1994;38:505–513.
11. Shaughnessy A, Slawson D, Bennett J. Becoming an information master: a guidebook to the medical information jungle. J Fam Pract 1994;39:489–499.
12. Fletcher R, Fletcher S. Keeping clinically up-to-date. Evidence-based approach to the medical literature. J Gen Intern Med 1997;12:S5–S14.
13. Lock S. Does editorial peer review work [editorial]? Ann Intern Med 1994;121:60–61.
14. Sonis J, Jones J. The quality of clinical trials published in The Journal of Family Practice, 1974–1991. J Fam Pract 1994;39:225–235.
15. Begg C, Cho M, Eastwood S, et al. Improving the quality of reporting of randomized controlled trials. The CONSORT statement. JAMA 1996;276:637–639.
16. Altman D. The scandal of poor medical research: we need less research, better research, and research done for the right reasons. BMJ 1994;308:283–284.
17. Reid M, Lachs M, Feinstein A. Use of methodological standards in diagnostic test research. Getting better but still not good. JAMA 1995;274:645–651.
18. Guyatt G, Rennie D. Users' guides to the medical literature [editorial]. JAMA 1993;270:2096–2097.
19. Department of Clinical Epidemiology and Biostatistics, McMaster University. How to read clinical journals. I: Why to read them and how to start reading them critically. CMAJ 1981;124:555–558.
20. Department of Clinical Epidemiology and Biostatistics, McMaster University. How to read clinical journals. II: To learn about a diagnostic test. CMAJ 1981;124: 703–710.
21. Department of Clinical Epidemiology and Biostatistics, McMaster University. How to read clinical journals. III: To learn the clinical course and prognosis of disease. CMAJ 1981;124:869–872.
22. Department of Clinical Epidemiology and Biostatistics, McMaster University. How to read clinical journals. IV: To determine etiology or causation. CMAJ 1981;124: 985–990.

23. Department of Clinical Epidemiology and Biostatistics, McMaster University. How to read clinical journals. V: To distinguish useful from useless or even harmful therapy. CMAJ 1981;124:1156–1162.

24. Oxman A, Sackett D, Guyatt G. Users' guides to the medical literature. I: How to get started. The Evidence-Based Medicine Working Group. JAMA 1993;270:2093–2095.

25. Guyatt G, Sackett D, Cook D. Users' guides to the medical literature. II: How to use an article about therapy or prevention? A. Are the results of the study valid? Evidence-Based Medicine Working Group. JAMA 1993;270:2598–2601.

26. Guyatt G, Sackett D, Cook D. Users' guides to the medical literature. II: How to use an article about therapy or prevention? B. What were the results and will they help me in caring for my patients? Evidence-Based Medicine Working Group. JAMA 1994;271:59–63.

27. Jaeschke R, Guyatt G, Sackett D. Users' guides to the medical literature. III: How to use an article about a diagnostic test. A. Are the results of the study valid? Evidence-Based Medicine Working Group. JAMA 1994;271:389–391.

28. Jaeschke R, Guyatt G, Sackett D. Users' guides to the medical literature. III: How to use an article about a diagnostic test. B. What are the results and will they help me in caring for my patients? The Evidence-Based Medicine Working Group. JAMA 1994;271:703–707.

29. Levine M, Walter S, Lee H, et al. Users' guides to the medical literature. IV: How to use an article about harm. Evidence-Based Medicine Working Group. JAMA 1994;271:1615–1619.

30. Laupacis A, Wells G, Richardson W, Tugwell P. Users' guides to the medical literature. V: How to use an article about prognosis. Evidence-Based Medicine Working Group. JAMA 1994;272:234–237.

31. Oxman A, Cook D, Guyatt G. Users' guides to the medical literature. VI: How to use an overview. The Evidence-Based Medicine Working Group. JAMA 1994;272:1367–1371.

32. Richardson W, Detsky A. Users' guides to the medical literature. VII: How to use a clinical decision analysis. A. Are the results of the study valid? Evidence-Based Medicine Working Group. JAMA 1995;273:1292–1295.

33. Richardson W, Detsky A. Users' guides to the medical literature. VII: How to use a clinical decision analysis. B. What are the results and will they help me in caring for my patients? Evidence-Based Medicine Working Group. JAMA 1995;273:1610–1613.

34. Hayward R, Wilson M, Tunis S, et al. Users' guides to the medical literature. VIII: How to use clinical practice guidelines. A. Are the recommendations valid? Evidence-Based Medicine Working Group. JAMA 1995;274:570–574.

35. Wilson M, Hayward R, Tunis S, et al. Users' guides to the medical literature. VIII: How to use clinical practice guidelines. B. What are the recommendations and will they help you in caring for your patients? Evidence-Based Medicine Working Group. JAMA 1995; 274:1630–1632.

36. Guyatt G, Sackett D, Sinclair J, et al. Users' guides to the medical literature. IX: A method for grading health care recommendations. Evidence-Based Medicine Working Group. JAMA 1995;274:1800–1804.

37. Naylor C, Guyatt G. Users' guides to the medical literature. X: How to use an article reporting variations in the outcomes of health services. The Evidence-Based Medicine Working Group. JAMA 1996;275:554–558.

38. Naylor C, Guyatt G. Users' guides to the medical literature. XI: How to use an article about a clinical utilization review. The Evidence-Based Medicine Working Group. JAMA 1996;275:1435–1439.

39. Guyatt G, Naylor C, Juniper E, et al. Users' guides to the medical literature. XII: How to use articles about health-related quality of life. The Evidence-Based Medicine Working Group. JAMA 1997;277:1232–1237.

40. Drummond M, Richardson W, O'Brien B, et al. Users' guides to the medical literature. XIII: How to use an article on economic analysis of clinical practice. A. Are the results of the study valid? The Evidence-Based Medicine Working Group. JAMA 1997;277:1552–1557.

41. O'Brien B, Heyland D, Richardson W, et al. Users' guides to the medical literature. XIII: How to use an article on economic analysis of clinical practice. B. What are the results and will they help me in caring for my patients? The Evidence-Based Medicine Working Group. JAMA 1997;277:1802–1806.

42. Dans A, Dans L, Guyatt G, Richardson S. Users' guides to the medical literature. XIV. How to decide on the applicability of clinical trial results to your patients. The Evidence-Based Medicine Working Group. JAMA 1998;279:545–549.

43. Richardson WS, Wilson MC, Guyatt GH, et al. Users' guides to the medical literature. XV. How to use an article about disease probability for differential diagnosis. The Evidence-Based Working Group. JAMA 1999;281:1214–1219.

44. Klassen T, Craig W, Moher D, et al. Nebulized budesonide and oral dexamethasone for treatment of croup: a randomized controlled trial. JAMA 1998;279:1629–1632.

45. Kassirer J, Campion E. Peer review—crude and understudied, but indispensable. JAMA 1994;272:96–97.

46. Abby M, Massey M, Galandiuk S, Polk H. Peer review is an effective screening process to evaluate medical manuscripts. JAMA 1994;272:105–107.

47. Goodman S, Berlin J, Fletcher S, Fletcher R. Manuscript quality before and after peer review and editing at Annals of Internal Medicine. Ann Intern Med 1994; 121:11–21.

48. Gardner M, Bond J. An exploratory study of statistical assessment of papers published in the British Medical Journal. JAMA 1990;263:1355–1357.

49. Justice A, Berlin J, Fletcher S, et al. Do readers and peer reviewers agree on manuscript quality? JAMA 1994;272:117–119.

50. Colaianni L. Peer review in journals indexed in Index Medicus. JAMA 1994;272:156–158.

51. Dickersin K, Min Y, Meinert C. Factors influencing publication of research results. Follow-up of applica-

tions submitted to two institutional review boards. JAMA 1992;267:374–378.

52. Jadad A, Rennie D. The randomized controlled trial gets a middle-aged checkup [editorial]. JAMA 1998;279: 319–320.

53. Rennie D, Flanagin A. Publication bias—the triumph of hope over experience. JAMA 1992;267:411–412.

54. Scherer R, Dickersin K, Langenberg P. Full publication of results initially presented in abstracts—a meta-analysis. JAMA 1994;272:158–162.

55. Ioannidis J. Effect of the statistical significance of results on the time to completion and publication of randomized efficacy trials. JAMA 1998;279:281–286.

56. Whitely W, Rennie D, Hafner A. The scientific community's response to evidence of fraudulent publication. The Robert Slutsky case. JAMA 1994;272:170–173.

57. Bero L, Galbraith A, Rennie D. The publication of sponsored symposiums in medical journals. N Engl J Med 1992;327:1135–1140.

58. Rochon P, Gurwitz J, Cheung M, et al. Evaluating the quality of articles published in journal supplements compared with the quality of those published in the parent journal. JAMA 1994;272:108–113.

59. Slawson D, Shaughnessy A, Ebell M, Barry H. Mastering medical information and the role of POEMs—patient-oriented evidence that matters. J Fam Pract 1997;45:195–196.

60. Greenhalgh T. How to read a paper: getting your bearings (deciding what the paper is about). BMJ 1997;315: 243–246.

61. Franks P. Clinical trials. Fam Med 1988;20:443–448.

62. Schulz K, Chalmers I, Grimes D, Altman D. Assessing the quality of randomization from reports of controlled trials published in Obstetrics and Gynecology journals. JAMA 1994;272:125–128.

63. Schulz K, Chalmers I, Hayes R, Altman D. Empirical evidence of bias. Dimensions of methodological quality associated with estimates of treatment effects in controlled trials. JAMA 1995;273:408–412.

64. O'Brien P, Shampo M. Statistics for clinicians: 1. Descriptive statistics. Mayo Clin Proc 1981;56:47–49.

65. Greenhalgh T. How to read a paper: statistics for the non-statistician. BMJ 1997;315:364–366.

66. Grimes D. The case for confidence intervals [editorial]. Obstet Gynecol 1992;80:865–866.

67. Simon R. Confidence intervals for reporting results of clinical trials. Ann Intern Med 1986;105:429–435.

68. Braitman L. Confidence intervals assess both clinical significance and statistical significance. Ann Intern Med 1991;114:515–517.

69. Gehlbach S. Interpreting the Medical Literature (3rd ed). New York: McGraw-Hill, 1993.

70. Detsky A, Sackett D. When was a "negative" clinical trial big enough? How many patients you needed depends on what you found. Arch Intern Med 1985; 145:709–712.

71. Raju R, Langenberg P, Sen A, Aldana O. How much "better" is good enough? The magnitude of treatment effect in clinical trials. Am J Dis Child 1992;146:407–411.

72. Moher D, Dulberg C, Wells G. Statistical power, sample size, and their reporting in randomized controlled trials. JAMA 1994;272:122–124.

73. Freiman J, Chalmers T, Smith H, Kuebler R. The importance of beta, the type II error, and sample size in the design and interpretation of the randomized control trial: survey of "negative" trials. N Engl J Med 1978;299:690–694.

74. Mengel M, Davis A. The statistical power of family practice research. Fam Pract Res J 1993;13:105–111.

Further Reading

Fletcher RH, Fletcher SW, Wagner EH. Clinical Epidemiology: The Essentials (3rd ed). Baltimore: Williams & Wilkins, 1996. A basic textbook written for clinicians and organized by clinical questions: diagnosis, treatment, and so forth.

Gelbach SH. Interpreting the Medical Literature (3rd ed). New York: McGraw-Hill, 1993. A basic introduction.

How to Keep Up with the Medical Literature. Ann Intern Med. A good series on the approach to keeping up with the medical literature.

Why try to keep up and how to get started. 1986;105: 149–153.

Deciding which journals to read regularly. 1986;105: 309–312.

Expanding the number of journals you read regularly. 1986;105:474–478.

Using the literature to solve clinical problems. 1986;105: 636–640.

Access by personal computer to the medical literature. 1986;105:810–816.

How to store and retrieve articles worth keeping. 1986; 105:978–984.

How to Read a Paper. BMJ. A great series that complements the user's guides.

The MedLine database. 1997;315:180–183.

Getting your bearings (deciding what the paper is about). 1997;315:243–246.

Assessing the methodological quality of published papers. 1997;315:305–308.

Statistics for the non-statistician. 1997;315:364–366.

Statistics for the non-statistician. II: "Significant" relations and their pitfalls. 1997;315:422–425.

Papers that report drug trials. 1997;315:480–483.

Papers that report diagnostic or screening tests. 1997;315:540–543.

Papers that tell you what things cost (economic analyses). 1997;315:596–599.

Papers that summarise other papers (systemic reviews and meta-analyses). 1997;315:672–675.

Papers that go beyond numbers (qualitative research). 1997;315:740–743.

How to Read Clinical Journals. Can Med Assoc J. The original McMaster University series; despite being published in 1981, this series still has some great information.

Why to read them and how to start reading them critically. 1981;124:555–558.

To learn about a diagnostic test. 1981;124:703–710.

To learn the clinical course and prognosis of disease. 1981;124:869–872.

To determine etiology or causation. 1981;124:985–990.

To distinguish useful from useless or even harmful therapy. 1981;124:1156–1162.

Hulley ST, Cummings SR. Designing Clinical Research: An Epidemiologic Approach. Baltimore: Williams & Wilkins, 1988. An excellent textbook on understanding research methods and statistics.

Riegelman RK, Hirsch RP. Studying a Study and Testing a Test: How to Read the Health Literature (3rd ed). Boston: Lippincott–Raven, 1996. A clear description of an approach to studies of diagnosis and treatment.

Sackett DL, Haynes RB, Guyatt GH, Tugwell P. Clinical Epidemiology: A Basic Science for Clinical Medicine (2nd ed). Boston: Little, Brown, 1991. A lively introduction to clinical epidemiology with special emphasis on diagnosis and treatment, by leading proponents of evidence-based medicine.

Shaughnessy AF, Slawson DC. Getting the most from review articles: A guide for readers and writers. Am Fam Phys 1997;55:2155–2160. Provides useful techniques on reading a review article.

Shaughnessy A, Slawson D, Bennett J. Becoming an information master: a guidebook to the medical information jungle. J Fam Pract 1994;39:489–499. An excellent article that reviews how to manage one's way through the medical information jungle without getting lost or eaten alive.

Slawson D, Shaughnessy A, Bennett J. Becoming a medical information master: feeling good about not knowing everything. J Fam Pract 1994;38:505–513. A superb article that addresses the concepts of POEMs (patient-oriented evidence that matters) and DOEs (disease-oriented evidence).

Users' Guides to the Medical Literature. The McMaster University series. JAMA. The "ultimate" series written from the perspective of a busy clinician who wants to provide effective medical care but is sharply restricted in time for reading.

How to get started. 1993;270:2093–2095.

How to use an article about therapy or prevention. A. Are the results of the study valid? 1993;270:2598–2601. B. What were the results and will they help me in caring for my patients? 1994;271:59–63.

How to use an article about a diagnostic test. A. Are the results of the study valid? 1994;271:389–391. B. What are the results and will they help me in caring for my patients? 1994;271:703–707.

How to use an article about harm. 1994;271:1615–1619.

How to use an article about prognosis. 1994;272:234–237.

How to use an overview. 1994;272:1367–1371.

How to use a clinical decision analysis. A. Are the results of the study valid? 1995;273:1292–1295. B. What are the results and will they help me in caring for my patients? 1995;273:1610–1613.

How to use clinical practice guidelines. A. Are the recommendations valid? 1995;274:570–574. B. What are the recommendations and will they help you in caring for your patients? 1995;274:1630–1632.

A method for grading health care recommendations. 1995;274:1800–1804.

How to use an article reporting variations in the outcomes of health services. 1996;275:554–558.

How to use an article about a clinical utilization review. 1996;275:1435–1439.

How to use articles about health-related quality of life. 1997;277:1232–1237.

How to use an article on economic analysis of clinical practice. A. Are the results of the study valid? 1997;277:1552–1557. B. What are the results and will they help me in caring for my patients? 1997;277:1802–1806.

How to decide on the applicability of clinical trial results to your patients. 1998;279:545–549.

How to use an article about disease probability for differential diagnosis. 1999;281:1214–1219.

Chapter 6

Applying a Meta-Analysis
to Daily Clinical Practice

William F. Miser

Case 1

You are seeing a cranky 4-year-old boy who has a low-grade fever and symptoms of an upper respiratory tract infection. On examination, he appears nontoxic but definitely has a left otitis media. He was previously healthy, with no history of an ear infection. You want to prescribe antibiotics, but family finances are tight (both parents are laid off from work), and the child hates to take any type of medicine. As you discuss the situation with the parents, you remember an article published recently that suggested children with otitis media can be effectively treated with a shorter course of antibiotics. You write a prescription for a 5-day course of amoxicillin and tell the parents you will call near the end of treatment to determine whether a longer course is needed. In the meantime, you find the article titled "Treatment of acute otitis media with a shortened course of antibiotics: a meta-analysis."[1] You have seen the term *meta-analysis* before but are unsure how to critique the article.

The ability to critically evaluate an article is a necessary skill for clinicians to maintain competency and to provide patients with the best possible care.[2] Although the first reported attempt at a meta-analysis was in 1904,[3] the actual methodologic technique was not defined until the mid-1970s.[4,5] Since then, the biostatistical method known as *meta-analysis* has gained popularity. The number of published articles using this technique rose from 109 in 1988 to 754 in 1998. Despite its widespread use, meta-analysis continues to be a controversial method.[6]

The intent of this chapter is to describe the purpose, strengths, and weaknesses of a meta-analysis and to provide the tools needed to critically evaluate an article that uses this methodology. Owing to space limitations, this chapter cannot cover everything in exhaustive detail, and the reader is encouraged to refer to the Further Reading section for several outstanding reviews.

In this chapter, using the article mentioned in the case as an example, you will learn how to use a worksheet that allows you to assess the validity of a meta-analysis. The ultimate goal is to enable you to determine whether you should apply the findings of a meta-analysis to the clinical problems you encounter daily.

Characteristics of a Meta-Analysis

The medical literature consists of two major types of studies: (1) those that report original research (analytic, primary studies) and (2) those that summarize or draw conclusions from this original research (integrative, secondary studies). Various types of integrative studies exist. The simplest, and least stringent study is a nonsystematic review written as a continuing medical education article by authors who are experts in a subject matter. These articles may be based solely on opinions and clinical experiences, with a cursory, if any, literature review performed. References used for support for review articles are primarily review articles as well. The authors pick and choose the studies that support their argument and ignore those that disagree. Oxman and Guyatt[7] found that the greater the expertise of the reviewer, the lower the quality of the review. For example, a review

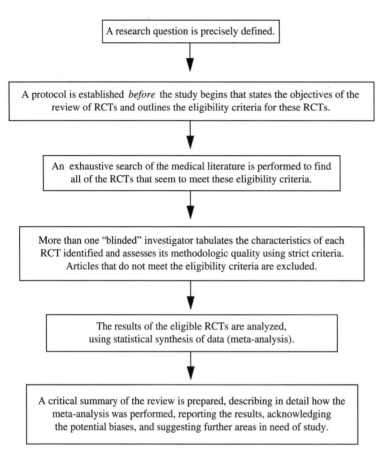

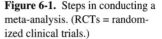

Figure 6-1. Steps in conducting a meta-analysis. (RCTs = randomized clinical trials.)

A research question is precisely defined.

A protocol is established *before* the study begins that states the objectives of the review of RCTs and outlines the eligibility criteria for these RCTs.

An exhaustive search of the medical literature is performed to find all of the RCTs that seem to meet these eligibility criteria.

More than one "blinded" investigator tabulates the characteristics of each RCT identified and assesses its methodologic quality using strict criteria. Articles that do not meet the eligibility criteria are excluded.

The results of the eligible RCTs are analyzed, using statistical synthesis of data (meta-analysis).

A critical summary of the review is prepared, describing in detail how the meta-analysis was performed, reporting the results, acknowledging the potential biases, and suggesting further areas in need of study.

article on screening for prostate cancer written by a urologist may reach a completely different conclusion than one written by a family physician, although the literature available to both is the same. This type of subjective review article is fraught with bias and may be misleading.[8]

A systematic review is a more precise, integrative study. This type of review article provides an overview of original research using a precise protocol with a statement of objectives and a literature review conducted according to a specific and reproducible methodology.[9–13] The authors provide a detailed description of how the articles were obtained and the methods by which articles were included or excluded for consideration. Much like conducting original research, the author follows a protocol in researching primary studies. When assessing such a review, the reader can judge the quality of science that went into the writing of the paper.

A meta-analysis is a type of systematic review of the literature that includes combining and analyzing the data of individual trials. Like any other research project, a meta-analysis should have a detailed, written protocol prepared in advance that includes a narrowly focused question to be answered. Original studies are found that address this question, their data are combined, statistical

tests are applied to these combined results, and the results are reported (Figure 6-1). It is a statistical procedure that integrates the results of several independent clinical trials considered by the analyst to be "combinable."[14] So, in addition to critically reviewing the primary research, the authors also statistically combine the results. It is literally a "study of studies."[15] A meta-analysis has been likened to an observational study of the evidence.[14] Most meta-analyses are applied to randomized clinical trials (RCTs), although some have attempted with varying degrees of success to apply this technique to nonrandomized trials and epidemiologic research.[16–18]

The potential benefits of meta-analyses are found in Table 6-1. As mentioned in Chapter 5, the sample in a RCT may be too small to detect a difference between groups when a difference actually exists (type II error). In a review of RCTs with negative results published between 1975 and 1990 in the *Journal of the American Medical Association* (*JAMA*), *Lancet*, and *New England Journal of Medicine*, the majority of these trials had too few patients, which led to insufficient power to detect a 25% or 50% difference.[19] A major advantage of a meta-analysis is that it may combine several smaller studies, thus increasing the number of subjects in the final analysis and improving the power to detect a treatment effect if one is present.

Another potential benefit of a meta-analysis is that it may answer questions about whether an overall study result differs among various subgroups (e.g., older and younger patients, men and women, or subjects with varying degrees of disease severity).[6] Also, if well performed, a meta-analysis is an excellent critical review of the literature that points out the strengths and weaknesses of prior research on a given topic. As such, it can generate research questions to be addressed in future studies, along with providing the sample size needed to answer these questions.

However, a meta-analysis is only as good as the research on which it is based; it is not an infallible tool.[6] Many authors view a meta-analysis as an easy way to get published, especially with the help of software programs that can rapidly perform statistical calculations.[20] Because of this, concern is growing about the quality of most meta-analyses.[16] The three main threats to the validity of a meta-analysis are (1) the combination of dissimilar studies, (2) publication bias, and (3) the inclusion of poor-quality studies in the analysis. Many meta-analyses are methodologically flawed because of these threats.[16,21,22] A classic example of a flawed meta-analysis is one that suggested that giving intravenous magnesium was beneficial to those who had myocardial infarctions.[23] However, a mega-trial involving 58,000 patients (International Study of Infarct Survival-4) found no benefit.[24] On further review, the meta-analysis was misleading because of publication bias and methodologic weaknesses in smaller trials.

In summary, meta-analyses have great potential to be useful for clinicians but not all are methodologically sound. It is important for clinicians to have the basic skills to be able to distinguish a well-designed meta-analysis from one that should be recycled.

Critical Appraisal of a Meta-Analysis

Assessing a meta-analysis involves two steps: (1) Conduct an initial validity and relevance screen, which was described in detail in Chapter 5, and if the article "passes," (2) perform a more in-depth evaluation of its validity.

Step One: Conduct an Initial Validity and Relevance Screen

The first step when assessing a meta-analysis is to ask yourself, "Is this article worth taking the time to review in depth?" This step can be quickly accomplished by examining the six simple questions outlined in Form 6-1. Using the article mentioned in the case and the questions in Form 6-1, you find these answers. The article you are assessing is published in *JAMA*. You are almost certain that this is a peer-reviewed journal, which is confirmed in the Instructions for Authors ("*JAMA* is an international, peer-

Table 6-1. Potential Benefits of a Meta-Analysis

Increases the number of subjects in an analysis, thus improving the statistical power to detect overall differences for primary end points within subgroups
Provides more objective appraisal of the literature, which may resolve uncertainty when reports disagree
Improves estimates of effect size or magnitude of association
Addresses research questions not posed at the start of individual trials
Assimilates large amounts of information
Improves the quality of primary research

Source: Adapted from M Egger, G Smith. Meta-analysis: potentials and promise. BMJ 1997;315:1371–1374; J Peipert, M Bracken. Systematic reviews of medical evidence: the use of meta-analysis in Obstetrics and Gynecology. Obstet Gynecol 1997;89:628–632; H Sacks, D Reitman, D Pagano, B Kupelnick. Meta-analysis: an update. Mount Sinai J Med 1996;63:216–223.

reviewed, general medical journal . . ."). You look at the end of the article to find that funding support was from two foundations, neither of which is a company that has commercial interests in the drugs mentioned in the study. Your attention now turns to the abstract. In the introduction, you read that the purpose of the meta-analysis is to determine whether treating children with a shorter course of antibiotics was comparable to treating them with a longer course. You then read this conclusion: "[F]ive days of short-acting antibiotic use is effective treatment for uncomplicated acute otitis media in children." You scan the rest of the abstract and find that the outcomes were treatment failures, relapses, or reinfections. Taking antibiotics for a shorter length of time reduces costs and lessens the chances of adverse reactions and drug resistance, outcomes of importance for you and your patients. As a primary care physician, otitis media is one of the most common problems seen in your practice, and you could easily write prescriptions for a shorter course of antibiotics. Because your practice is to treat a child with otitis media with at least 10 days of antibiotics, using this information requires you to change your current practice.

In only a few seconds, you have quickly answered yes to six pertinent questions that allow you to decide whether you want to take the time to critically review this meta-analysis. This "weeding" tool allows you to recycle those articles that are not relevant to your practice, thus allowing more time to examine the validity of those few articles that may have an impact on the care of your patients. Based on the information you have found from this screen, you may be tempted to already begin writing for a shorter course of antibiotics for otitis media. Before you make a drastic change in your prescribing pattern for this common problem, however, you want assurances that the authors of the paper conducted a valid meta-analysis.

Step Two: Determine the Validity of the Meta-Analysis

You decide to critically assess this *JAMA* article based on your initial screen. Using the questions found in Form 6-1, you turn your attention to the Methods section.

1. *Was the literature search done well?* The strength of a meta-analysis depends on the quality of the medical literature search. The search must be thorough and objective, using multiple computerized literature databases and various techniques.[25] A poorly conducted literature search often results in a meta-analysis that yields invalid conclu-sions. The authors should attempt to do more than a simple MEDLINE search; even the best MEDLINE search misses as much as 20–70% of articles pertinent to the topic.[16,26–28] In addition to a computerized literature search, the authors should review the references for each of the articles found through the search. Looking up citations of these references often yields useful articles not identified in the original search.

Publication bias is a considerable threat to the validity of a meta-analysis.[29] Studies showing statistically significant (positive) results and having larger sample sizes are more likely to be written and submitted by authors and subsequently accepted and published

---

Form 6-1. Steps in Determining the Validity of a Meta-Analysis

1. Was the literature search done well?		
a. Was it comprehensive?	Yes	No
b. Were the search methods systematic and clearly described?	Yes	No
c. Were the key words used in the search described?	Yes	No
d. Was the issue of publication bias addressed?	Yes	No
2. Was the method for selecting articles clear, systematic, and appropriate?		
a. Were there clear, pre-established inclusion and exclusion criteria for evaluation?	Yes	No
b. Was selection systematic?	Yes	No
Was the population defined?	Yes	No
Was the exposure/intervention clearly described?	Yes	No
Were all outcomes described and were they comparable?	Yes	No
c. Was selection done blindly and in random order?	Yes	No
d. Was the selection process reliable? (Were at least two independent selectors used?)	Yes	No
Was the extent of selection disagreement evaluated?)		
3. Was the quality of the primary studies evaluated?		
a. Did all studies, published or not, have the same standard applied?	Yes	No
b. Were at least two independent evaluators used, and was the inter-rater agreement assessed and adequate?	Yes	No
c. Were the evaluators blinded to the authors, institutions, and results of the primary studies?	Yes	No
4. Were results from the studies combined appropriately?		
a. Were the studies similar enough to combine results? (Were the study designs, populations, exposures, outcomes, and direction of effect similar in the combined studies?)	Yes	No
b. Was a test for heterogeneity done and was its *P* value nonsignificant?	Yes	No
5. Was a statistical combination (meta-analysis) done properly?		
a. Were the methods of the studies similar?		
b. Was the possibility of chance differences statistically addressed? (Was a test for homogeneity done?)	Yes	No
c. Were appropriate statistical analyses performed?	Yes	No
d. Were sensitivity analyses used?	Yes	No
6. Are the results important?		
a. Was the effect strong?	Yes	No
Was the odds ratio large?	Yes	No
Were the results reported in a clinically meaningful manner, such as the absolute difference or the number needed to treat?	Yes	No
b. Are the results likely to be reproducible and generalizable?	Yes	No
c. Were all clinically important consequences considered?	Yes	No
d. Are the benefits worth the harm and costs?	Yes	No

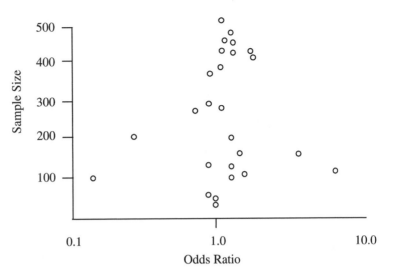

Figure 6-2. Funnel plot of the odds ratio versus sample size for studies included in the meta-analysis.

than are nonsignificant (negative) studies.[30–33] For example, in one study of publication bias, 85% of studies with significant results compared with 65% of negative studies had been published after 10 years.[34] The median time to publication was 4.8 years for the studies with significant results compared with 8.0 years for those with negative results.

To avoid this bias, investigators should decide whether the search should include unpublished data, known as the *gray literature*.[11] Talking to experts in the research community and reviewing research data that have not yet been published may yield results different from those published. Obtaining and including data from unpublished data may avoid publication bias, but not completely.[35] The inclusion of this gray literature into a meta-analysis is still controversial. In 150 meta-analyses from January 1989 to February 1991, most investigators had searched for unpublished material, although only 31% included this material.[36] The best approach is to carry out an extensive search for unpublished data and obtain them if possible. The subsequent analysis should then be performed with and without the unpublished data; if the conclusions change based on the inclusion or exclusion of this data, the results of either approach should be viewed cautiously.

Restricting the literature search to only the English language also may introduce a "Tower of Babel" bias.[37] Meta-analyses published in English language journals often restrict their search to the English language.[29] Investigators working in a non–English speaking country may be more likely to report positive findings in an international, English language journal and negative findings in their local, non–English language journal. To reduce this bias, a meta-analysis should not place a limit on the type of language searched.[38]

Funnel plots, which are simple scatterplots of the trials' odds ratios against their sample size, are useful in

detecting publication bias in a meta-analysis. Typically, results from small studies scatter widely at the bottom of the graph; this spread narrows as precision increases among larger studies.[29,39] In the absence of bias, the plot should resemble a symmetric inverted funnel, as seen in Figure 6-2.

In the article you are assessing, you find the authors focused on RCTs comparing different durations of antibiotic treatment in children with acute otitis media. They used four different databases (MEDLINE, EMBASE, Current Contents, and Science Citation Index) with no language restrictions and reviewed the reference lists of relevant articles to find further trials. Key words that were used are listed. The authors do not specifically mention looking at the gray literature. Although not mentioned in the Methods section, you find later in the article that the authors address the possibility of publication bias in their search by doing a "funnel plot." You are assured that the authors performed a thorough literature search and proceed with your assessment.

2. *Was the method for selecting articles clear, systematic, and appropriate?* Once a comprehensive literature search has been done, the investigators should have a systematic way to evaluate which of the articles should be included in the analysis. Eligibility criteria should be clearly documented in the protocol. The population should be well defined and the intervention and all outcomes clearly described. When the eligibility criteria for a meta-analysis are strict, the final number of studies included in the analysis is much fewer in comparison with the number of studies identified in the literature search.[18] To improve the selection process, at least two independent selectors should be used, and an evaluation should be performed on how closely they agreed on which articles should be selected and which should be discarded. A log should be maintained of the excluded articles to allow the reader to assess the quality of the screen.

In the Methods section, you read that the investigators clearly identified the eligibility criteria (age 4 weeks to 18 years, clinical diagnosis of acute otitis media not on antibiotics, randomized to fewer than or more than 7 days of treatment, and an assessment of clinical resolution). Using these strict criteria for selection, seven investigators independently evaluated those articles found in the literature search. They then applied a statistical test (kappa statistic) to document this close agreement. You answer yes to this question.

3. *Was the quality of the primary studies evaluated?* The criteria used to reject articles as flawed must be explicit and independent of the results of those trials. The investigators should have a list of criteria, including generic (i.e., common to all research studies) and particular (i.e., specific to the area in question) aspects of quality, used to judge each trial. All of the articles should have the same standard applied. Ideally, investigators should consider including only controlled trials with proper randomization of patients in a double-blinded manner who are analyzed on an intention-to-treat basis using objective measures of outcomes.[14] Assessing the quality of a study can be subjective unless strict quality criteria are used, such as those found in the Jadad scale.[40] Also, to decrease the possibility of bias, at least two independent evaluators should be used, and inter-rater agreement should be assessed. To obtain more consistent quality scores of the studies, the investigators should evaluate the articles "blindly" (i.e., remove information such as author names, journal names, and study locations).[41]

In the article you are critiquing, the investigators used an accepted quality score (the Jadad scale) and applied this standard to all articles. At least two independent investigators were used to assess the quality of the articles, with a high degree of inter-rater agreement. The "majority of trials" were blindly evaluated. Of the 41 articles originally selected, 12 were excluded. Reasons for their exclusion are outlined. You also note that the overall quality score for the RCTs for treating acute otitis media is 2.7 out of 5 possible points, which suggests that quality studies on such a common condition are lacking. You answer yes to this question.

4. *Were results from the studies combined appropriately?* Once the articles are identified and their quality assessed, the next step in a meta-analysis involves combining the data from these studies. The studies should be similar enough in terms of design, population, and outcomes to permit the data to be combined. If the end points being studied are binary (e.g., relapse versus no relapse, survival versus death), odds ratios are often calculated. The odds ratio, an estimate of relative risk, has mathematical properties that allow one to easily combine the data and to test for the overall effect of significance.[14]

It would be inappropriate to combine the results if the studies differed greatly. A test for heterogeneity (dissimilarity) across the studies allows one to statistically examine the degree of similarity in the outcomes of the studies. Averaging the odds ratios from all of the studies would give misleading results, as smaller studies are more subject to chance. To acknowledge the variability of the results between studies and to give larger trials more influence in the overall result, meta-analyses use one of two different techniques to test for heterogeneity. The "fixed effects" model attributes the variability between studies to random variation. Thus, if all the studies were large enough, they would yield the same results. In contrast, the "random effects" model considers the samples from each study to be drawn from a different population. The odds ratio, therefore, varies from study to study; thus, differences are due to experimental error and differences in the populations.[16]

You see in Table 1 of the article you are assessing that the investigators grouped the studies by the pharmacokinetic behavior of the antibiotic. They performed a test for heterogeneity (random effects) and found that the studies were similar and the results could be combined. You answer yes to this question and proceed with your assessment.

5. *Was a statistical combination (meta-analysis) done properly?* The next step is the actual statistical combination (meta-analysis) of the data. The investigators should address the possibility that chance differences did not occur (a test for homogeneity). Homogeneity means that the results of each individual trial are mathematically compatible with the results of any of the others.[11]

Homogeneity can be quickly assessed by reviewing a graphic display of the numerical data with their odds ratios and 95% confidence intervals (Figure 6-3). The horizontal line for each trial shows the odds of successful treatment. The vertical line in the middle of each of these lines represents the point estimate of the difference between the groups. The width of each line represents the 95% confidence interval of this point estimate (i.e., the true answer falls within the boundaries 95% of the time). A bold horizontal line (odds ratio of 1.0) is known as the *line of no effect.* When the confidence interval of the result (horizontal line) crosses the line of no effect (vertical line), the difference in the effect of treatment is not significant at $P > .05$. In Figure 6-3, the confidence interval of all but two of the trials (a, c) cross this line, indicating that the treatment effects were not significant. The summary odds ratio, using either the fixed effects or random effects model, is also found in Figure 6-3. The vertical dashed line crosses the horizontal lines of all individual studies except one (c). This indicates a fairly homogeneous set of studies.

In addition to a test for homogeneity, the investigators should also perform a sensitivity analysis (Table 6-2). Depending on the test chosen, the same set of data may be combined to give different conclusions. If one finds that "fiddling" with the data in various ways makes little or no difference to the review's overall results, one can assume that the review's conclusions are accurate. In the sensitivity analysis used as an example in Table 6-2,

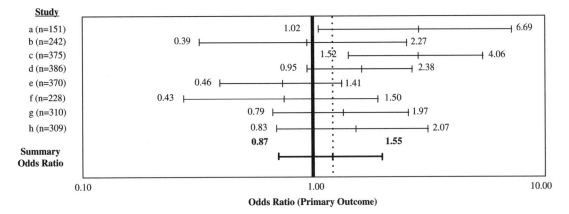

Figure 6-3. Display of treatment outcomes (odds ratio [OR]) and 95% confidence intervals. An OR greater than 1 favors treatment.

the data were analyzed based on quality score, adequacy of treatment allocation, and presence or absence of chronic disease.

In the article you are reviewing, you find in Figure 1 a test for homogeneity. The investigators also used a statistical test (Peto fixed-effects model) that allowed them to calculate the summary odds ratio. They also performed a sensitivity analysis by excluding trials of lower methodologic quality, trials involving patients with recurrent or chronic otitis media, and trials comparing different antibiotics; none made a difference in the overall results. Assured that the investigators appropriately performed the meta-analysis, you answer yes.

6. *Are the results important?* This final question forces us to consider the cost benefit and risks of the therapy. The investigators should demonstrate a strong effect manifested by a "large" (2.0 or greater) odds ratio. They should also address the number needed to treat, which takes into consideration the likelihood of an outcome or side effect. As you review this question, you would also like to see that all clinically important consequences are considered and that the benefits are worth the risks and costs.

In the meta-analysis you are evaluating, the odds ratio was not large, which means that no statistical difference was present in treating a child with a shorter or longer course of antibiotics. You see that you would have to treat 44 children with a 10-day course to prevent one treatment failure at 30 days using a shorter course of antibiotics.

Conclusion of Case

After a thorough assessment of this article, you conclude that it is well designed with valid results. You now feel confident that a shorter course of antibiotics for children with uncomplicated acute otitis media is just as beneficial as a longer course. As you institute this as a standard within your practice, however, you also make a commit-

ment to monitor its benefits and risks to your patients and to scan the literature for future articles that may offer additional information about length of therapy for acute otitis media. Consistency of the results in your practice, as well as across multiple published studies, is one characteristic of the scientific process that leads to acceptance and implementation.

With some practice and the use of the worksheet, one can quickly (within a few minutes) perform a critical assessment of a meta-analysis. While performing this appraisal, it is important to keep in mind that few meta-analyses are perfect. Only you can determine the exact shade of gray that you are willing to accept when deciding to apply the results of the study to your practice. By applying the knowledge, principles, and techniques presented in this chapter, however, you can more confidently recognize the various shades of gray and reject those meta-analyses that are seriously flawed.

Table 6-2. An Example of a Sensitivity Analysis Based on 13 Trials (a–m)

Description	Included Trials	8- to 30-Day Summary Odds Ratio (95% Confidence Interval)
All trials	a, b, d, h–m	1.38 (1.15–1.66)
Quality score >2	a, d, l	1.20 (0.83–1.75)
Quality score ≤2	b, h–k, m	1.44 (1.17–1.78)
Adequate concealment	h, i, l	1.14 (0.88–1.47)
Inadequate concealment	a, b, d, j, k, m	1.68 (1.39–2.19)
Chronic disease excluded	h, j, k	1.29 (0.76–2.20)
Chronic disease included	a, b, d, i, l, m	1.39 (1.15–1.70)

References

1. Kozyrskyj A, Hildes-Ripstein G, Longstaffe S, et al. Treatment of acute otitis media with a shortened course of antibiotics: a meta-analysis. JAMA 1998;279:1736–1742.
2. Miser W. Critical appraisal of the literature: how to assess an article and still enjoy life. J Am Board Fam Pract 1999; in press.
3. Pearson K. Report on certain enteric fever inoculation statistics. BMJ 1904;3:1243–1246.
4. Glass G. Primary, secondary and meta-analysis of research. Educ Res 1976;5:3–9.
5. Chalmers T, Matta R, Smith JJ, et al. Evidence favoring the use of anticoagulants in the hospital phase of acute myocardial infarction. N Engl J Med 1977;297:1091–1096.
6. Egger M, Smith G. Meta-analysis: potentials and promise. BMJ 1997;315:1371–1374.
7. Oxman A, Guyatt G. Guidelines for reading literature reviews. CMAJ 1988;138:697–703.
8. Shaughnessy A, Slawson D. Getting the most from review articles: a guide for readers and writers. Am Fam Physician 1997;55:2155–2160.
9. Goodman S. Have you ever meta-analysis you didn't like? Ann Intern Med 1991;114:244–246.
10. Sacks H, Berrier J, Reitman D, et al. Meta-analyses of randomized clinical trials. N Engl J Med 1987;316: 450–455.
11. Greenlaugh T. How to read a paper: papers that summarise other papers (systematic reviews and meta-analyses). BMJ 1997;315:672–675.
12. Thompson S, Pocock S. Can meta-analyses be trusted? Lancet 1991;338:1127–1130.
13. Peipert J, Bracken M. Systematic reviews of medical evidence: the use of meta-analysis in *Obstetrics and Gynecology*. Obstet Gynecol 1997;89:628–632.
14. Egger M, Smith G, Phillips A. Meta-analysis: principles and procedures. BMJ 1997;315:1533–1537.
15. Kassirer J. Clinical trials and meta-analysis: What do they do for us? N Engl J Med 1992;327:273–274.
16. Sacks H, Reitman D, Pagano D, Kupelnick B. Meta-analysis: an update. Mount Sinai J Med 1996;63:216–223.
17. Egger M, Schneider M, Smith G. Meta-analysis: spurious precision? Meta-analysis of observational studies. BMJ 1998;316:140–144.
18. Petitti D. Meta-analysis and endocrinology. Endocrin Metab Clin North Am 1997;26:31–44.
19. Moher D, Dulberg C, Wells G. Statistical power, sample size, and their reporting in randomized clinical trials. JAMA 1994;272:122–124.
20. Yusof S. Meta-analysis of randomized trials: looking back and looking ahead. Control Clin Trials 1997; 18:594–601.
21. Jadad A, Cook D, Jones A, et al. Methodology and reports of systematic reviews and meta-analyses: a comparison of Cochrane Reviews with articles published in paper-based journals. JAMA 1998;280:278–280.
22. Bailar J. The practice of meta-analysis. J Clin Epidemiol 1995;48:149–157.
23. Magnesium, myocardial infarction, meta-analysis and mega-trials [review]. Drug Ther Bull 1995;33:25–27.
24. Egger M, Smith D. Misleading meta-analysis: lessons from "an effective, safe, simple" intervention that wasn't. BMJ 1995;310:752–754.
25. Greenhalgh T. The Medline database. BMJ 1997;315: 180–183.
26. Dickersin K, Scherer R, Lefebvre C. Identifying relevant studies for systematic reviews. BMJ 1994;309:1286–1291.
27. Fox R, Ventura M. Efficiency of automated literature search mechanisms. Nurs Res 1984;33:174–177.
28. Hersh W, Hickam D. How well do physicians use electronic information retrieval systems? A framework for investigation and systematic review. JAMA 1998;280: 1347–1352.
29. Egger M, Smith G. Meta-analysis: bias in location and selection of studies. BMJ 1998;316:61–66.
30. Chalmers T, Frank C, Reitman D. Minimizing the three stages of publication bias. JAMA 1990;263:1392–1395.
31. Rennie D, Flanagin A. Publication bias: the triumph of hope over experience. JAMA 1992;267:411–412.
32. Scherer R, Dickersin K, Langenberg P. Full publication of results initially presented in abstracts: a meta-analysis. JAMA 1994;272:158–162.
33. Dickersin K, Min Y, Meinert C. Factors influencing publication of research results. Follow-up of applications submitted to two institutional review boards. JAMA 1992;267:374–378.
34. Stern J, Simes R. Publication bias: evidence of delayed publication in a cohort study of clinical research projects. BMJ 1997;315:640–645.
35. Smith G, Egger M. Meta-analysis: unresolved issues and future developments. BMJ 1998;316:221–225.
36. Cook D, Guyatt G, Ryan G, et al. Should unpublished data be included in meta-analyses? Current convictions and controversies. JAMA 1993;269:2749–2753.
37. Gregoire G, Derderian F, LeLorier J. Selecting the language of publications included in a meta-analysis: is there a Tower of Babel bias? J Clin Epidemiol 1995;48:159–163.
38. Moher D, Fortin P, Jadad A, et al. Completeness of reporting of trials published in languages other than English: implications for conduct and reporting of systematic reviews. Lancet 1996;347:363–366.
39. Egger M, Smith G, Schneider M, Minder C. Bias in meta-analysis detected by a simple, graphical test. BMJ 1997;315:629–634.
40. Moher D, Jadad A, Nichol G, et al. Assessing the quality of randomized controlled trials: an annotated bibliography of scales and checklists. Control Clin Trials 1995;16:62–73.
41. Jadad A, Moore A, Carroll D, et al. Assessing the quality of reports of randomized clinical trials: is blinding necessary? Control Clin Trials 1996;17:1–12.

Chapter 7

Using Outcomes to Improve Quality of Research and Quality of Care*

Richard A. Deyo

Case 1

Your clinic decided to undertake a quality improvement initiative for patients with low back pain. A steering committee recommended implementing a set of evidence-based guidelines developed under the sponsorship of the Agency for Health Care Policy and Research. Strategies are now in place to modify your and your colleagues' prescribing practices with regard to bedrest, use of imaging studies, and days off from work. Always the skeptic, you ask your medical director, "How will we know if following these guidelines has done any good?"

For a growing number of clinicians and health care administrators, the answer to this question is that we should examine patient "outcomes." But what does this mean, and why has "outcomes research" become a buzz-word of the 1990s?

Several pressures have led to interest in studying outcomes of care and also to the growing importance of evidence-based medicine in general. Perhaps the most obvious pressure has been the rapid increase in health care costs, which leads health care purchasers, employers, the public, and the government to ask, "Are we getting our money's worth?" This question is especially relevant because despite higher health care costs paid by Americans, many public health statistics regarding morbidity and mortality are worse in the United States than in many other developed countries.[1] Second, accumulating evidence demonstrates enormous geographic variations in the style of medical care[2] and even specialty variations in management of patients with apparently similar conditions.[3] This finding suggests to many

observers that some clinical practices and their resultant costs are idiosyncratic, based on variations in training, local habits, and differing opinions, rather than on firm evidence of what produces the best patient results. The implication of the wide variations is that some care may be unnecessary. The questions from those outside the medical profession are, "If clinicians know what they are doing, why does such wide variation in care exist? And why should we pay for care that exceeds some average?" Such questions constitute a call for accountability by health care providers to justify their high costs in terms of good outcomes.

What Are Outcomes?

Traditionally, physicians have thought of outcomes in terms of physiologic phenomena. For example, suppression of cardiac arrhythmias might be an appropriate outcome for antiarrhythmic drug therapy in a patient with ischemic heart disease. A decrease in the erythrocyte sedimentation rate might be seen as an outcome for patients with rheumatoid arthritis who are receiving disease remitting therapy. Reduction in prostate size might be seen as the appropriate goal of drug therapy for benign prostatic hypertrophy. Ultimately, however, these physiologic and

*Supported in part by grant No. HS-08194 from the Agency for Health Care Policy and Research. Reprinted with permission from RA Deyo. Using outcomes to improve quality of research and quality of care. J Am Board Fam Pract 1998;11:465–473.

Table 7-1. Examples of Dissociations between Surrogate Outcomes and End Results

Treatment	Surrogate Outcomes	End Results
Encainide, flecainide for ventricular arrhythmia after myocardial infarction	90% Suppression of complex ventricular ectopy	Mortality twice as high as placebo
Clofibrate for hypercholesterolemia	Lower cholesterol levels, fewer ischemic heart disease events	Mortality 25% greater than with placebo
Plasmapheresis for rheumatoid arthritis	Lower erythrocyte sedimentation rate, complement levels	No improvement in pain relief, function, or number of inflamed joints
Finasteride for benign prostatic hyperplasia	Shrinkage of prostate size	No improvement in urinary frequency or urgency
Biofeedback for low back pain	Reduced electromyographic activity in paraspinous muscles	No significant reduction in pain

anatomic end points are often termed *surrogate outcomes.* We presume that they are closely linked with the ultimate outcomes of greatest interest to patients and to society, such as symptom relief, the ability to perform normal daily activities, and survival. However, many sobering examples exist of surrogate outcomes that were poor markers for these ultimate outcomes of interest. Some examples are shown in Table 7-1.[4–8]

All of these examples illustrate the hazard of depending on surrogate outcomes to judge the effects of therapy. They support the argument that if we regard symptom relief, daily functioning, and survival as the major goals of therapy, we must measure them directly rather than inferring them from physiologic changes. However, clinical research historically has focused on just physiologic outcomes, and only recently have investigators incorporated measures of symptoms and function into many clinical trials.

These considerations partially explain the growth of questionnaire measures for assessing patient symptoms, function, and "health-related quality of life." The latter term has been adopted because of the recognition that quality of life depends on many factors beyond the control of medical care, including income; safe housing; job opportunities; and many other features of the social, political, and economic

environment. The current generation of questionnaires for measuring health status or health-related quality of life fuse social science methodology and clinical expertise to quantify important but subjective phenomena.

A common complaint about questionnaire data is that they are "soft" as opposed to the "harder" outcomes of physiologic measures. However, the boundary between hard and soft data is often indistinct. We may judge the hardness of data by their objectivity (e.g., physician report vs. patient observation), preservability (e.g., x-ray or histologic specimen), or dimensionality (e.g., a hematocrit vs. the observation of paleness). However, some methodologists argue that reproducibility of a result is the crucial attribute of "hardness," and by this yardstick many questionnaire measures are at least as hard as widely accepted clinical measures.[9] Table 7-2 illustrates some examples in which the reproducibility of questionnaire measures actually exceeded the reproducibility of expert clinical judgments.[10–15]

Reproducibility aside, we can demonstrate that questionnaire results correlate with other health phenomena of obvious importance. For example, Figure 7-1 shows survival curves among middle-aged men in a national survey who responded at baseline to a question regarding their overall health.[16] It can be seen that 10-year

Table 7-2. Studies of the Reproducibility of Patient Reports and Expert Evaluations

Subjective Reports	Kappa*	Expert Evaluation	Kappa*
Cough	0.87	Abnormal throat examination	0.37
Runny nose	0.75	Abnormal tympanic membranes	0.42
Health history questionnaire	0.79	Dorsalis pedis pulse, present or not	0.51
Function: Sickness Impact Profile	0.87	Ankle reflexes normal	0.50
Pain: visual analogue scale	0.94	Radiologist agreement whether lumbar spine x-rays are normal	0.51

*The kappa statistic quantifies agreement between two observers or replicate measurements after adjusting for chance agreements. Scores range from −1 (perfect disagreement) to 0 (no better than random agreement) to +1 (perfect agreement).

Figure 7-1. Male mortality in National Health and Nutrition Examination Survey-I Epidemiologic Follow-Up Study by levels of self-rated health. (Reprinted with permission from EL Idler, RJ Angel. Self-rated health and mortality in the NHANES-I Epidemiologic Follow-Up Study. Am J Public Health 1990;30:446–452.)

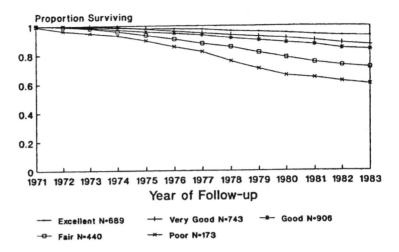

mortality was strongly associated with the respondent's own judgment about whether his health was excellent, very good, good, fair, or poor. Furthermore, the survival differences were substantial, ranging from approximately 60% to 95%. Although we know little about how the respondents made these health judgments at baseline, this simple subjective report obviously had substantial prognostic power. Associations of this kind provide evidence for the validity of many widely used health status questionnaires.

Outcomes Management

Most observers make a distinction between *outcomes management* and *outcomes research. Outcomes management* refers to the use of outcome measures in the course of routine clinical care. For example, outcome measures might be used for quality improvement purposes and to evaluate changes in the organization or content of clinical care. This use of outcome measurement is illustrated by Case 1. Use of outcome measures for such purposes is increasingly advocated by accrediting organizations that deal with large ambulatory care systems.

In some cases, hospitals or health plans have advocated using outcome measures to compare individual physicians or different treatments. For example, a hospital in Portland, Oregon, used a popular health status questionnaire, the short form with 36 items (SF-36), to examine outcomes of hip replacement surgery.[17] As shown in Figure 7-2, these studies permitted comparisons between individual orthopedic surgeons and also between different prosthetic devices. Several points were apparent from these studies. First, rapid improvement after surgery was generally observed, although the longer-term results were somewhat less favorable. Second, although differences were found between surgeons and between prosthetic devices, at least some of the differences could be accounted for by differences in the baseline severity of the patients' conditions, as suggested by differences in SF-36 scores at the preoperative measurement. Nonetheless, it is easy to visualize how data of this kind allow individual providers to compare notes or to choose a standard approach that appears to optimize patient outcomes.

Outcome data might also be used to evaluate large system changes by a hospital, a health care system, or a new health policy. If, for example, a health care system chose to alter its mix of generalist and specialist physicians, it might ask whether the end results in terms of patient outcomes were better or worse after the change. At one time, the state of Washington anticipated a major health policy reform (including universal coverage in a system similar to the "Clinton Plan") that ultimately was reversed by the state legislature. Had the plan gone forward, the state's department of health anticipated developing a statewide outcome tracking system to determine whether the overall health impact on the citizens of Washington was favorable, unfavorable, or neutral.

To use outcome data in routine care, better data systems are necessary. Some have suggested that the use of very brief health status questionnaires could be accomplished routinely at clinic visits, much as vital signs are routinely collected.[18] Nonetheless, manipulating the data, entering it into a computerized database, and analyzing the results all impose important burdens and costs. Many health care providers have information systems that routinely collect information on patient use of services, amounts billed, diagnoses, and insurance coverage. These information systems, however, typically have no data concerning patient symptoms, dysfunction, or satisfaction, nor do they have the kind of clinical detail that is necessary to interpret these outcomes. Thus, realizing the full potential of outcome measures likely requires greater attention to their incorporation into large computerized databases. In the meantime, even small, repeated patient

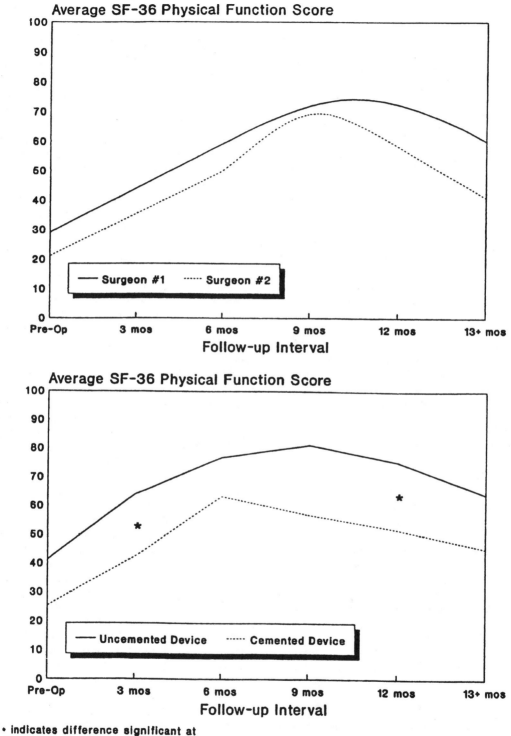

* indicates difference significant at
.05 level.

Figure 7-2. Examples of the use of health-related quality-of-life measures for outcomes management. These data from a single hospital compared baseline status and outcomes for patients undergoing total hip replacement. (Reprinted with permission from D Lansky, JBV Butler, FT Waller. Using health status measures in the hospital setting: from acute care to "outcomes management." Med Care 1992;30:MS57–MS73.)

surveys may provide useful information for quality improvement purposes.[19]

Outcomes Research

Outcomes research refers to investigation aimed at understanding what works and what does not work in clinical care. Typically, such research is focused on the end results of patient care in terms of symptoms, disability, and survival rather than the surrogate outcomes of physiology, laboratory results, or imaging. The term is generally applied to studies of the "effectiveness" of various clinical approaches, meaning their success in routine clinical practices. This is in contrast to studies of treatment "efficacy" that typically are randomized clinical trials conducted among highly selected patient populations, often in academic centers, often with leading experts providing the care, and with closer monitoring and follow-up than is generally the case in routine settings. Efficacy studies address whether a treatment *can* work under ideal circumstances, not whether it *does* work as generally applied in routine care. Effectiveness in routine care is a function of efficacy, but also of diagnostic accuracy, a physician's skill in applying a treatment, patient compliance, and perhaps other factors that are artificially optimized in the clinical trial setting. Some would include randomized trials of treatment impact under the rubric of "outcomes research," however, if the trials incorporated patient-relevant outcome measures and were conducted in routine clinical settings.

More commonly, however, *outcomes research* refers to the analysis of large administrative databases, such as insurance claims, to learn about the costs, complications, and utilization of services associated with certain clinical strategies, or it refers to the use of observational designs, such as cohort studies, which follow patients receiving different treatments for the same condition but with the treatments determined by the course of usual care rather than the intervention of a randomization schedule or investigator. Outcomes studies using these designs have, in some cases, added greatly to our understanding of the patient experience of various outcomes, unexpected consequences of therapy, and important gaps in our clinical knowledge.

A series of studies conducted by our patient outcome research team on low back pain may serve as examples. Back pain was chosen for study because of its high prevalence, high costs, and wide variability in styles of practice. One aspect of the project focused on outcomes of lumbar spine surgery, beginning with a synthesis of published literature on outcomes.[20–22] This synthesis demonstrated that fair evidence exists from randomized trials to support the efficacy of conventional lumbar diskectomy but not the newer percutaneous techniques. The cost-effectiveness of diskectomy compared favorably with other widely accepted treatments, such as treatment of mild hypertension.[23] The evidence on spinal fusion suggested that this procedure offers little advantage when used in conjunction with simple diskectomy for patients with herniated disks. No controlled trials were found of spinal fusion for degenerative disks in the absence of herniation.

Subsequent analyses of insurance claims databases demonstrated that lumbar spine operations involving fusion procedures were associated with higher costs and complication rates than diskectomy or laminectomy alone.[24,25] They also demonstrated that reoperation rates after spinal fusion were at least as high as reoperation rates after laminectomy or diskectomy without fusion. In the absence of randomized trials, these studies provided important descriptive information that supplemented the results of the literature syntheses.

We also conducted a prospective cohort study that tracked patients with sciatica or spinal stenosis in the offices of orthopedic surgeons, neurosurgeons, or occupational medicine physicians. This study provided richer detail regarding patient outcomes than was previously available and, like the only randomized trial, suggested that after controlling for important confounding variables, surgery offered an advantage in many 1-year outcomes for patients with herniated disks and spinal stenosis.[26–28] However, return to work after 1 year and 4 years were virtually the same with or without surgery.

We used the outcome data from our literature syntheses and claims analyses to develop an interactive computer-based video program for patients considering low back surgery. The intent of the program was to provide the best available information on outcomes of surgical or nonsurgical care, tailored specifically to diagnosis and patient age.[29] Thus, the program provides outcome data to patients in an effort to involve them more directly in decisions about their own care.

Some data from these studies were also incorporated into clinical guidelines for managing low back pain.[30] These guidelines have had important impacts on quality and costs of care in some large health care organizations, and the research data may have contributed (with several other factors) to a national decrease in spinal fusion rates in 1994.

Commonly Used Instruments for Studying Health Outcomes

A wide variety of questionnaires are available for measuring symptoms and functional outcomes. These typically measure outcomes in separate dimensions, such as physical functioning, emotional functioning, and role functioning. Some of these instruments are generic, meaning that they could be used for a wide variety of patients with a wide variety of conditions.[31] Examples include the SF-36 (adapted from the Medical Outcomes Study)[32] and its shorter version, the SF-12.[33] These instruments are currently in very wide use. Other examples are the Sickness Impact Profile,[34] Duke University Health Profile,[35,36] the Dartmouth COOP charts,[37] and the Quality of Well-Being Scale.[38] The latter instrument and the EuroQoL (European Quality of Life Scale)[39] not only measure patient symptoms and functioning, but also attach preference weights derived from interviews with large numbers of laypersons to each outcome state. These instruments permit the calculation of a single "utility" score for any outcome condition, which could theoretically be used in decision analysis and cost-effectiveness analysis.

In contrast to generic, health-related, quality-of-life instruments, disease-specific questionnaires focus more closely on the types of symptoms and dysfunctions that occur with particular disease conditions. Examples are available for studying the outcomes of asthma,[40] back pain,[41,42] heart disease,[43,44] arthritis,[45,46] diabetes,[47] and many other conditions. Examples of studies using such instruments are our cohort studies of back pain outcomes and studies of outcomes of different treatments for hypertension,[48] rheumatoid arthritis,[49] acquired immunodeficiency syndrome,[50] and many others.

Generic questionnaires are needed when comparing the impacts of treatments for different diseases, including their cost-effectiveness. Disease-specific questionnaires are often more sensitive to subtle but clinically important changes and may identify very specific health improvements that would not be apparent with a generic instrument. For research purposes, many investigators advocate including both a generic and a disease-specific measure.

Barriers and Hazards of Outcomes Analysis

Unfair Outcome Comparisons

A major problem with the use of outcomes for comparing providers or health care systems is that incentives to "game" the results may be present. One destructive way in which this could occur would be if certain providers simply declined to take the most difficult or severely ill patients. Accepting only healthier patients at the beginning of treatment assures having healthier patients at the end, and it has been suggested, for example, that cardiac surgeons might "shun the tough cases."

More generally, making fair comparisons among physicians or hospitals based on their outcomes requires careful adjustment for "case mix," so that providers with more sick or demographically disadvantaged patients are not unfairly penalized. Strategies for adjusting risk have been developed, generally incorporating at least patient age, gender, and comorbid conditions, all of which are available in most large automated databases.[51] In some cases, adjustment for disease severity or complications is included, although such information is less consistently available. If health status or quality-of-life questionnaires were in widespread routine

use, they could offer a powerful additional method for adjusting for baseline characteristics, in addition to providing measures of outcome. Such adjustment techniques can help to "level the playing field," but it is unlikely they will ever completely adjust for important differences among populations (indeed, this is the reason for the ascendancy of random allocation in comparing treatment efficacy).

Factors Other Than Medical Management That Affect Outcomes

Many factors other than medical care affect the outcomes of a particular illness. For example, patients with multiple, comorbid, chronic diseases are likely to have worse outcomes than patients with just a single condition. Homeless persons may have worse outcomes from many diseases than patients who are more affluent. Patients who are compliant with drug therapy or with physical treatments are likely to have better success than those who are not. Genetic endowment may have important influences on outcomes regardless of the quality of care. Thus, it is important to identify outcomes that are truly sensitive to the quality and effectiveness of the medical care delivered.

Difficulties in Measurement

For many conditions, the optimal timing or duration of follow-up for outcome assessments is unclear. The timing may be quite different for acute versus chronic diseases and even among chronic conditions. Different measures may be necessary for different settings and different populations, providing challenges for decision makers and for efforts to standardize measurement.[52] Patient reading ability and language fluency have important effects on the feasibility of measuring health-related quality of life. Similarly, cognitive impairments may make it difficult or impossible to collect data from certain patients, and the validity of surrogate responses is variable.

Costs and Burdens

The costs associated with collecting and analyzing outcomes data may be substantial and may not be offset by immediate or obvious savings in other areas. The respondent burden for patients may be substantial, depending on the length or frequency of measures.

Conclusions

Variations in care and cost pressures have combined to create ever-increasing calls for accountability on the part of the health care professions. In many cases, this has required not only attention to the process of care, but also to the results. Recognition is growing that physiologic, laboratory, and imaging outcomes are sometimes poorly associated with symptomatic, functional, and survival outcomes and, thus, the latter must be measured directly.

Symptoms, function, and quality of life can be quantified in a meaningful way, and a wide variety of well-validated instruments are available for use. Their adoption and widespread use in routine care settings for outcomes management requires additional resources and far better data systems than are currently available. In the research arena, we hope that patient-centered outcomes are increasingly incorporated into clinical trials. Outcomes research in the traditional sense, including large database analysis and cohort studies, are complementary to, rather than in competition with, randomized controlled trials. Finally, clinicians and investigators should be aware that outcomes research may, in some cases, precipitate political, legal, and media attacks and controversies because such research focuses on clinical strategies that already have some credibility and a share in the marketplace.[53]

We should not expect magic from outcomes assessment because of the many problems and pitfalls described earlier. Nevertheless, the current focus on outcomes may substantially improve the quality of care and research in our health care system.

References

1. Geyman JP. Evidence-based medicine in primary care: an overview. J Am Board Fam Pract 1998;11:46–56.
2. Wennberg JE, McPherson K, Caper P. Will payment based on diagnosis-related groups control hospital costs? N Engl J Med 1984;311:295–300.
3. Cherkin DC, Deyo RA, Wheeler K, Ciol MA. Physician variation in diagnostic testing for low back pain. Who you see is what you get. Arthritis Rheum 1994;37:15–22.
4. Echt DS, Liebson PR, Mitchell LB, et al. Mortality and morbidity in patients receiving encainide, flecainide, or placebo. The Cardiac Arrhythmia Suppression Trial. N Engl J Med 1991;324:781–788.
5. Oliver MF, Heady JA, Morris JN, Cooper J. World Health Organization. Cooperative trial on primary prevention of ischemic heart disease using clofibrate to lower serum cholesterol: mortality follow-up. Lancet 1980;2:379–385.
6. Dwosh IL, Giles AR, Ford PM, Pater JL. Plasmapheresis therapy in rheumatoid arthritis: a controlled, double-blind, crossover trial. N Engl J Med 1983;308:1124–1129.
7. Lepor H, Williford WO, Bary MJ, et al. The efficacy of terazosin, finasteride, or both in benign prostatic hyperplasia. Veterans Affairs Cooperative Studies Benign Prostatic Hyperplasia Study Group. N Engl J Med 1996;335:533–539.
8. Nouwen A. EMG biofeedback used to reduce standing levels of paraspinal muscle tension in chronic low back pain. Pain 1983;17:353–360.
9. Feinstein AR. Clinical biostatistics XLI. Hard science, soft data, and challenges of choosing clinical variables in research. Clin Pharmacol Ther 1977;22:485–498.
10. Deyo RA, Andersson G, Bombardier C, et al. Outcome measures for studying patients with low back pain. Spine 1994;19:2032S–2036S.
11. Wood RW, Diehr P, Wolcott BW, et al. Reproducibility of clinical data and decisions in management of upper respiratory illnesses: comparison of physician and non-physician providers. Med Care 1979;17:767–779.
12 Koran LM. The reliability of clinical methods, data, and judgements. N Engl J Med 1975;293:642–646, 695–701.
13. Deyo RA, Rainville J, Kent DL. What can the history and physical examination tell us about low back pain? [see comments]. JAMA 1992;268:760–765.
14. Pecoraro RE, Inui TS, Chen MS, et al. Validity and reliability of a self-administered health history questionnaire. Public Health Rep 1979;94:231–238.
15. Deyo RA. Measuring the functional status of patients with low back pain. Arch Phys Med Rehabil 1988;69:1044–1053.
16. Idler EL, Angel RJ. Self-rated health and mortality in the NHANES-I Epidemiologic Follow-up Study. Am J Public Health 1990;30:446–452.
17. Lansky D, Butler, JBV, Waller FT. Using health status measures in the hospital setting: from acute care to "outcomes management." Med Care 1992;30:MS57–MS73.
18. Ellwood PM. Shattuck lecture—outcome management: a technology of patient experience. N Engl J Med 1988;318:1549–1556.
19. Langley GJ, Nolan KM, Nolan TW, et al. The Improvement Guide: A Practical Approach to Enhancing Organizational Performance. San Francisco: Jossey-Bass, 1996;109–112.
20. Hoffman RM, Wheeler KJ, Deyo RA. Surgery for herniated lumbar discs: a literature synthesis. J Gen Intern Med 1993;8:487–496.
21. Turner JA, Ersek M, Herron L, Deyo R. Surgery for lumbar spinal stenosis. Attempted meta-analysis of the literature. Spine 1992;17:1–8.
22. Turner JA, Ersek M, Herron L, et al. Patient outcomes after lumbar spinal fusions. JAMA 1992;268:907–911.
23. Malter AD, Larson EB, Urban N, Deyo RA. Cost-effectiveness of lumbar discectomy for the treatment of herniated intervertebral disc. Spine 1996;21:1048–1054.
24. Deyo RA, Cherkin DC, Loeser JD, et al. Morbidity and mortality in association with operations on the lumbar spine. The influence of age, diagnosis, and procedure. J Bone Joint Surg Am 1992;74:536–543.
25. Deyo RA, Ciol MA, Cherkin DC, et al. Lumbar spinal fusion. A cohort study of complications, reoperations, and resource use in the Medicare population. Spine 1993;18:1463–1470.
26. Keller RB, Atlas SJ, Singer DE, et al. The Maine Lumbar Spine Study, Part I. Background and concepts. Spine 1996;21:1769–1776.
27. Atlas SJ, Deyo RA, Keller RB, et al. The Maine Lumbar Spine Study, Part II. 1-year outcomes of surgical and non-

surgical management of sciatica. Spine 1996;21: 1777–1786.

28. Atlas SJ, Deyo RA, Keller RB, et al. The Maine Lumbar Spine Study, Part III. 1-year outcomes of surgical and nonsurgical management of lumbar spinal stenosis. Spine 1996;21:1787–1795.

29. Spunt BS, Deyo RA, Taylor VM, et al. An interactive videodisc program for low back pain patients. Health Educ Res 1996;11:535–541.

30. Bigos S, Bowyer O, Braen G, et al. Clinical Practice Guideline No. 14: Acute Low Back Problems in Adults. Rockville, MD: U.S. Department of Health and Human Services, Agency for Health Care Policy and Research; December 17, 1994. AHCPR Publication 95-0642.

31. Patrick DL, Deyo RA. Generic and disease-specific measures in assessing health status and quality of life. Med Care 1989;27:S217–S232.

32. Ware JE, Sherbourne CD. The MOS 36-item short-form survey (SF-36). I: Conceptual framework and item selection. Med Care 1992;30:473–483.

33. Ware JE, Kosinski, Keller SD. A 12-item short form health survey. Med Care 1996;34:220–233.

34. Bergner M, Bobbitt RA, Carter WB, Gilson BS. The Sickness Impact Profile: development and final revision of a health status measure. Med Care 1981;19:787–805.

35. Parkerson GR, Broadhead W, Tse CKJ. The Duke health profile: a 17-item measure of health and dysfunction. Med Care 1990;28:1056–1072.

36. Blake RL Jr, Vandiver TA. The reliability and validity of a ten-item measure of functional status. J Fam Pract 1986;23:455–459.

37. Nelson EC, Landgraf JM, Hays RD, et al. The functional status of patients. How can it be measured in physicians' offices? Med Care 1990;28:1111–1126.

38. Kaplan RM, Bush JW, Berry CC. Health status; type of validity and the Index of Well Being. Health Serv Res 1976;11:478.

39. EuroQoL Group. EuroQoL—a new facility for the measurement of health-related quality-of-life. Health Policy 1990;16:199–208.

40. Juniper EF, Guyatt GH, Feffie PJ, Griffith LE. Measuring quality of life in asthma. Am Rev Respir Dis 1993;147:832–838.

41. Roland M, Morris R. A study of the natural history of back pain. Part I: Development of a reliable and sensitive measure of disability in low back pain. Spine 1983;8:141–144.

42. Patrick DL, Deyo RA, Atlas SJ, et al. Assessing health-related quality of life in patients with sciatica. Spine 1995;20:1899–1909.

43. Spertus JA, Winder JA, Dewhurst TA, et al. Development and evaluation of the Seattle Angina Questionnaire: a new functional status measure for coronary artery disease. J Am Coll Cardiol 1995;25:333–341.

44. Guyatt GH, Nogradi S, Halcrow S, et al. Development and testing of a new measure of health status for clinical trials in heart failure. J Gen Intern Med 1989;4:101–107.

45. Fries JF, Spitz PW, Krainos RG, Holman HR. Measure of patient outcome in arthritis. Arthritis Rheum 1980; 23:137–145.

46. Meenan RF, Gertman PM, Mason JH. Measuring health status in arthritis: the arthritis impact measurement scales. Arthritis Rheum 1980;23:146–152.

47. Boyer JG, Earp JL. The development of an instrument for assessing the quality of life of people with diabetes. Diabetes 39. Med Care 1997;35:440–453.

48. Beto JA, Bansal VK. Quality of life in treatment of hypertension: a meta-analysis of clinical trials. Am J Hypertens 1992;5:125–133.

49. Bombardier C, Ware J, Russell IJ, et al. Auraofin therapy and quality of life in patients with rheumatoid arthritis. Results of a multicenter trial. Am J Med 1986;81:565–578.

50. Weissman JS, Cleary PD, Seagl GR, et al. The influence of health-related quality of life and social characteristics on hospital use by patients with AIDS in the Boston health study. Med Care 1996;34:1037–1054.

51. Wray NP, Hollingsworth JC, Peterson NJ, Ashton CM. Case-mix adjustment using administrative databases: a paradigm to guide future research. Med Care Res Rev 1997;54:326–356.

52. Deyo RA, Patrick DL. Barriers to the use of health status measures in clinical investigation, patient care, and policy research. Med Care 1989;27:S254–S268.

53. Deyo RA, Psaty BM, Simon G, et al. The messenger under attack: intimidation of researchers by special-interest groups. N Engl J Med 1997;336:1176–1180.

Chapter 8

Understanding the Choices
That Patients Make*

Thomas R. Taylor

A number of developments in health care have focused increasing attention on the patient's role in his or her own health care. Patients are demanding greater participation in the decision making that surrounds their care as more and more of the financial responsibility for their care falls on their own shoulders. Drug companies "pitch their wares" directly to patients via the media over the heads of physicians. The intention is to create demand by changing patients' preferences for the benefits offered by companies' products. The role of health maintenance organizations in limiting access to specialists, expensive investigations, and high-tech treatments such as bone marrow transplantation is under legislative assault as patients demand that their reasonable preferences be met.

It is important to emphasize that this chapter does not focus on the population-level policy decisions described above but on the individual health care choices made by patients. In practice, physicians make decisions all day as they choose tests and treatments, select screening tests, and help patients to manage chronic and life-threatening diseases. Most decisions are made in the face of uncertainty, in the sense that the outcome of the action they select is unknown.

Patient Decision Making

The two key elements in any decision are (1) what is likely to happen, and (2) the value of the outcome to the decision maker. A patient's preference of one outcome over another is a direct reflection of the information available and the values of the decision maker. Because the response to treatment is not absolutely guaranteed, these decisions are seen as being made under uncertainty, in which the outcome may or may not be the desired one.

Physicians repeatedly make the same kinds of decisions. They develop a relatively stable understanding of risks and benefits in their area of expertise and of the information needed to make satisfactory choices. When the decision making is controlled by the patient, however, a completely new set of circumstances comes into play.

Patients make health care decisions relatively infrequently and thus cannot build up a stable understanding of the key elements of most of the decisions they make. Patients make most health care decisions with little preparation or repetition. Thus, in thinking about an illness and its treatment in the context of making advance directives for themselves or their parents, patients are usually starting from scratch. The ways in which the choices are described, including the language chosen to describe possible outcomes, have a profound effect in "framing" such decisions and in influencing which options are eventually chosen. It is critically important that patients be provided with relevant, accurate information in a form that is amenable to influencing their preferences.

Role of Preferences

A woman with an intraductal carcinoma of the breast faces two main choices for its treatment: a simple mastectomy or a "lumpectomy" with radiation. In choosing one or the other, the patient is demonstrating a preference for life after a simple mastectomy or life after a lumpectomy with radiation. Therefore, the preference of one treatment over the other is a combination of how likely one or the other is to be successful and how the patient values the likely outcome of each treatment. According to the literature, the probability of survival is approximately the same with each treatment. Because the outcome in either case is uncertain, the patient's preferences in this case are called *utilities*, because they reflect the patient's risk attitude or preference in the face of uncertainty.

*Reprinted with permission from TR Taylor. Understanding the choices that patients make. J Am Board Fam Pract 2000;13:(in press).

By contrast, if the outcomes of a choice can be predicted with certainty, then the preferences are called *values*. Thus, a patient with a hematologic malignancy might be asked if he or she prefers 4 years without treatment to 8 years with repeated cycles of chemotherapy and transfusions. The patient is asked to assume that each outcome would occur with certainty. Again, the patient is choosing one length and quality of life over another in light of his or her relevant values.

Do Preferences Really Exist?

Another fundamental problem with eliciting patient preferences is the assumption that preferences already exist in the patient's mind, and that by presenting him or her with data in a particular way, clinicians can elicit preferences. This concern has been raised by a number of authors.[1] Lenert and colleagues,[2] compared the ways in which the preference elicitation task was presented to the subjects. Two approaches were compared, namely, titration (i.e., steadily changing one option) versus "ping-pong" (i.e., going back and forth between options). They found that, on repeated testing, these two methods produced significantly different preference measurements, suggesting that preferences are strongly influenced by the elicitation process and, indeed, they may even be created during the process of elicitation.

Importance of Risk in Preference

Decision making is acknowledged to be a process of balancing competing risks—for example, loss versus gain.[3] Tversky and Kahneman[4] have similarly shown that decisions involving uncertainty are influenced by whether the alternatives are perceived as gains or losses. Patients who shy away from more risky alternatives in favor of less risky alternatives are *risk averse*; if they are indifferent, they are *risk neutral*; and if they prefer risky situations, they are *risk seeking*.

The impact of differences in risk preferences within a family can be illustrated by a study of prostate cancer screening by Volk and colleagues.[5] Screening for prostate cancer is a "utility-sensitive decision," because the apparent gain in life expectancy from screening is small, and patients may attach unusual importance to certain outcomes of treatment, such as impotence or incontinence. This is one of the classes of decision that Kassirer[6] identifies as appropriate for incorporating patient preferences.

The issue of who is the decision maker was also critical in the study by Volk and colleagues.[5] In some cases, the husband had the final say, whereas in others, the wife insisted (over her husband's wishes to avoid unpleasant complications) that time together mattered more than anything. This latter stance reflects the value that quantity of life is more important than quality of life. It also reflects differences in risk perception between husbands and wives. In the above study, known evidence for and against prostate screening was assembled based on a recent decision analysis.[7] The evidence summary (or balance sheet) covered both short- and long-term complications of prostate cancer treatment. These included complete impotence, urinary incontinence, urethral stricture, rectal injury, and hormonal therapy–related complications. Short-term complications included gastrointestinal tract complications, thromboembolism, lymphedema, and radiation cystitis.

Preferences were assessed using the time trade-off method (discussed later). The periods of time attached to each outcome reflected trade-offs between quantity and quality of life. Preferences were estimated separately for orchiectomy, because subjects associated particular importance to this procedure.

The study found that nine out of 10 wives preferred screening for their husbands, whereas seven out of 10 husbands preferred no screening at all. A majority of husbands have a higher risk tolerance for this choice than their wives. Wives associated little burden with the complications of treatment and preferred to maximize their husbands' quantity of life, regardless of the complications. The issue of who is the decision maker is paramount in the case of prostate screening, and optimal screening strategies may differ from the perspectives of husbands and wives.

The importance of risk preference for physicians has also been demonstrated in a number of clinical situations. No doubt exists that similar effects could be demonstrated on patients' choices.

Physicians have been shown to exhibit variations in preferences for avoiding harmful medical actions. Some physicians are more sensitive to losses than to gains. Nightingale[8] showed that physicians in a general medical clinic who were categorized as *loss averse* on a risk-preference scale ordered twice as many laboratory tests in hypothetical cases as their colleagues who were not as sensitive to loss. The more loss averse an emergency room physician is, the more cases he or she admits to intensive care units and the longer he or she continues resuscitation efforts after spontaneous contractions have ceased.[8]

Effect of Framing on How Patients Use Information

In the process of eliciting patient preferences, information should be provided on the costs, benefits, complications, and outcomes of each treatment. A critically important feature of presenting choices to patients is the effect of framing.[4,9] Thus, choices can be presented to patients within a neutral, positive, or negative framework. For example, clinicians can provide patients with information about the probable outcomes of chemotherapy versus surgery for cancer and about side effects and their impact on a patient's ability to function.

Using the same wording, a positive presentation emphasizes how many patients would be free of side effects and which patients would survive. By contrast, the negative presentation emphasizes those patients who would experience significant side effects and those who would not survive. The neutral presentation gives equal emphasis to both good and bad outcomes.

Outcomes that are described positively, in terms of ability to function and interaction with one's family even for a short period of time, are more attractive to patients than a longer life limited by side effects such as nausea, bleeding, fatigue, or anorexia. Depending on the context in which a choice is presented, patients make very different choices.[10]

Importance of Clarifying the Individual Values of Patients

Because preferences directly reflect the underlying values of the patient, a real possibility exists that individual patients differ widely on which values are considered relevant to a particular decision.

The importance of exploring the perspectives of patients before presenting them with choices was illustrated in a study by Pierce.[11] In the context of selecting treatment for early-stage breast cancer, she focused on the attributes of the treatment outcomes that best reflected the values considered by women who are confronted with this choice. The options considered were simple mastectomy versus lumpectomy and radiation. The subjects were actual patients in this situation. It was assumed (for the sake of this comparison) that survival was comparable between the two options.

In the study, 48 women were interviewed while making the choice between simple mastectomy and lumpectomy with radiation in a real-life situation and were asked what the attractive or unattractive features were of each option. The results of this value-clarification exercise revealed five principal dimensions of value in this choice between simple mastectomy and lumpectomy with radiation. These dimensions were:

Expediency: Was it quick and easy?
Safety: Was eradication of the cancer thorough?
Survival: How much did it extend the length of the patient's life?
Health: To what degree was the patient returned to normalcy?
Body integrity: How much was the breast or body kept intact?

The literature on patients' choices for breast cancer management does not address these individual attributes of the outcomes. Any attempt to elicit patients'

preferences for these two procedures that did not explicitly address them would be unlikely to result in patient satisfaction. It is unknown whether another sample of patients with breast cancer would identify the same attributes.

Preference Elicitation and the Role of the Balance Sheet

It is important not to oversimplify the process by which human beings make decisions. Decisions are not made in a vacuum. Whereas many day-to-day decisions have to be made with very little information, most of us would agree that as much relevant information as possible should be available before making an important health-related decision. Patient interest is increasing for using information sources on the Internet to help choose treatments, drug regimens, or surgical procedures. The emergence of many patient decision support systems is an indication of this trend.

The process of eliciting preferences from a particular decision maker (whether patient or physician) begins by assembling an evidence-based summary (i.e., balance sheet) of the relevant information linking the options to the anticipated outcomes. The more personally involved the patient is in understanding the evidence, the more likely that the preferences elicited represent the patient's values and intentions.

One study of primary care patient preferences for methods of screening for colon cancer[12] illustrates the role of an evidence-based information summary in the form of a balance sheet (Table 8-1) for assembling the evidence that a patient may consider in the rational examination of clinical preferences. The balance sheet organizes the information summary around five screening options. The balance sheet in this study was prepared using MEDLINE search references and data from the 1995 Office of Technology Assessment publication, "Cost-Effectiveness of Colorectal Cancer Screening in Average-Risk Adults."[13] The screening options were those proposed by the American Gastroenterological Association.

In that study, patients from the offices of primary care physicians listened to a scripted oral presentation while viewing a table supplemented by pie charts describing five screening methods and their outcomes. The patients were asked the following questions:

Considering the risks and benefits of colorectal cancer screening, if you were asked to select one of these options, which one would you choose?
Considering the risks and benefits of colorectal cancer screening, please evaluate how likely you would be to undergo each of the following (with each option listed to be ranked on a 5-point Likert scale).

Table 8-1. A Balance Sheet of Colon Cancer Screening Tests Used in the Study of Patient Preferences

Event	Without Screening	Fecal Occult Blood Test	Flexible Sigmoidoscopy	Barium Enema	Colonoscopy
Description of test	No test	You place two samples of stool onto special cards for 3 consecutive days and then mail them to your doctor for analysis.	A flexible tube with a television camera at the tip is placed into your rectum and can examine approximately half of your colon.	You are given an enema of a liquid that can be seen on x-ray films. Multiple x-ray films are taken with you lying in different positions.	A flexible tube with a television camera at the tip is placed into your rectum and examines your entire colon. If polyps are found, they can be removed and a biopsy can be performed on them.
Preparation required for the test	None	For 5 days, you must alter your diet so as not to eat any red meat, certain fruits and vegetables, or vitamin C.	You must give yourself two enemas 1 hr before the procedure.	You must drink a laxative solution the evening before the test, which causes diarrhea to clear your colon.	You must drink a laxative solution the evening before the test, which causes diarrhea to clear your colon. You cannot take aspirin or non-steroidal anti-inflammatory medicines for 1 wk before the procedure.
Intravenous sedation for test	No	No	No	No	Yes
Time required for test	None	A few mins	15 mins	30 mins	45 mins
Time missed from work for test	None	None	2–3 hrs	2–3 hrs	Entire day
How often test should be repeated	Not applicable	Every yr	Every 3–5 yrs	Every 5 yrs	Every 5–10 yrs
Likely discomfort associated with the test	None	Process associated with obtaining stool samples from toilet	Mild sensation of urge to have bowel movement, and possibly crampy abdominal pain	Mild abdominal pain	Mild sensation of urge to have bowel movement, and possibly crampy abdominal pain
Risk of making hole in the colon, which requires hospitalization and may result in surgery or death	0	0	0–4/10,000	0–4/10,000	10–20/10,000
Probability of developing colon cancer over the rest of one's life	53/1,000	49/1,000	38/1,000	22/1,000	18/1,000

Event	Without Screening	Fecal Occult Blood Test	Flexible Sigmoidoscopy	Barium Enema	Colonoscopy
Probability of dying as a result of colon cancer over the rest of one's life	25/1,000	19/1,000	14/1,000	7/1,000	6/1,000
Colorectal cancers prevented (%)	None	10–38	45	40–70	58–87
Decrease in colorectal mortality as a result of screening procedure (%)	0	20–33	45–70	45–70	70–80
Chance that the screening test will be positive and result in the need for a colonoscopy over 10 yrs (%)	0	40	8–13	30–40	Not applicable
Unit cost per procedure ($)	None	5–10	80–135	131–200	285–500

(Reprinted with permission from LE Leard, MD Savides, TG Geniats. Patient preferences for colorectal cancer screening. J Fam Pract 1997;45:213.)

I would want/I would not want to have this test if it were recommended by my physician (asked for each option).

The scaling methods used in this study were a Likert scale for one question, a choice of best test, and response to physician's recommendation for each option in turn. All of these approaches fall into the direct category scaling method (described later).

The important feature of this study is that it links the evidence, in the form of the literature reviews used in developing a guideline to the patients' process of preference elicitation by the mechanism of the balance sheet (see Table 8-1). The study showed that 38% of subjects chose colonoscopy as a preferred method of screening, 31% chose fecal occult blood test, 40% chose barium enema, and 13% chose flexible sigmoidoscopy.

The balance sheet is a list of possible outcomes that assists the patient or provider in making an informed decision regarding alternative interventions.[14,15] An outcome is a benefit or harm to the patient, such as a potential complication, change in life expectancy, or the pain or discomfort resulting from a procedure. The balance sheet presents this information, along with the probability that the outcome occurs for each option. By condensing the pertinent information onto a single, structured balance sheet, the patient or provider is able to consider more easily the possible outcomes before

making a decision. The Agency for Health Care Policy and Research used a similar balance sheet to summarize the evidence from the literature reviews on benign prostatic hyperplasia from which the guideline was developed.[16]

Role of Time and Time Trade-Offs in Patient Preferences

For some patients, time in the context of making choices is not a uniform dimension. For example, they may be willing to put up with a great deal in the way of complications and side effects from a cancer treatment that would allow them to stay alive long enough to attend a daughter's wedding or the birth of a grandchild.

Perhaps one of the best examples of time trade-offs is in the prevention of the complications of a chronic disease, such as diabetes. It is not easy to convince patients that a lifetime dedicated to very tight control over their diabetes has a conjectured improvement in outcomes such as small-vessel disease. For example, a very tightly controlled diet with large amounts of exercise and strict use of either an insulin pump or multiple daily shots of insulin results in tight diabetes control with blood sugars kept well within or near the normal range. Trade-offs are that if the diabetes is controlled too tightly, a real danger exists of hypoglycemia that is, in many ways, a more serious short-term complication than hyperglycemia. All of this is directed at minimizing the progression of small-vessel disease manifested by renal failure, diabetic polyneuropathy, and ischemic heart disease.

Patients differ in how much they take current account of the long-term consequences of their actions and the degree to which they can defer gratification, for example, by a tightly controlled diet to gain long-term benefits. Time and the length of the interval between the proximal actions and the distal outcomes is a very important part of patient preferences.

The effect of time on patients' preferences can be illustrated in another context. Christensen-Szalanski[17] studied 18 pregnant women and their attitudes toward avoiding pain and avoiding the use of anesthesia during childbirth at three time periods. One month before labor, they were consistently against pain avoidance. During early labor, they were still consistently against pain avoidance. During active labor, however, a shift to favoring pain avoidance occurred. One month postpartum, they were again against pain avoidance. An important feature of this study was that the patients held opinions on outcomes that they had never experienced, and they changed their preferences in the light of experience only to revert to previous preferences as memory of the labor pain faded. The study is useful in emphasizing the distinction between current and longer-term values.

How Are Preferences Measured?

All research on measuring patient preferences has been conducted in highly structured experimental settings. Even in these settings, the process of measurement is fraught with difficulties. A few studies (described earlier) tried to move the measurement process into the real world of clinicians' offices, but the problems of translation are formidable. The kind of precision demanded by the techniques described later are very difficult to sustain in the real-world interaction in a physician's office.

It is likely that techniques and instruments will be developed for specific common clinical problems (e.g., the colon or prostate cancer screening described earlier) and then be adapted for use in physicians' offices. Following is a description of the methods and techniques that have emerged in the research world; the aim is to illustrate the complexities of preference measurement rather than provide a blueprint for practice.

The process of eliciting preferences (e.g., for colon cancer screening) begins with the identification of the key options (fecal occult blood test, flexible sigmoidoscopy, colonoscopy, barium enema) followed by the assembling and framing of the evidence in a form that is accessible and acceptable to patients. It culminates in the measurement and quantification of the preferences.

Three approaches are widely used for measuring or quantifying preferences: the *standard gamble*, the *time trade-off*, and the *rating scale*. The standard gamble is the only approach that measures utilities in the sense that the risk attitude of the patient is included. The time trade-off and the variants of the rating scale approach are used to measure values.

The standard gamble is the best-known method and is derived directly from expected utility theory. Utility theory proposes, among other assumptions, that the rational decision maker acts so as to achieve the maximum expected overall utility or benefit. The standard gamble poses a choice between a certain outcome and a gamble; for example, patients are asked to consider themselves as having congestive heart failure (American Heart Association classification II). They are asked to consider a choice between staying at their current level of disability and accepting a gamble of a 40% chance of cure and a 40–100% chance of sudden death. The probability of cure is systematically varied until decision makers are indifferent between their current level of disability and a specific probability of cure.[18] The probability level of cure at the point of indifference is a reflection of the utility that the decision maker attaches to cure. The standard gamble always poses a choice between a gamble and an outcome, in which the certain outcome is intermediate in desirability between the best (cure) and worst (death) gamble outcomes.

The time trade-off method was developed by Torrance and colleagues[19] as a more easily understood alternative to the standard gamble. In this approach, patients are asked to choose between two certain outcomes (i.e., the element of the gamble is omitted, thus, the preferences measured are values and not utilities because no risk is involved). They are asked how many years in a healthy state would be equivalent to X years in a poorer state of health. In this case, time is used as the unit of comparison; by comparing the two times, the utility or value for each outcome can then be calculated.

The third approach is the category rating scale. It is derived from the field of psychometrics and uses a scale anchored at each end. The patient identifies the best (i.e., perfect health) and worst (i.e., death) states of health for either end of the scale. The patient then rates the desirability of the health states in question as points between the two extremes. For example, an interval scale of 10 categories is frequently used. The category rating scale is the most widely used method for measuring health state preferences.[20]

Three much less widely used category rating techniques have been adopted to measure health states. They are aimed at improving on the category rating scale. One is *magnitude estimation*,[21] in which one outcome is taken as the standard and other outcomes are compared with this standard. For example, the standard is given a value of 10, and the others are rated above or below it. Studies using this approach have produced inconsistent results.[22] The second method is called *equivalence*,[23] in which patients are asked how many patients in state A are equivalent to 100 patients in state B. The third approach is called *willingness to pay*.[24] In this exercise, patients are told that a state of health, such as arthritis, is to be compared with perfect health. The patients are then asked what proportion of their household income they would be willing to pay to get from the state of having arthritis to being in perfect health.

Evaluation of the Different Methods

The standard gamble is very difficult to explain to physicians, let alone to patients, and it is not intuitively obvious to most people. A number of studies, including those of Llewellyn-Thomas and colleagues,[1] have shown that changes in the gamble outcome significantly influenced the reported utilities for health states. This finding indicates that the standard gamble is internally inconsistent. Schoemaker[25] also presented extensive evidence to support this view. He found that people using the standard gamble tend to provide utilities that are biased in the direction of risk aversion (i.e., minimizing risk in their choices), leading to higher utility values than those derived from methods that do not involve gambles of any kind, such as time trade-off or category scaling.

An extensive review of studies by Froberg and Kane[22] compared the six methods described earlier (standard gamble, time trade-off method, category rating scale, magnitude estimation, equivalence, willingness to pay). They reviewed a large number of studies comparing various permutations of the six methods and concluded that none of the methods is strictly comparable to another. They concluded that the most promising methods are category scaling, magnitude estimation, and time trade-off. The category scaling method is the easiest to administer, is the least expensive, and appears to yield scale values that are as valid as any other method. Thus, those authors recommend this method as a first choice, especially in large-scale studies. They advocate a more limited place for magnitude estimation and time trade-off approaches for studies that focus on decision making and are smaller in scale. The time trade-off approach is more difficult to administer and more expensive but has good validity levels. These findings reflect the fact that there is no way of knowing which elicitation method represents the gold standard. At this point, the most direct and straightforward technique, namely, the category scaling method, appears to be most attractive.

More standardized approaches have emerged because of the complex and time-consuming nature of the approaches described earlier to eliciting preferences and attempting to quantify them. They are based on multiattribute utility theory,[26] regarded as being easy to understand and theoretically robust. This theory focuses on the utilities of decision makers rather than on probabilities. Multiattribute utility theory helps decision makers to break down the decision-making process into manageable segments, to evaluate the segments separately, and then to systematically recombine these segments to reach a decision.

The set of approaches described below use prescored multiattribute health status measures in which the key attributes are already identified and have been standardized on a random sample of the public with scores derived for each response.

The following are three well-known systems:

1. The Quality of Well-Being Scale is scale based and, therefore, measures values. The respondents are asked to rate a single day on four attributes: mobility, physical activity, social activity, and symptom or problem. If the patient has multiple symptoms or problems, then the patient rates the one that is most undesirable.[27]
2. The European Quality of Life Scale uses five attributes: mobility, self-care, usual activity, pain/discomfort, and anxiety/depression. This instrument was developed using a time trade-off technique and, therefore, yields values rather than utilities. It was standardized with a random sample of 3,000 adults in the United Kingdom.[28]
3. The Health Utilities Index is based in part on the Quality of Well-Being Scale. This instrument was developed using a time trade-off technique and, therefore, yields values rather than utilities. It was standardized on a random sample of residents of Hamilton, Ontario. A pediatric version has also been developed.[29]

All three approaches were developed for evaluating treatments and health care systems, such as neonatal intensive care (Health Utilities Index). Drummond and colleagues[30] have critically reviewed this set of approaches in some detail.

When Should Patient Preferences Be Explicitly Assessed?

Although eliciting the preferences of patients is a desirable goal, it is not practical in every clinical encounter, so some selectivity is appropriate. Choosing where to invest the effort is important. This issue has been dealt with in some detail by Kassirer.[6] Among the most important decisions in which patient preferences should be explicitly assessed are (1) when major differences exist in the kinds of possible outcome (e.g., death vs. disability), (2) when major differences exist between treatments and the likelihood and impact of complications, (3) when choices involve trade-offs between near-term and long-term outcomes, (4) when one of the choices can result in a small chance of a grave outcome, (5) when the apparent differences between options is marginal, (6) when a patient is particularly adverse to taking risks, and (7) when a patient attaches unusual importance to certain possible outcomes.

Physician and Patient Participation in Patient Preferences

A sizable literature exists on the way in which decisions are made by patients in relation to their physicians. Wide differences exist among both physicians and patients as to the degree of control that patients should expect from their physicians in critically important decision making. Thus, there is a long tradition of a paternalistic approach to decision making in which the physician "knows best" and advises the patient what should happen, with the patient merely concurring with the physician's analysis of the problem and the presentation of choices. The choices in this context are those of the physician and not of the patient. Although patients may be allowed to choose, they are choosing from a menu of choices arrived at by physicians. Some physicians see themselves as technocrats or experts and believe that the reason patients come to see them is to be advised as to how they should proceed.

Some patients value this approach and are comfortable with it, whereas other patients find it intolerable. A collaborative form of decision making involves the physician presenting the options to the patient, examining the situation with the patient to see whether other options are available, and then presenting enough information for the patient to make his or her choice.

Understanding a patient's priorities and perspectives on important decisions is not only good clinical care, but also has been shown to result in better outcomes and improvements in patient satisfaction with care.[31] In a study of 117 patients in a health maintenance organization–based general internal medicine practice, 47% of patients reported playing an active role in decision making whereas 53% played a passive role. When compared with passive patients 1 week after a clinic visit, active patients described less discomfort, significantly greater reduction in symptoms, and more improvement in their general medical condition. When interviewed 7 days after the visit, active patients reported less concern with their illness, greater sense of control of their illness, and more satisfaction with its management.

Mort[32] advocates a norm of collaborative decision making and cites studies of outcomes in breast cancer management, peptic ulcer disease, and diabetes to show that better participation leads to better outcomes. Peters[33] has shown that the move away from medical paternalism necessitates the matching of information-gathering styles and decision-making styles of patients and their physi-

cians. Patients vary in their perceived information needs; in their ability to acquire, process, and understand relevant medical information; and in their need for control over medical decisions.

Conclusion

Patient preferences are implicit to most of the practice of medicine. With the increasing degree of patients' participation in their own health care and their increasing financial responsibility, it becomes more important to understand how these preferences are generated, how they can be elicited, and how they can be brought to bear on important decisions in preventive and therapeutic medicine.

Almost all of the applications in this chapter have been developed for use in the evaluation of health systems or for research studies on how patients make important decisions. The studies by Leard et al.[12] and by Volk et al.[5] are the beginning of a move away from the research arena towards the day-to-day practice of medicine. Because the quantification of preferences by the techniques described earlier is only the end-stage of a process of decision making, it is likely that balance sheets and easily scored instruments will gradually emerge to help physicians participate with their patients in the informed decision making that more and more patients demand.

References

1. Llewellyn-Thomas H, Sutherland HJ, Tibshirani R. The measurement of patients' values in medicine. Med Decis Making 1982;2:449–462.
2. Lenert LN, Cher DL, Goldstein MK, et al. The effect of search procedures on utility elicitations. Med Decis Making 1998;18:76–83.
3. Eraker SA, Sox HC. Assessment of patient preferences for therapeutic outcomes. Med Decis Making 1981;1:29–39.
4. Tversky A, Kahneman D. The framing of decisions and the psychology of choice. Science 1981;211: 453–458.
5. Volk RJ, Cantor SB, Spann SJ. Preferences of husbands and wives for prostate cancer screening. Arch Fam Med 1997;6:72–76.
6. Kassirer JP. Incorporating patient preferences into medical decisions. N Engl J Med 1994;330:1995–1996.
7. Cantor SB, Spann SJ, Volk RJ, et al. Prostate cancer screening: a decision analysis. J Fam Pract 1995;41: 33–34.
8. Nightingale SD. Risk preference and laboratory test selection. J Gen Intern Med 1987;2:25–28.
9. McNeil BJ, Pauker SG, Sox HC, Tversky A. On the elicitation of preferences for alternative therapies. N Engl J Med 1982;306:1259–1262.
10. Siminoff LA, Fetting JH. Effects of outcome framing on treatment decisions in the real world: impact of

framing on adjuvant breast cancer decisions. Med Decis Making 1989;9:262–271.

11. Pierce PF. Defining and Measuring Personal Values in Breast Cancer Treatment Decisions. In Proceedings of the 18th Annual Meeting of the Society of Medical Decision Making 1996;23.

12. Leard LE, Savides MD, Geniats TG. Patient preferences for colorectal cancer screening. J Fam Pract 1997;45:211–218.

13. Office of Technology Assessment. Cost-Effectiveness of Colorectal Cancer Screening in Average-Risk Adults. Washington DC: Government Printing Office, 1995. Publication OTA-BP-H-146.

14. Eddy DM. Comparing benefits and harms: the balance sheet. JAMA 1990;263:2493–2505.

15. Eddy DM. Clinical decision-making: from theory to practice. Designing a practice policy: standards, guidelines, and options. JAMA 1990;263:3077.

16. McConnell JD, Barry MJ, Bruskewitz RC. Benign Prostatic Hyperplasia: Diagnosis and Treatment. Quick Reference Guide for Clinicians. Agency for Health Care Policy and Research, 1994. Rockville, MD: AHCPR publication 94-0583.

17. Christensen-Szalanski J. Discount functions and the measurement of patients' values: women's decisions during childbirth. Med Decis Making 1984;4:47–58.

18. von Neumann J, Morgenstern O. Theory of Games and Economic Behavior. New York: John Wiley, 1953.

19. Torrance GW, Thomas WH, Sackett DL. A utility maximization model of evaluation of health care programs. Health Serv Res 1972;7:118–133.

20. Torrance GW. Utility approach to measuring health-related quality of life. J Chron Dis 1987;40:593–600.

21. Stevens SS. Issues in psychophysical measurement. Psychol Rev 1971;78:426–450.

22. Froberg DG, Kane RL. Methodology for measuring health-state preferences. II: Scaling methods. J Clin Epidemiol 1989;42:459–471.

23. Patrick DL, Bush JW, Chen MM. Methods for measuring levels of well-being for a health status index. Health Serv Res 1973;8:228–245.

24. Thompson MS. Willingness to pay and accept risk to cure chronic disease. Am J Public Health 1986;76:392–396.

25. Schoemaker PJ. The expected utility model: its variants, purposes, evidence and limitations. J Econ Lit 1982;20:529–563.

26. Keeney R, Raiffa H. Decisions with Multiple Objectives: Preferences and Value Trade-Offs. New York: Wiley, 1976.

27. Kaplan RM, Anderson JP. The General Health Policy Model: An Integrated Approach. In B Spiker (ed), Quality of Life and Pharmacoeconomics in Clinical Trials (2nd ed). Philadelphia: Lippincott–Raven, 1996;309–322.

28. Brooks R, with the EuroQual Group. EuroQuol: the current state of play. Health Policy 1996;37:53–72.

29. Gold MR, Seigel JE, Russell LB, Weinstein MC. Cost Effectiveness in Health and Medicine. New York: Oxford University Press, 1996.

30. Drummond MF, O'Brien B, Stoddart GL, Torrance GW. Methods for the Economic Evaluation of Health Care Programs (2nd ed). New York: Oxford University Press, 1997.

31. Brody D, Miller S, Lerman C, et al. Patient perception of involvement in medical care. J Gen Int Med 1989;4:506–511.

32. Mort EA. Clinical decision-making in the face of scientific uncertainty: hormone replacement therapy as an example. J Fam Pract 1996;42:147–151.

33. Peters RM. Matching physician practice style to patient informational issues and decision-making preferences. An approach to patient autonomy and medical paternalism issues in clinical practice. Arch Fam Med 1994;3:760–763.

Chapter 9
Assessing Accuracy of Diagnostic and Screening Tests

Joann G. Elmore and Edward J. Boyko

Case 1

A 55-year-old man presents with substernal chest pain of 1-month duration. The pain occurred on five occasions while awake without any precipitating factor, including exercise. The pain resolved spontaneously within approximately 1 hour on each occasion. No history of heart disease, hypercholesterolemia, hypertension, or diabetes mellitus is present. The patient reports approximately 20 pack-years of smoking, none for the past 10 years. Physical examination reveals a blood pressure of 146/90, a pulse of 72 with regular rhythm, and a normal cardiac examination. Electrocardiogram reveals normal sinus rhythm without evidence of ischemia. You are concerned about the possibility that the chest pain was due to coronary artery disease and order a diagnostic exercise treadmill test. During this treadmill test, the patient reaches his target heart rate with no evidence of ischemia on electrocardiogram or symptoms during exercise. How does this test result affect your estimate of the probability of ischemic heart disease in this patient?

The evaluation of diagnostic and screening tests using an evidence-based approach involves several different considerations.[1,2] The first relates to the ability of the test to assist the clinician in deciding whether a symptomatic or asymptomatic patient has the disease of interest or is at risk for the disease. This point involves attention to test sensitivity and specificity and the clinician's estimate of the probability of disease before obtaining the test. Diagnostic tests are done when patients are symptomatic, whereas screening tests are done on asymptomatic individuals. One also must critically evaluate the evidence regarding the test's ability to accurately classify individuals as having or not having a disease or condition of interest by focusing on whether an appropriate, unbiased study design was used. Ultimately, a test must be shown to have an overall net benefit for the patient. This chapter focuses on these issues as well as others that are important in assessing the published evidence on diagnostic and screening tests.

Diagnostic Tests

Disease Probability: Pre- and Post-Test Estimates

Clinicians have access to a large diagnostic armamentarium to assist in identifying the cause of a patient's problem. Regardless of the particular diagnostic test, certain principles apply to the interpretation of results. These principles apply to diagnostic tests regardless of their cost or level of technical sophistication. For example, these principles would apply to the interpretation of clinical examination findings or the results of a "high-tech" test, such as dipyridamole-thallium imaging for coronary artery disease.

Diagnostic tests, however, cannot be interpreted as 100% perfect, with a positive test meaning disease is definitely present and a negative test meaning disease is definitely absent. Instead, diagnostic tests alter the probability of disease being present and always require that the clinician formulate an impression of the chance that disease is present before the test is ordered. This impression is

---

Case 2

A 67-year-old woman presents with a 6-month history of joint pain involving the hands and wrists. The pain is worse in the morning and subsides throughout the day. She denies skin rash or nodules. She has been in good health throughout her life, with no previous history of surgery, blood transfusions, or hepatitis. She reports that her mother had rheumatoid arthritis. Physical examination reveals a blood pressure of 138/86 and a pulse of 84 with regular rhythm; no heart murmur is present, and skin examination is negative for rash or subcutaneous nodules. Examination of the joints reveals bilateral swelling of the first and second metacarpal-phalangeal joints and the wrists bilaterally. You believe that rheumatoid arthritis is very likely the cause of the patient's symptoms. On diagnostic laboratory evaluation, the erythrocyte sedimentation rate is 90, and the rheumatoid factor and antinuclear antibody are both negative. Should you discard rheumatoid arthritis as the working diagnosis?

---

referred to as the *pretest disease probability*. The means by which a clinician develops a pretest disease probability in response to a given clinical situation is not entirely clear but appears to result mainly from training and experience. For example, clinicians learn during training that several infectious agents may cause lobar pneumonia. Through experience in caring for multiple patients who present with lobar pneumonia, clinicians develop a ranking of the most- to least-likely common infectious agents that produce this condition. A combination of information from published literature and personal experience enables the clinician to develop a clinical impression or "pretest probability" of a particular condition based on the initial history and physical examination.

In many clinical encounters, the clinician does not order any diagnostic tests after completing the initial history and physical examination. Why is this? Because the initial history and physical examination lead the clinician to believe that a certain problem is either (1) very likely to be present, (2) very unlikely to be present, or (3) in no need of further evaluation owing to prognostic considerations.

The "threshold" approach to clinical decision making is a useful construct to explain the clinician's decision whether to order a diagnostic test.[3] This heuristic postulates that clinicians take action when the disease probability crosses a certain threshold. The left half of Figure 9-1 demonstrates this construct. The black area indicates a range of pretest disease probabilities in which no particular clinical action is indicated. To proceed further, the disease probability must cross the upper or lower threshold before additional treatment, diagnostic action, or no action can occur. The left half of Figure 9-1 demonstrates a decision that requires a high upper threshold of disease probability. Such decisions are often characterized by a treatment that is associated with a high risk of morbidity and mortality. The upper probability threshold is very high to avoid the possibility of making a diagnosis in a patient who does not have the illness, thereby exposing this patient to the risks of treatment without any possibility of potential benefit. For example, the probability of acute myelocytic leukemia must be very high before treatment is initiated because of the morbidity and mortality associated with treatment of this condition.

The right half of Figure 9-1 demonstrates a clinical decision with a low upper probability threshold for action. For example, the upper threshold probability for admission to the intensive care unit to rule out myocardial infarction in a patient presenting with chest pain is 15–20%. When clinicians believe that the probability of myocardial infarction exceeds this boundary, they admit the patient to rule out myocardial infarction. The threshold for this decision is determined by multiple factors, including the benefits and risks of treatment weighed against the benefits and risks of nontreatment. The threshold for the "rule out myocardial infarction" diagnosis is rather low, because the risks of nontreatment are great, whereas the risks of ruling out persons without myocardial infarction are costly but not likely to adversely affect health or survival. If the initial evaluation yielded a very low probability of disease, the clini-

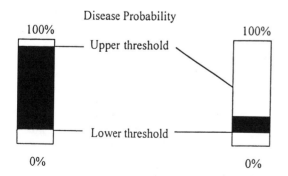

Figure 9-1. The threshold approach to medical decision making.

cian concludes that the diagnosis of myocardial infarction had been ruled out sufficiently with just the history and examination, and that further diagnostic or therapeutic steps were not indicated.

For certain conditions, no diagnostic threshold can be said to exist. Lack of effective treatment or benign course seems to characterize this clinical scenario. For example, clinicians do not attempt to diagnose the cause of mild diarrhea in an otherwise healthy patient, because in nearly all cases, the illness runs a self-limited course, and treatment has no effect on illness duration or outcome.

Between the upper and lower probability thresholds for clinical action lies a range of disease probability in which insufficient grounds exist for a particular clinical action (gray areas in Figure 9-1). If the history and physical examination place the disease probability in this range, the clinician usually orders a diagnostic test in an attempt to cross a threshold for further clinical action (e.g., treatment if the upper probability threshold is surpassed or watchful waiting or pursuit of another diagnosis if the lower probability threshold is crossed).

A diagnostic test allows a clinician to revise his or her pretest disease probability estimate. This revised estimate is referred to as the *post-test probability*. The *post-test disease probability* refers to the chance of disease being present, taking into consideration both the pretest disease probability and the result of the diagnostic test. Some basic mathematical analysis is required to obtain the post-test disease probability given the results of the diagnostic test and the estimate of pretest probability. Certain concepts related to test accuracy must be defined to proceed with this discussion.

Test Accuracy

An ideal or "gold standard" diagnostic test would have 100% sensitivity, such that all persons with the disease would have a positive test result, and it would have 100% specificity, such that all nondiseased persons would have a negative test result. No diagnostic test known to these authors exhibits these characteristics. Consider death, a diagnosis that one might assume can be made with complete accuracy. If one chooses to define the diagnostic test for death as positive if pulse, respirations, and blood pressure were absent, this definition would have a sensitivity of less than 100%, because it would not detect patients who have experienced brain death. If one defines the diagnostic test for death as positive if electroencephalographic brain activity is absent, then this definition would also have a specificity of less than 100%, because a small number of persons who later woke up would be falsely classified as having died by this criterion (Figure 9-2).

Although diagnostic test characteristics are expressed in terms of sensitivity and specificity, these are not the most useful parameters for guiding clinical decisions. The post-test disease probabilities are needed for these

	Disease Present	Disease Absent	Total
Diagnostic Test Positive	A	B	A + B
Diagnostic Test Negative	C	D	C + D
Total	A + C	B + D	N = (A + B + C + D)

Definitions

Sensitivity: A/(A + C)
Specificity: D/(D + B)
False-negative rate: C/(C + A)
False-positive rate: B/(B + D)
Positive predictive value: A/(A + B)
Negative predictive value: D/(C + D)
Pretest disease probability: (A + C)/(A + B + C + D)
Post-test disease probability, positive result: A/(A + C)
Post-test disease probability, negative result: (C/C + D)

	Disease Present	Disease Absent	Total
Test Positive	100	0	100
Test Negative	0	100	100
Total	100	100	200

Calculations

Sensitivity: 100/(100 + 0) = 100%
Specificity: 100/(100 + 0) = 100%
Positive predictive value: 100%
Post-test disease probability, negative test: 0%

Figure 9-2. Definitions and calculations for a perfect ("gold standard") diagnostic test. Definitions of sensitivity, specificity, predictive values, and post-test disease probability.

circumstances. The post-test disease probabilities may be calculated from a diagnostic test's sensitivity, specificity, and an estimate of pretest disease probability. These test characteristics are defined in Figure 9-2.

As a concrete demonstration of disease probability revision using the results of a diagnostic test, post-test disease probabilities are calculated in Figure 9-3 for the example of the 55-year-old patient with chest pain presented in Case 1. The clinical impression or pretest probability of coronary artery disease based on the patient's clinical presentation is estimated to be 0.33. This pretest probability is high enough that the clinician orders an exercise treadmill test with a sensitivity of 0.7 and specificity of 0.8. To determine post-test disease probabilities, a 2 × 2 table is constructed with 300 simulated subjects with the same clinical presentation as described in Case 1. Each member of this population selected at random has

	Disease Present	Disease Absent	Total
Test Positive	70	40	110
Test Negative	30	160	190
Total	100	200	300

Calculations
Sensitivity: 70/100 = 0.7
Specificity: 160/200 = 0.8
Pretest disease probability: 100/300 = 0.33
Post-test disease probability, positive test: 70/110 = 0.64
Post-test disease probability, negative test: 30/90 = 0.16

Interpretation: The diagnostic test provides useful information whether negative or positive. In either case, the post-test disease probability differs substantially from the pretest value and may result in a clinician crossing a decision "threshold," as described in the text.

Figure 9-3. Results for 55-year-old men (n = 300) with a history of chest pain who undergo exercise treadmill testing.

a 0.33% chance of having coronary artery disease. Among the 110 patients in this simulated sample who test positive by the exercise treadmill test, 70 have coronary artery disease, which means that the post-test disease probability of having coronary artery disease given a positive test result is 0.64. Among the 190 patients in this sample who test negative, 30 have coronary artery disease, for a post-test disease probability of 0.16 associated with a negative exercise treadmill test. So the result of the diagnostic test, whether positive or negative, substantially changes the initial or pretest disease probability. The positive test result in this case would likely lead to medical treatment for angina or possibly catheterization, whereas the negative result of the case scenario might lead to exploration of other causes of chest pain or watchful waiting (see Figure 9-3).

The same analysis could be performed using Bayes' theorem to revise pretest probability. Interested readers may refer to other texts for additional information regarding Bayes' theorem.[4]

It is important to understand that the post-test disease probability depends not only on diagnostic test sensitivity and specificity, but also the clinician's estimate of pretest disease probability. Note what happens to the example of the 55-year-old man with chest pain if the pretest disease probability is increased or decreased dramatically, given the same sensitivity and specificity as in Figure 9-3:

Pretest Disease Probability	Post-Test Probability	
	Negative Test	**Positive Test**
0.05	0.02	0.16
0.33	0.16	0.64
0.95	0.88	0.99

When the pretest disease probability is only 5%, a positive test result increases the post-test disease probability, but the chance of coronary artery disease being present remains small. When coronary artery disease pretest probability is quite high, such as 95%, a negative exercise treadmill test is still associated with a very high coronary artery disease probability (88%). In general, diagnostic tests result in greater change in pretest disease probability when the pretest estimates are nearer to 0.5 (i.e., a 50/50 chance of having the disease) than to the boundary values (i.e., 0% and 100%).

Case 2 demonstrates this characteristic of diagnostic test interpretation, as shown in Figure 9-4. This woman meets the 1987 American Rheumatism Association revised criteria for the classification of rheumatoid arthritis, so we assume for this example that her pretest probability of having rheumatoid arthritis is quite high at 0.9, or 90%.[5] The rheumatoid factor test sensitivity and specificity are assumed to be 0.66 and 0.91 in this example.[6] A positive test for rheumatoid factor tells us little, because the disease probability increases from 0.9 pretest probability to 0.99 post-test probability. A negative test result is associated with a probability of this disorder of 0.77, well above 50%! It would not be reasonable to assume that rheumatoid arthritis is unlikely given a negative test for rheumatoid factor in this clinical scenario (see Figure 9-4).

Readers with an interest in diagnostic testing may wish to explore further the issue of disease probability revision using multiple diagnostic tests performed serially or in parallel.[4] Disease probability revision also can be performed using likelihood ratios for diagnostic tests and a variant of Bayes' theorem.[4] Likelihood ratios take sensitivity and specificity into consideration. Interested readers may refer to Table 9-1 for definitions of likelihood ratios for positive and negative diagnostic test results. The values of likelihood ratios of certain magnitudes for disease diagnosis are shown in this table, along with the formulas used to estimate post-test disease probability using likelihood ratios and the clinician's estimate of pretest disease probability.

Diagnostic tests may be ordered so that the highest (or lowest) post-test probability is achieved, thereby effectively "ruling in" disease when the highest disease probability is obtained or "ruling out" disease when the opposite is true. Although others have written that tests with the highest specificity best rule *in* disease, whereas those with the highest sensitivity best rule *out* disease, the best indicator of a diagnostic test's ability to rule in or rule out disease is obtained from the likelihood ratio.[7] The higher the likelihood ratio, the better the test's ability to rule in disease, whereas the lower the likelihood ratio, the better the test's ability to rule out disease.

Evaluating the Design of Studies of Diagnostic Tests

Principles of study design have been developed for the assessment of diagnostic tests. Much less work has been performed on these principles than for study designs used to assess risk factors for disease or the possible benefits of a therapeutic intervention. The most valid studies of a diagnostic test contain the following elements: (1) consecutive recruitment of study subjects presenting with predefined clinical symptoms and signs suggesting the disease of interest, (2) performance of the candidate diagnostic test and the gold standard test in all study subjects, and (3) assessment of diagnostic test results occurring while blinded to the results of the gold standard. The first element protects from bias in estimation of test sensitivity and specificity. For example, some studies of diagnostic tests have selected diseased subjects with very advanced illness and nondiseased subjects from persons with no symptoms or signs suggestive of the disease. This methodology likely overestimates both sensitivity and specificity. The second element guards against workup bias. For example, some studies have referred only diagnostic test–positive subjects for the gold standard test, which can lead to the underestimation of test specificity.[8] The third element guards against bias in diagnostic test interpretation owing to knowledge of the better gold standard test result. For example, a radiologist interpreting a chest radiograph might be more likely to interpret it as suggestive of cancer if the radiologist knows the results of a lung biopsy that reveals cancer.

Many biases may enter into the interpretation of studies of diagnostic test sensitivity and specificity. "Spectrum" bias may result if the test is evaluated in patients with a level of disease severity that differs from those in whom it is applied clinically.[9] An imperfect gold standard test (as defined in Figure 9-2) leads to under- or overestimation of diagnostic test sensitivity and specificity.[10] Performance of the gold standard test among only patients who test positive by the candidate diagnostic test results in workup bias. Bias might also occur owing to inaccuracy of pretest prob-

	Disease Present	Disease Absent	Total
Test Positive	594	9	603
Test Negative	306	91	397
Total	900	100	1,000

Calculations
Sensitivity: 594/900 = 0.66
Specificity: 91/100 = 0.91
Pretest disease probability: 900/1,000 = 0.90
Post-test disease probability, positive test: 0.99
Post-test disease probability, negative test: 0.77

Interpretation: The post-test disease probability differs to a smaller degree from the pretest value. The presence of disease is very likely even if the diagnostic test is negative.

Figure 9-4. Symmetric distal arthritis in 67-year-old women (n = 1,000) who underwent a test for rheumatoid factor.

ability estimation or generalization of published diagnostic test sensitivity and specificity to populations in which such tests perform differently. Despite these problems, the Bayesian approach to diagnostic test interpretation remains the most widely respected and taught system.

Many diagnostic tests are ordered for reasons other than those developed in this chapter. For example, nonprobabilistic considerations, such as concern about malpractice liability or clinical inexperience, have been reported to affect the frequency with which clinicians use diagnostic tests.[11,12]

Diagnostic Tests and Medical Decision Making

The decision of when to perform a diagnostic test and which test to use is not solely based on considerations

Table 9-1. Definition and Use of Likelihood Ratios in Clinical Diagnosis

A. Definitions
    Likelihood ratio with a positive test result (LR+) = sensitivity/(1 − specificity)
    Likelihood ratio with a negative test result (LR−) = (1 − sensitivity)/specificity
B. Effect of the LR+ and LR− on pretest disease probability

LR+	LR−	Test Value
1.0	1.0	Useless (pretest disease probability = post-test disease probability)
1.0–2.0	0.5–1.0	Usually none to small
2.0–5.0	0.2–0.5	Small to moderate
5.0–10.0	0.1–0.2	Moderate to large
>10.0	0.0–0.1	Large

C. Use of the LR+ and LR− to calculate post-test disease probability
    Post-test disease odds = (LR+ or LR−) × (pretest odds)
    Probability to odds conversion (and vice versa)
    Odds = probability/(1 − probability)
    Probability = odds/(1 + odds)

Case 3

A 58-year-old man with a 100 pack-year history of smoking, 4 months of weight loss, and a new productive cough wants a screening test, such as a chest radiograph, for lung cancer. How do you counsel this patient?

---

regarding change in disease probability. Also at play are patient and clinician values, (sometimes referred to as *utilities*), economic considerations, and the potential for providing effective treatment for conditions that are identified. For example, some patients might not tolerate the uncertainty associated with noninvasive tests for coronary artery disease and insist on cardiac catheterization for more definitive diagnosis. Other patients with chest pain might refuse further evaluation or treatment of coronary artery disease, thereby removing the rationale for noninvasive testing for this diagnosis. These are extreme examples to indicate the important role that patient values play in the selection and use of diagnostic tests. Less extreme examples require complex analysis and discussion that is beyond the scope of this chapter. Although many of the issues discussed above regarding diagnostic tests apply to interpreting the evidence for or against screening tests, important differences do exist, as discussed in the next section.

Screening Tests

Definition and Requirements of Screening Tests

Screening tests should be differentiated from diagnostic tests; the key difference is that individuals being screened are *not* known to have the disease or even to be at higher risk of having the disease at the time of the screening. The aim of screening is to identify individuals at high risk for having asymptomatic disease or those with risk factors that put them at high risk for developing a disease. Screening is an initial examination only, and individuals with positive screening test results usually require additional diagnostic examinations to verify that they have the disease.

The 58-year-old man described above in Case 3 is not eligible for screening because he is symptomatic, with weight loss and productive cough. Because he has symptoms suggestive of lung cancer, a chest radiograph would be a diagnostic test, not a screening test.

Cases 4 and 5 are common examples taken from outpatient visits—in both of these cases, the patients would likely appreciate their clinician being able to describe the benefits and the risks of the screening.

In general, the benefits of screening should outweigh the risk of the test, including the subsequent evaluations if the screening test is positive. Benefits can include a longer life or a better quality of life. In addition, some individuals get a sense of confidence with screening that makes them feel they are "doing all they can do" to prevent a cancer.

Certain specific requirements should be met before a screening program is considered for a specific disease. These requirements relate to the disease itself, the treatment for the disease, and the screening tests as described below (Table 9-2):

1. The disease should be severe, with a high burden of suffering. The disease should have a high amount of the "six d's": death, disease, disability, discomfort, dissatisfaction, and destitution.[10] It is helpful if the natural history of the disease is understood and a long asymptomatic time period exists in which early detection of the disease might make a difference in the outcome. We have identified many rare medical diseases (e.g., those with fewer than 10 case reports in the entire published literature); screening all U.S. citizens for these rare diseases would obviously not be worthwhile, as the yield of cases detected from screening would be too low. In addition, you would probably have too many false-positive test results from this type of screening program. False-positive tests generate anxiety, financial costs, and morbidity.

Case 4

A 42-year-old woman with no family history of breast cancer comes to your office and asks if she should get a screening mammogram. She tells you that she has heard it is controversial. She asks you why the controversy exists and what the risks and benefits of mammography would be for her. What should you do? How do you counsel this patient?

Case 5

A 53-year-old male patient asks you, "Doctor, should I get a prostate-specific antigen test?"

---

2. Effective treatment should exist before a screening program is designed to detect a disease. Treatment should be something that patients can tolerate and, therefore, should be something with which they will comply. Treatment also should improve their outcome, either in terms of longer real survival time or less pain and suffering from the disease. We would not want to screen individuals for the presence of beta-thalassemia because this is not a severe, life-threatening disease and effective treatment is not currently available. We have new genetic markers for many diseases, but screening individuals for diseases such as Huntington's chorea can lead to difficult personal issues for patients because we have no effective treatment to offer them.

3. The screening test itself should be good in terms of accuracy, cost, safety, simplicity, and acceptability to patients. Screening tests can include clinical histories, such as the CAGE questions we ask our patients to screen for alcoholism (Have you ever felt the need to *c*ut down or tried to quit? Have others been *a*nnoyed at your use? Have you felt *g*uilty about your use or behavior when using? Have you taken a morning drink or pill [*e*ye opener] to feel better?) Screening tests also can be laboratory tests (e.g., screening serum cholesterol), a physical examination (e.g., clinical breast examination), or a procedure (e.g., flexible sigmoidoscopy to screen for colon cancer). Although we have developed many medical tests, not all are useful for general screening programs. Bone marrow biopsies or exploratory laparotomies are examples of tests that are not commonly used in screening the general population, as these procedures can be expensive, time consuming, and painful for the patients.

In deciding what screening program is best for our patients, we should take into consideration specific characteristics of our patients and their previous screening results. Screening programs may be effective in one gender or specific age group. Other programs may be best for individuals who are already known to be at high risk for the disease (e.g., those with a strong family history of the disease). For older patients and those with severe comorbid disease, we should think carefully about whether they will live long enough to benefit from the screening (i.e., they should have a life expectancy of at least 8 years to be considered for screening of some cancers, such as breast and colon).

A positive screening test may result in a much lower post-test disease probability than one would think. For example, the positive predictive value of a positive hemoccult test is only 2–11% for colon cancer,[11] yet this test has been shown to reduce colon cancer mortality.

Critically Evaluating the Published Literature

General Issues in Study Design

Randomized clinical trials are the best study design to assess the utility and accuracy of screening tests. By randomly assigning study participants into screening versus control (no screening) groups, the randomized clinical trial design helps to eliminate self-selection bias. Self-selection bias occurs when the screening programs attract younger, more educated, wealthier individuals who are in better general health than those who do not seek screening. These people would often have better outcomes regardless of the screening and would tend to overestimate the benefits of screening if a nonrandom assignment to treatment was used.

Whereas randomized clinical trials are the best-quality study design to evaluate screening tests, they are not perfect. For example, participants in clinical trials do not always do what they are supposed to do. Participants have been noted to seek out screening when in the control group; in one screening mammography trial, 35% of individuals in the control groups received screening. In

Table 9-2. Requirement for Ideal Screening Programs

General requirements
    The benefit of testing outweighs the harm.
Disease requirements
    The disease is serious with a high burden of suffering.
    The natural history of the disease is understood.
    The disease occurs frequently.
Treatment requirements
    Effective treatment exists, and early treatment is more
        effective than late treatment.
Screening test requirements
    The test is easy to administer.
    The test is inexpensive.
    The test is safe.
    The test is acceptable to participants.
    The sensitivity, specificity, and other operating characteristics of the test are acceptable.

Source: Adapted with permission from J Jekel, JG Elmore, D Katz. Epidemiology, Biostatistics, and Preventive Medicine. Philadelphia: Saunders, 1996;216–218.

NO SCREENING

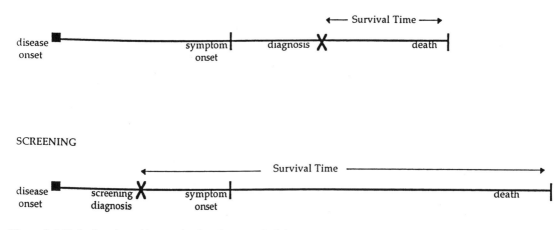

Figure 9-5. Early detection with screening lengthens survival time.

addition, participants do not always comply with the study recommendations when assigned to the screening group; in one mammography trial, only 61% of the intervention group actually received screening. The "intention to treat" analysis is often used in these studies; this approach analyzes data from the two groups (intervention and control) by initial treatment assignment, without taking into consideration whether they did or did not get the intervention.

Unfortunately, these randomized clinical trials are hard to do: They can take many thousands (and even hundreds of thousands) of study subjects and a long follow-up period (e.g., 10–15 years of follow-up to assess mortality rates). For example, to evaluate the effectiveness of screening women 40–49 years of age with mammography, you could not rely on only 10,000 women being screened over 3 years. You would need many hundreds of thousands of women, who would be screened repeatedly over at least 5–10 years of follow-up. Breast cancer is less common in younger women than in older women. Therefore, you have to screen almost 1,000 women between the ages of 40 and 49 years before you detect just one new breast cancer, as opposed to having to screen just 500 women aged 50–59 years.

Lead-Time and Length Bias

A few types of methodologic bias can affect study results and thus should be considered when thinking about screening tests. Figure 9-5 shows the usual progression of a disease from the onset of detectable disease in the asymptomatic phase to the development of symptoms and, ultimately, death from the disease. Our aim with screening is to detect disease early in the asymptomatic state, when early treatment can be given that improves the outcome for the patient.

The biases described in the following paragraphs may occur when those screened are compared with those not screened. These biases require that investigations of screening use the randomized control trial or similar methods to obtain an estimate of screening benefit that is not upwardly biased (Figure 9-6).

Lead-time bias occurs when the diagnosis made with screening is earlier than it would have been without screening, making the apparent survival seem longer. Remember, survival is calculated as the time from the date of disease diagnosis to the date of the death. With lead-time bias, the amount of time that the patient actually knows that they have the disease is longer, but you don't actually help the patient to live longer.

Length bias (or *time bias*) occurs when screening programs more frequently detect patients with longer periods of disease. Some patients with the disease have slow rates of disease progression and others have fast rates of progression (e.g., patients with slow-growing vs. fast-growing tumors). Patients with fast rates of progression are not going to be in the asymptomatic phase of disease very long, whereas the slow progressers usually are in this phase for a very long time, and these patients also usually have a better prognosis. Screening likely detects more cases of the slowly progressing disease. Screening, therefore, can appear to be working better than it actually is.

Risks of Screening

According to our Hippocratic oath, we must "first do no harm." This directive is extremely important to consider when we are planning a screening program. In these screening programs, we are looking for disease in individuals who are, in general, healthy. Many possible types of "risks" have been associated with screening programs in addition to the possible benefits. For exam-

LEAD-TIME BIAS

Unscreened

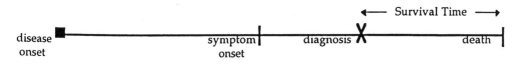

Screened (patient has a longer "survival time" period with the disease, but does <u>not</u> live longer)

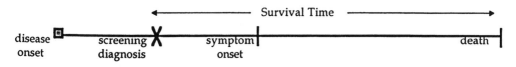

LENGTH BIAS

Slow Progression (more likely to be detected with a screening program)

Fast Progression (shorter presymptomatic period, therefore less likely to be detected with a screening program)

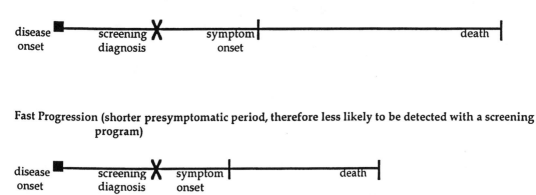

Figure 9-6. Disease progression and the possible sources of bias in studies of screening programs.

ple, the screening test should be painless (or as painless as possible), and it should not be unduly expensive. It should not lead to additional psychological harm, either through the individual worrying about the diagnostic workups after the false-positive tests or from an early diagnosis of cancer (Table 9-3).

Screening women in their forties with mammography can lead to many false alarms—test results in which the woman is told that she has an abnormality that might be breast cancer when, in fact, she does not have cancer. If we screen 40-year-old women for breast cancer every year with mammography, they have a 50% chance of having at least one false-positive test result before they reach 50 years of age (Figure 9-7).[13]

False-negative test results also should be considered. Approximately 25% of all breast cancers in women younger than 50 years cannot be detected on mammograms; these women would have "normal" readings.[14] A possibility exists that these women might be falsely reassured by the "normal" reading and not seek evaluation if they subsequently note a breast abnormality.

Screening programs are detecting many early preinvasive lesions, such as ductal carcinoma in situ of the breast. These lesions are not the same as invasive breast cancer. Some women with ductal carcinoma in situ go on to have invasive breast cancer (approximately 50%), but some do not.[14] Currently, most women who have ductal carcinoma in situ diagnosed are undergoing treat-

Table 9-3. Possible Benefits and Risks of Screening Programs

Possible benefits
Early detection could lead to early treatment with better outcomes (less morbidity and/or longer mortality).
Less need for extensive surgery and/or treatment if disease is detected in early stages.
Patient confidence that they are doing "everything they can."
Possible risks
Discomfort or pain with test procedure (e.g., blood draw).
Personal inconvenience (e.g., time off work, travel to test site).
Morbidity and mortality associated with test itself or subsequent diagnostic tests done to evaluate "positive" screens.
Anxiety.
Cost (test itself and all diagnostic workups).
Incorrect readings (false-positive and false-negative readings).
Detection of clinically insignificant lesions (e.g., in situ lesions).
Other (e.g., radiation exposure).

ment, often with lumpectomy or mastectomy, to prevent subsequent invasive cancer. The possibility that we are overdiagnosing lesions of uncertain future clinical significance should be considered.

The risks and benefits of screening should be discussed with each patient. For some individuals, the risks of screening are too high. For others, a sense that they are actively involved in trying to screen for a disease is enough benefit.

Guidelines on Screening Tests

Guidelines for a screening test are often available from different organizations with divergent recommendations. Screening mammography for women 40–49 years of age is an example: The U.S. Preventive Services Task Force states that inadequate data exist to recommend routine screening for women 40–49 years of age and, thus, they do not recommend it, whereas the American Cancer Society recommends screening every year. How does this disagreement in guidelines occur? First, not all of the data (or evidence) needed to completely assess the efficacy of screening women in their forties are available. To definitively answer this question would require hundreds of thousands of women participating in randomized clinical trials that would follow the women for many years. Second, the two groups are looking at the same published data and coming to different conclusions. These groups use different approaches to review the literature: The American Cancer Society uses a "consensus" panel of experts in the field, whereas the U.S. Preventive Services Task Force uses an evidence-based medicine approach. The U.S. Preventive Service Task Force members perform detailed literature reviews, follow debates, and collect critical comments from expert reviewers. They rate the quality of the evidence supporting each recommenda-

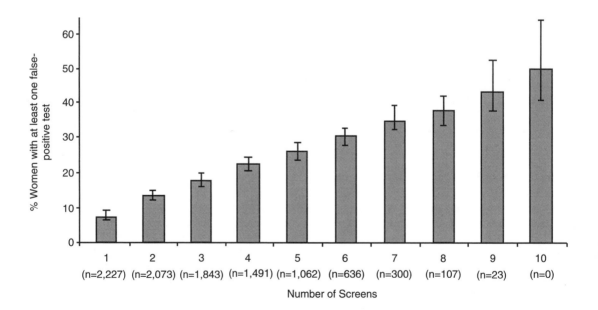

Figure 9-7. A woman's estimated risk of having at least one false-positive screening mammogram according to the total number of screening mammograms obtained. (Adapted with permission from JG Elmore, Barton MB, Moceri VM, et al. Ten-year risk of false positive screening mammograms and clinical breast examinations. N Engl J Med 1998;338:1093. Copyright © 1998, Massachusetts Medical Society. All rights reserved.)

Table 9-4. Rating of Quality of Evidence Used by the U.S. Preventive Service Task Force

Quality of Evidence Rating	Source of Evidence
I	At least one properly designed randomized controlled trial
II-1	Well-designed controlled trials without randomization
II-2	Well-designed cohort or case-control analytic studies, preferably from more than one center or research group
II-3	Multiple time series with or without the intervention
III	Opinions of respected authorities, based on clinical experience; descriptive studies and case reports; or reports of expert committees

Source: Adapted with permission from U.S. Preventive Service Task Force, Guide to Clinical Preventive Services (2nd ed). Alexandria, VA: International Medical Publishing, 1996;862.

tion. Their summary recommendations on 53 screening tests are published in their *Guide to Clinical Preventive Services*.[11] Their recommendations are often grouped by age, gender, and other risk factors. In addition, this guide cites the recommendations of other authorities (e.g., the American Cancer Society) wherever possible, so that readers may judge for themselves whether they think specific recommendations are appropriate (Table 9-4).

Summary

Clinicians must use the available evidence regarding the value of diagnostic and screening tests to assess whether these are of value in a given clinical setting. For each, two types of evidence must be weighed: (1) the design of the test evaluation and (2) the ability of the test to guide clinical decision making. The latter consideration differs somewhat for diagnostic and screening tests, in that diagnostic tests are mainly judged by their ability to alter disease probability, whereas screening tests are judged by this criterion as well as improved outcomes for persons with the condition of interest. Hopefully this chapter has demonstrated the importance of taking an evidence-based approach to make best clinical use of available and soon-to-be-developed diagnostic and screening modalities.

Acknowledgments

This work was supported by the Robert Wood Johnson Foundation Generalist Physician Faculty Award (J. G. Elmore).

References

1. Jaeschke R, Guyatt F, Sackett DL. Users' Guides to the Medical Literature. III: How to Use an Article About a Diagnostic Test. A. Are the Results of the Study Valid? JAMA 1994;271:389–391.
2. Jaeschke R, Guyatt F, Sackett DL. Users' Guides to the Medical Literature. III: How to Use an Article About a Diagnostic Test. B. What Are the Results and Will They Help Me in Caring for My Patients? JAMA 1994;271:703–707.
3. Pauker S, Kassirer J. The threshold approach to clinical decision making. N Engl J Med 1980; 302:1109–1117.
4. Sackett D, Hayes RB, Guyatt GH, et al. Clinical Epidemiology: A Basic Science for Clinical Medicine (2nd ed). Boston: Little, Brown, 1991.
5. Arnett F, Edworthy SM, Bloch DA, et al. The American Rheumatism Association 1987 revised criteria for the classification of rheumatoid arthritis. Arthritis Rheum 1988;31:315–324.
6. Visser H, Gelinck LB, Kampfraath AH, et al. Diagnostic and prognostic characteristics of the enzyme-linked immunosorbent rheumatoid factor assays in rheumatoid arthritis. Ann Rheum Dis 1996;55:157–161.
7. Boyko E. Ruling out or ruling in disease with the most sensitive or specific diagnostic test—short cut or wrong turn? Med Decis Making 1994;14:175–179.
8. Rozanski A, Diamond GA, Berman D, et al. The declining specificity of exercise radionuclide ventriculography. N Engl J Med 1983;309:518–522.
9. Ransohoff D, Feinstein A. Problems of spectrum and bias in evaluating the efficacy of diagnostic tests. N Engl J Med 1978;299:926–930.
10. Fletcher RI, Fletcher SW, Wagner EH. Clinical Epidemiology. The Essentials (3rd ed). Baltimore: Williams & Wilkins, 1996.
11. U.S. Preventive Services Task Force. Guide to Clinical Preventive Services (2nd ed). Alexandria, VA: International Medical Publishing, 1996.
12. Jekel J, Elmore JG, Katz D. Epidemiology, Biostatistics, and Preventive Medicine. Philadelphia: Saunders, 1996.
13. Elmore JG, Barton MB, Moceri VM, et al. Ten-year risk of false positive screening mammograms and clinical breast examinations. N Engl J Med 1998;338: 1089–1096.
14. Ernster VL, Barclay J, Kerlikowske K, et al. Incidence of and treatment for ductal carcinoma in situ of the breast. JAMA 1996;275:913–918.

Chapter 10
Evaluating Evidence from a Decision Analysis*

Scott D. Ramsey

Case 1

A 28-year-old man presented to your office with a 6-month history of recurrent attacks of arthritis in his left knee. During each episode the knee was tender, slightly swollen, and mildly red. He denied fevers, chills, gastrointestinal symptoms, or morning stiffness. Each attack lasted approximately 2–3 weeks, then slowly subsided. Approximately 1 month before the onset of symptoms, the patient went on a 1-week backpacking trip in the mountains. He did not recall seeing a tick on his body or his clothing during the trip, nor did he notice a rash during his outing or after he returned. Your examination today is unremarkable. You consider Lyme disease in your differential diagnosis, remembering that one of your colleagues treated a patient empirically for Lyme disease early last fall when the patient presented with a rash that resembled erythema migrans. You consider testing the patient for Lyme disease but are uncertain about the best approach to take, so a brief review of the literature is in order.

Searching the literature, you come across a decision analysis of test-treatment strategies for patients with suspected Lyme disease.[1] The article presented three common clinical scenarios in which Lyme disease is considered in the differential diagnosis: (1) myalgic symptoms, (2) rash resembling erythema migrans, and (3) recurrent oligoarticular inflammatory arthritis. For inflammatory arthritis symptoms (your patient), the article recommends no testing or empirical treatment for Lyme disease. Because this is a decision analysis and not a report from a high quality clinical trial, you question whether the findings are valid and should guide your clinical approach to the patient.

Practitioners of evidence-based medicine seek evidence from high quality studies (e.g., randomized, controlled trials) to inform the decisions they make in day-to-day practice. Direct evidence, however, is often unavailable to guide clinical decision making. Decisions must then be made with only partial or incomplete evidence. In these cases, one would still like to make the best possible estimate of the impact of the therapy on outcomes rather than an estimate based on a "best guess" or the vague concept of a "standard of care."

Decision analysis is the systematic, quantitative approach to addressing clinical decision making under uncertainty.[2] In theory, it is an extremely attractive way to address these situations. It explicitly integrates the best external evidence, clinical expertise, and individual patient choice[3] to help inform decisions. It can improve decision making when the database is incomplete. Decision analysis has been used to guide decisions for individual patients and for policy development for groups of patients, and it is often the first step in a cost-effectiveness analysis. As a result, many advocate more widespread use of decision analysis in all aspects of medicine.[4,5] In practice, however, many barriers exist to using decision analysis, both "at the bedside" and in guiding clinical policy.

*Reprinted with permission from SD Ramsey. Evaluating evidence from a decision analysis. J Am Board Fam Pract 1999;12:(in press).

This chapter is directed toward readers who have considered the merits of decision analyses but are not particularly familiar with the techniques of this discipline. First, it reviews the strengths and limitations of clinical decision analysis. Next, it identifies several areas in which decision analysis may be of most use to practicing clinicians. Finally, it identifies the elements that readers should look for to help them determine whether the decision analysis has been performed properly. Excellent reference articles and texts are available for those who want to read more about this technique.[2,6–8]

Strengths of Decision Analysis

Decision analysis can be a powerful tool to address questions that have clinical relevance but have not yet been subjected to high quality clinical trials. In cases in which controlled trials are not feasible (e.g., trials of pacemakers for life-threatening arrhythmias) or in which the risks and benefits of the intervention are uncertain (perhaps because preliminary studies have yet to be published), decision analysis may be the only way to address the problem systematically. Even when "definitive" studies have been done on one population, they do not directly address the relative benefits of the intervention for a related but somewhat dissimilar population of interest. For example, lowering cholesterol with 3-hydroxy-3-methylglutaryl coenzyme A reductase inhibitors has clearly been shown to be effective in reducing morbidity and mortality for patients with known coronary artery disease and elevated low-density lipoprotein cholesterol. Strong evidence does not exist, however, of the degree of benefit in those whose only substantial risk for coronary artery disease is an elevated low-density lipoprotein cholesterol level. In such cases, decision analysis can weigh the risks, benefits, and costs of interventions of cholesterol lowering in populations in which definitive studies have not been done. Finally, decision analysis can provide timely information about a clinical problem that otherwise would take years to address through the mechanism of a clinical trial. For example, the Coronary Heart Disease Policy Model was used to estimate the impact of risk-factor modification (e.g., cholesterol reduction) on morbidity, mortality, and costs of coronary heart disease years before definitive randomized trials were published.[9] In the example above, Goldman and colleagues used the Coronary Heart Disease Policy Model to demonstrate that cholesterol reduction for individuals without known coronary artery disease was only likely to be cost-effective for individuals with multiple risk factors.[10]

Although decision analysis cannot definitively resolve clinical controversies when data from clinical trials are unavailable, it can convey several important pieces of information regarding an intervention for a particular clinical problem. First, it can determine whether a beneficial effect is likely. Second, it can determine the likely degree of benefit. Third, it can identify "holes" in the evidence chain. *Holes* refer to points in the clinical management pathway where the evidence is weak or lacking. When a decision analysis identifies such holes in the evidence chain, it can be illuminating and a justification for funding high quality clinical trials. For example, although dual-energy x-ray absorptiometry nuclear medicine scans are sensitive and specific for detecting osteoporosis and evidence exists that treatment of women with osteoporosis reduces the incidence of hip and vertebral fractures, no direct evidence exists that screening asymptomatic women with the dual-energy radiography absorptiometry technology improves outcomes compared with usual practice.[9–15] A cost-effectiveness study that contained a decision analysis identified that the clinical policy for or against dual-energy radiography absorptiometry screening may be highly sensitive to data informing this weak link in the evidence chain, and the researchers called for further study of the issue.[16]

Limitations of Decision Analysis

Despite the real and potential advantages of decision analysis, even ardent advocates of the discipline admit that its use in clinical decision making and policy analysis is limited. There are two important reasons for this. With regards to clinical decision making, decision analyses are much more time consuming to create than those who are unfamiliar with the discipline usually are aware. Well-built decision analyses of complex problems can take months or years to complete. Even "simple" problems can take 2–3 days of work, even for those who are trained in the process. As a result, ad hoc decision analyses have not been adopted for day-to-day clinical practice and probably will not be adopted in the future. Rather, the primary role of decision analysis probably will be to inform clinical practice policy,[17] such as whether to test dyspeptic patients for *Helicobacter pylori*.[18,19]

Another limitation of decision analyses is that they usually require integrating pieces of information from different studies, none of which directly addresses the problem at hand. The information can vary widely, not only in quality, but also in applicability to the clinical problem. O'Brien has referred to this issue as the *Frankenstein's monster problem*, because the analyst patches together the model with disparate information, hoping it behaves in a predictable way.[20] In addition, when holes in the evidence chain are found, analysts often have to rely on educated guesses or expert opinion to complete one or more sections of the analysis. This guesswork, however, is exactly the type of surrogate information that evidence-based medicine seeks to avoid! As a result, decision analysis (like medicine) will always be part art and part science. Nevertheless, adhering to certain principles vastly

Table 10-1. Possible Lyme Disease Scenarios

Scenario	Presentation	Clinical Features
A	Myalgic symptoms	Fatigue Stiffness Diffuse muscular aches Tenderness
B	Rash resembling erythema migrans	Slowly expanding rash Malaise Fatigue Intermittent fever Headache Mild stiff neck Arthralgia or myalgia
C	Recurrent oligoarticular inflammatory arthritis	Recurrent attacks of marked, painful swelling One or more large joints affected Episodes last 2 wks at a time Episodes occur every 3 mos Long episodes of complete remission

Source: Reprinted with permission from G Nichol, DT Dennis, AC Steere, et al. Test-treatment strategies for patients suspected of having Lyme disease: a cost-effectiveness analysis. Ann Intern Med 1998;128:37–48.

improves the quality of a decision analysis. Readers should satisfy themselves that these issues are in order before accepting the results of these studies.

Critical Appraisal of a Decision Analysis

In providing a guide for evaluating a decision analysis, it is assumed that the reader is searching for evidence that can help guide his or her management of a particular clinical problem for a given type of patient. In Case 1, for example, the physician who sees a patient with recurrent oligoarticular inflammatory arthritis should know if obtaining Lyme disease serologies is warranted. A search of the literature revealed a paper entitled, "Test-Treatment Strategies for Patients Suspected of Having Lyme Disease: A Cost-Effectiveness Analysis." The article contains a decision analysis–type evaluation of the problem. The key questions this doctor must ask of the study are the following: (1) Does the study apply to my patient or patient group? (2) Are the methods used to address the problem appropriate? (3) Do the results help me improve the care of my patient or patient group compared with what I would have done before I read the article? These questions are addressed in the sections that follow.

Does the Study Apply to My Patient or Patient Group?

This is a fundamental question that should be addressed before reading further into the article. The two elements to this question are the patient and the clinical problem. Because the authors of a decision analysis essentially fab-

ricate the patient population and clinical situation, it is important that the patient and clinical scenario be defined clearly and precisely. The patient group that is the subject of the decision model should be well described and as specific as possible. Age range, gender, and medical history should be described whenever changing these details would alter the testing or treatment pathway. The clinical history and examination findings (if necessary) should be detailed in a way that is easily recognizable to the reader or clinician. In the article on Lyme disease, three patient scenarios were detailed in tabular format (Table 10-1). If, however, one of the patient scenarios outlined in the article on Lyme disease was "presents with rash," it would be difficult to know if it applied to the situation that the doctor faces because the history is so vague and nonspecific. Case 1 contains elements that most closely fit scenario C, but it is not an exact fit (as is typical). Ultimately, the reader must judge whether the scenario(s) described in the decision analysis are "close enough" to their clinical situation to inform the decision.

Are the Methods Used to Address the Problem Appropriate?

Clinical Decision Pathway

After describing the patient, clinical history, and examination, the details of the analysis must be described clearly and systematically. First, the decision pathway must be clearly explained and justified. The pathway usually is represented graphically in the form of a decision tree. The decision pathway often begins with two or more options that the clinician can choose. On the deci-

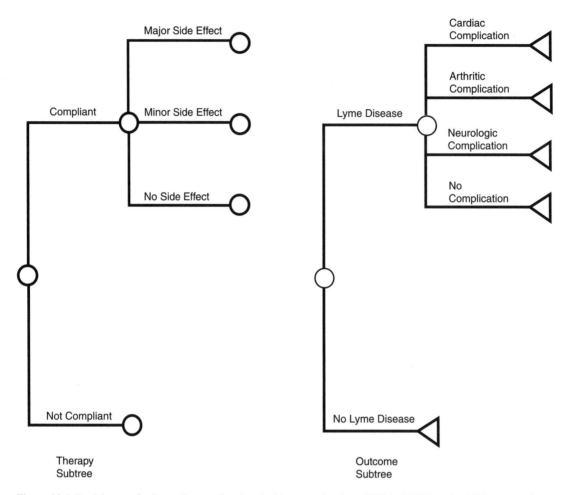

Figure 10-1. Decision tree for Lyme disease. (Reprinted with permission from G Nichol, DT Dennis, AC Steere, et al. Test-treatment strategies for patients suspected of having Lyme disease: a cost-effectiveness analysis. Ann Intern Med 1998;128:37–48.)

sion tree, these options are represented by small squares, called *decision nodes*. In the Lyme disease example, four initial options exist: (1) treat all, (2) test using enzyme-linked immunosorbent assay, (3) two-step testing, and (4) no testing or treatment (Figure 10-1). The options should be mutually exclusive, include all choices that are typical for the situation and, if applicable, include the new (atypical) option of interest.

A chain of events on the decision tree follows the decision node. The events begin with two or more outcomes, each of which occurs with a given probability. Small circles, called *chance nodes*, represent the range of outcomes. The outcomes after a chance node should include all that are possible for the patient; in other words, the probabilities for all outcomes included after the chance node should add up to one. In the Lyme disease example, choosing the enzyme-linked immunosorbent assay testing option brings the decision maker to a chance node with two outcomes: positive or negative

(note that if an "equivocal" outcome was possible for this test, then this chance node would be incomplete). The outcomes can be intermediate, in which case other decision nodes or chance nodes follow, or final, representing end points in the clinical pathway. A final outcome is usually referred to as a *terminal node*. In Case 1, terminal nodes include no Lyme disease and Lyme disease with one of four sequelae: cardiac, arthritic, neurologic, or no complications. The total group of terminal nodes should be mutually exclusive and represent all major end points related to the condition of interest. Note that the outcomes for the patient who has Lyme disease are not exclusive. This is problematic because values must be attached to each outcome (one of the next issues for evaluating the model). If the outcomes are not comprehensive and exclusive, then it is difficult for the decision maker to judge whether including the missing outcomes would change the preferred choice for the initial decision node. It is important that all major clinical decisions and impor-

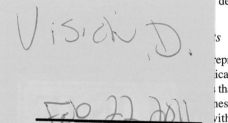

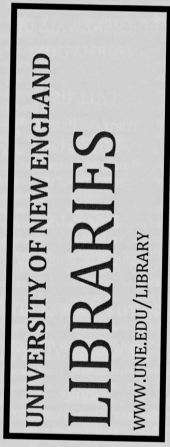

ibly valued. The valuation of costs is discussed extensively in Chapter 11. In general, the costs should reflect the value of the resources used rather than what is charged for those resources. This is particularly important for interventions that potentially will be applied to large numbers of individuals (e.g., screening tests or immunizations). Inappropriate over- or underpricing may adversely influence policy decisions regarding these technologies.

Deriving and Comparing Results for the Alternative Decisions

The summary outcome for each decision option for the initial decision node at the beginning of the decision analysis is derived by "folding back" the tree to that decision point. This is done by multiplying from right to left the outcomes and probabilities throughout the tree, summing at the branch points. The result is a number representing the expected outcome for each decision. It is important to note that this outcome represents an average for many patients rather than the likely outcome for any one patient. The authors should state that the outcomes for each decision node reflect the average outcome for a population of patients relative to the alternative decisions in the tree.

Accounting for Uncertainty

A final issue that the reader of a decision analysis must evaluate is how the analysts address uncertainty in the model. Uncertainty can be an issue for the structure of the decision tree itself or in the estimates for the probabilities and outcomes that are used to inform the tree. Decision analysts systematically explore uncertainty in the model with a technique called *sensitivity analysis*. The basic approach involves varying a particular parameter value (e.g., the cost of a test) between the best (low cost) and worst (very high cost) cases and then rerunning the calculations to determine how the variation affects the ultimate outcome of the model. Inputs can be varied individually (one-way sensitivity analysis) or simultaneously (two- through *n*-way sensitivity analysis). In practice, it is very hard for a reader to interpret the sensitivity analysis when more than two inputs are varied simultaneously. A newer technique for estimating uncertainty involves varying several parameters simultaneously, given a probability distribution for all inputs. Multiple iterations are performed using a technique such as Monte Carlo simulation until a confidence interval is created around the estimate.[24] The analyst can then state the degree of confidence in the results in probabilistic manner, such as, "a 5% probability exists that the true cost-effectiveness of the new treatment is more than $100,000 per life-year gained."

In addition to conveying uncertainty, sensitivity analysis also is important because the primary findings of decision analyses represent the average outcome based on the input parameters that the authors consider "typical" for the clinical situation. Individual patients invariably differ from these averages. Sensitivity analysis allows the reader to identify outcomes for parameters that more closely match the reader's own "typical" patient.

Ultimately, sensitivity analysis is part art as well as part science. Thus, evaluating the robustness of the sensitivity analysis involves judgement. The author follows a few rules to judge the sensitivity analysis of a decision model. These involve determining whether (1) all clinically important variables were subjected to sensitivity analysis, (2) the best and worst cases met or exceeded the author's own judgement of the range of possible outcomes for the parameter, (3) for parameters that alter the outcome of the analysis when varied, more than one form of sensitivity analysis (e.g., one-way and probabilistic) was used to evaluate the estimate, and (4) tables or figures display the range of results for parameters in cases in which varying the results alters the outcome of the analysis.

The Lyme disease model used only one-way sensitivity analysis of the parameters in the model. The clinical variables varied only as far as the range of values that were recorded in published studies. Because most of the cited studies had rather small numbers of patients, the range is probably too narrow to be fully robust. The authors note that "extreme" values for the sensitivities and specificities of the diagnostic tests influenced which strategy was the most economically attractive for certain scenarios, but they did not provide graphic or tabular data showing which scenarios change.

Do the Results Help Me Improve the Care of My Patient or Patient Group Compared with What I Would Have Done Before I Read the Article?

Clinicians read the literature to improve the care they deliver to their patients. A decision analysis should provide information that allows the reader to improve the way they diagnose and manage health problems. Thus, even if the methods are sound, the study is not useful unless the results and the implications of the results are described in a way that provides useful, practical information.

Three questions to consider when evaluating the clinical usefulness of a decision analysis include the following: (1) Was the recommended strategy for addressing the clinical problem clear and unequivocal? (2) What was the magnitude of the difference between the recommended strategy and the next best alternative? (3) Is the recommended strategy feasible in the reader's clinical practice?

Complex, multilayered clinical practice guidelines are difficult to adhere to in practice compared with simpler guidelines.[25] Similarly, the reader of a decision analysis needs a clearly stated "bottom line" to act on it in clinical practice. The recommendation should include a description of the patient, clinical problem, and preferred management strategy in relation to the alternatives. A rationale for the recommended strategy should be given

(e.g., less expensive, fewer morbid end points, greater life expectancy or QAL expectancy). All of this should take place in the space of one or two short paragraphs. The authors of the Lyme disease paper do a nice job of succinctly stating their findings. For example, they state for two of the three clinical scenarios outlined in Table 10-1:

> For a patient with myalgic symptoms or oligoarticular arthritis, two-step testing was economically attractive compared with no testing–no treatment if other features suggestive of Lyme disease were present. Other strategies were either more costly and less effective or were associated with incremental cost-effectiveness ratios of more than $50,000 per QALY.

Even if the analysis identifies a single "best" course of action, the differences in outcome and cost between the preferred strategy and the next best strategy should be large enough to make them clinically meaningful. How large must the difference be to be important? This depends on the outcome and the opinion of the reader. For life expectancy, some authors suggest that a difference of 2 months or longer is clinically meaningful.[26,27] Although no similar systematic review of differences in QAL expectancy have been performed, 2 months of relatively good health (utility weight of at least 0.8) would translate to 0.13 QALYs.[28] Other ad hoc outcomes (e.g., number of strokes prevented) are more subjective. In all cases, it is important to remember that a decision analysis gives the expected average difference between groups and rarely is able (except when using the confidence interval technique above) to give a sense of the true variability around the average. If the variability is high, clinicians see a large number of patients whose outcomes are much better or much worse than the number stated in the model. In the Lyme disease model, the differences ranged from 0.003 to 0.019 QALYs. This might not be considered a clinically meaningful difference.

If one considers cost and outcome simultaneously (i.e., the incremental cost-effectiveness of the alternative interventions), then different thresholds may apply. Some have proposed that $20,000 and $100,000 per QALY are reasonable boundaries for determining whether a technology is cost-effective (less than $20,000 per QALY [grade B]), moderately cost-effective ($20,000 to $100,000 per QALY [grade C]), or relatively cost-ineffective (more than $100,000 per QALY [grade D]).[29] In this case, the recommended strategies for Lyme disease in each clinical scenario are cost-effective.

Finally, the reader must decide whether the strategies recommended by the decision analysis are feasible to implement in his or her own clinical practice. Often, the decision problem has several implicit but unstated assumptions that are critical to the reader's own situation. For example, the author and a colleague used decision analysis to determine whether computed tomographic (CT) scanning of the cervical spine is preferred over the standard practice of plain radiographs for screening examinations of patients who present to the emergency department with head trauma.[30] Although CT scanning was found to be effective and cost-effective, it is not a feasible alternative for those who work in emergency departments without ready access to CT scanners (unless safely transferring the patient to a facility with a CT scanner is an option). Decision analyses that involve cost-effectiveness often ignore the "start-up" costs of acquiring the technology of interest. If the start-up costs are great, the cost-effectiveness for the clinician who does not have ready access to the technology may be very different from what has been presented in the decision model.

In the case of the decision analysis for Lyme disease, the author found that the recommended two-step approach for diagnosing those with oligoarticular arthritis was clearly stated and the magnitude of the difference between strategies compelling enough to warrant using this approach in his clinical practice. The laboratory in which the author practices is able to perform all the tests included in the decision analysis, so the strategy is feasible. Because the patient with oligoarthritis did not present with other features suggestive of Lyme disease (e.g., history of tick bite or rash), the strategy of no testing and no empirical treatment was adopted.

Decision analysis can be used to guide individual patient decision making and policy development about managing groups of patients, and it is often the first step in a cost-effectiveness analysis. The decision analysis on Lyme disease illustrates that the distinction between a decision analysis that is purely clinical and one that includes economic end points is often blurry. Economic arguments often influence clinical recommendations in decision analyses. Readers are cautioned that decision analyses in which the economic outcomes "drive" the recommendations may not be appropriate for patient-level decision making.

Conclusions

Decision analysis can be a useful tool for guiding clinical practice policy and clinical decision making. Decision analysis can help guide practice in situations in which direct evidence from clinical trials is unavailable or in which the studies do not pertain directly to patient or patient group of interest. When reading a published decision analysis, it is important to consider how the study applies to the clinician's patient or patient group, whether the methods used to address the problem are appropriate, and whether the results provide information that can help the reader improve the care of a particular patient or patient group. Although decision analyses are not a substitute for high quality clinical trials, their systematic approach to synthesizing the evidence can help clinicians make more informed choices regarding the care of their patients.

References

1. Nichol G, Dennis DT, Steere AC, et al. Test-treatment strategies for patients suspected of having Lyme disease: a cost-effectiveness analysis. Ann Intern Med 1998;128:37–48.
2. Petitti, Diana B. Meta-Analysis, Decision Analysis, and Cost-Effectiveness Analysis: Methods for Quantitative Synthesis in Medicine. New York: Oxford University Press, 1994.
3. Sackett DL, Richardson WS, Rosenberg W, Haynes RB. Evidence-Based Medicine: How to Practice and Teach EBM. Edinburgh: Churchill Livingstone, 1997.
4. Dowie J. Evidence based medicine. Needs to be within framework of decision making based on decision analysis. BMJ 1996;313:170.
5. Dowie J. "Evidence based," "cost-effective" and "preference-driven" medicine: decision analysis based medical decision making is the pre-requisite. J Health Serv Res Policy 1996;1:104–113.
6. Richardson WS, Detsky AS. Users' guides to the medical literature. VII: How to use a clinical decision analysis. B. What are the results and will they help me in caring for my patients? Evidence Based Medicine Working Group. JAMA 1995;273:1610–1613.
7. Richardson WS, Detsky AS. Users' guides to the medical literature. VII: How to use a clinical decision analysis. A. Are the results of the study valid? Evidence Based Medicine Working Group. JAMA 1995;273:1292–1295.
8. Weinstein MC, Fineberg HV. Clinical Decision Analysis. Philadelphia: Saunders, 1980.
9. Weinstein MC, Coxson PG, Williams LW, et al. Forecasting coronary heat disease incidence, mortality, and cost: the Coronary Heart Disease Policy Model. Am J Public Health 1987;77:1417–1426.
10. Goldman L, Weinstein MC, Goldman PA, Williams LW. Cost-effectiveness of HMG-CoA reductase inhibition for primary and secondary prevention of coronary heart disease. JAMA 1991;265:1145–1151.
11. Wimalawansa SJ. A four-year randomized controlled trial of hormone replacement and bisphosphonate, alone or in combination, in women with postmenopausal osteoporosis. Am J Med 1998;104: 219–226.
12. Lips P, Graafmans WC, Ooms ME, et al. Vitamin D supplementation and fracture incidence in elderly persons. A randomized, placebo-controlled clinical trial. Ann Intern Med 1996;124:400–406.
13. Ensrud KE, Black DM, Palermo L, et al. Treatment with alendronate prevents fractures in women at highest risk: results from the Fracture Intervention Trial. Arch Intern Med 1997;157:2617–2624.
14. Black DM, Cummings SR, Karpf JC, et al. Randomised trial of effect of alendronate on risk of fracture in women with existing vertebral fractures. Fracture Intervention Trial Research Group. Lancet 1996;348:1535–1541.
15. Hailey D, Sampietro Colom L, Marshall D, et al. The effectiveness of bone density measurement and associ-

ated treatments for prevention of fractures. An international collaborative review. Int J Technol Assess Health Care 1998;14(Spring):237–254.

16. Tosteson AN, Rosenthal DI, Melton LJ, Weinstein MC. Cost effectiveness of screening perimenopausal white women for osteoporosis: bone densitometry and hormone replacement therapy. Ann Intern Med 1990;113: 594–603.

17. Eddy DM. Designing a practice policy: standards, guidelines, and options. JAMA 1990;263:3077, 3081, 3084.

18. Sonnenberg A. Cost-benefit analysis of testing for *Helicobacter pylori* in dyspeptic subjects. Am J Gastroenterol 1996;91:1773–1777.

19. Briggs AH, Sculpher MJ, Logan RP, et al. Cost effectiveness of screening for an eradication of *Helicobacter pylori* in management of dyspeptic patients under 45 years of age [published erratum appears in BMJ 1996;312:1647]. BMJ 1996;312:1321–1325.

20. O'Brien BJ. Economic evaluation of pharmaceuticals: Frankenstein's monster or vampire of trials? Med Care 1996;34(Suppl):DS99–DS108.

21. Irwig L, Tosteson AN, Gatsonis C, et al. Guidelines for meta-analyses evaluating diagnostic tests. Ann Intern Med 1994;120:667–676.

22. Dickersin K, Berlin JA. Meta-analysis: state-of-the-science. Epidemiol Rev 1992;14:154–176.

23. DerSinonian R, Laird N. Meta-analysis in clinical trials. Control Clin Trials 1986;7:177–188.

24. Gold MR, Siegel JE, Russell LB, Weinstein MC. Cost-Effectiveness in Health and Medicine. New York: Oxford University Press, 1996.

25. Siegel D, Lopez J. Trends in antihypertensive drug use in the United States: do the JNC V recommendations affect prescribing? Fifth Joint National Commission on the Detection, Evaluation, and Treatment of High Blood Pressure. JAMA 1997;278:1745–1748.

26. Naimark DM, Naglie G, Detsky AS. The meaning of life expectancy: what is a clinically significant gain? J Gen Intern Med 1994;9:702–707.

27. Tsevat J, Weinstein MC, Williams LW, et al. Expected gains in life expectancy for various coronary heart disease risk factor modifications. Circulation 1991;83:1194–1201.

28. Torrance GW. Utility approach to measuring health-related quality of life. J Chron Dis 1987;40:593–603.

29. Laupacis A, Feeny D, Detsky AS, et al. How attractive does a new technology have to be to warrant adoption and utilization? Tentative guidelines for using clinical and economic evaluations. CMAJ 1992;146:473–481.

30. Blackmore CC, Ramsey SD, Frederick AM, Deyo RA. Cervical spine screening with computed tomography in trauma patients: a cost-effectiveness analysis. Radiology 1999 (in press).

Chapter 11

Weighing the Economic Evidence: Guidelines for Critical Assessment of Cost-Effectiveness Analyses*

Scott D. Ramsey and Sean D. Sullivan

Introduction

Evidence-based medicine is concerned with the conscientious, explicit, and judicious use of current best evidence in making decisions about the care of individual patients.[1] Increasingly, health care providers are being asked to weigh economic evidence alongside clinical evidence when making decisions about the care of their patients. Although the idea that physicians *should* consider economics in their decision making is viewed as an anathema to many,[2] this chapter takes the position that today's environment makes some consideration of economics inevitable. If one accepts the notion that economic considerations are unavoidable in clinical decision making, it seems reasonable to then take a position that only high quality economic evidence should be used, in the spirit that evidence-based medicine is used to weigh clinical evidence. This chapter is devoted to giving clinicians the tools to evaluate economic evidence and determine whether that evidence is suitable for consideration in their clinical practice.

This chapter is written for clinicians who are not well-versed in the purposes and methods of cost-effectiveness analysis (CEA). Cost-effectiveness studies have much in common with the clinical literature that most physicians are comfortable reading and critically appraising. Thus, the authors highlight important similarities and differences between sound economic and sound clinical evaluations. Some of the subtler aspects of CEA (e.g., discounting of future costs and benefits, comparative measures of benefit) are not emphasized here. The interested reader can find greatly expanded discussions of these issues, along with the major themes discussed later, in several excellent reference texts.[3–5]

Before discussing the major issues that should be addressed when evaluating an article that provides economic evidence, it is useful to outline the important similarities and differences between clinical evidence and economic evidence. We begin with the similarities. Both evidence-based medicine and CEA take a "population" viewpoint for decision making. This viewpoint involves basing decisions on evidence gathered from studies of populations rather than on evidence gathered on a case-by-case basis. For example, the clinician who is deciding whether a particular treatment is appropriate for an asthmatic patient would look to the literature reporting results from randomized controlled trials rather than assess how this treatment worked on his or her last patient (or even his or her colleague's patients). Similarly, CEA is designed to inform resource allocation decisions in health care based on evidence gathered from studies of populations, including the study types that are familiar to clinical readers (e.g., randomized controlled trials, case-control studies, cohort studies).

Although evidence-based medicine and CEA have much in common, important differences exist between the two methodologies. First, the perspective is generally different. Clinical decisions are usually made from the perspective of what is best for the patient. Economic analyses are generally conducted from the perspective of society—that is, including all costs and benefits that are attributable to the intervention, even if they do not necessarily involve the patient directly. Taking a societal perspective is important in CEA because costs and benefits from medical treatments often "spill over" to others beyond the person receiving treatment. For example, when a child is vaccinated against chickenpox, not

*Reprinted with permission from SD Ramsey and SD Sullivan. Weighing the economic evidence: guidelines for critical assessment of cost-effectiveness analyses. J Am Board Fam Pract 1999;12:(in press).

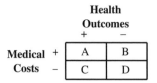

Figure 11-1. Depiction of possible outcomes of pharmacoeconomic studies. (A = higher costs, improved outcomes [trade-off]; B = high costs, worsened outcomes [reject]; C = lower costs, improved outcomes [accept]; D = lower costs, worsened outcomes [trade-off].) (Adapted from P Ellwood. Outcomes management: a technology of patient experience. N Engl J Med 1988;318:1549–1556.)

only does the child benefit from the vaccine, but also other children who would have been exposed to the child if he or she was not vaccinated and contracted the disease. Sometimes, taking the societal perspective leads to different conclusions than when one takes the perspective of the patient. In addition, although clinical effectiveness is necessary for a therapy to be cost-effective, a treatment can have clinical effectiveness and still not be cost-effective. Thus, the clinical information provided from evidence-based medicine does not necessarily help with economic decisions. This fact has not been lost on the proponents of evidence-based medicine, who note that practicing evidence-based health care is at least as likely to increase medical care costs as it is to decrease costs. Third, economic analyses are conducted under the assumption that the decision maker operates within a budget constraint. Decisions to spend more on one program mean spending less on other programs. As a result, CEAs almost always involve a comparison between alternative therapies to ascertain which therapy offers the best health value per dollar expended. Clinical evidence, more commonly, compares a new therapy with placebo care, even when placebo care (i.e., no care) is not the standard of practice in the community.

For those who wish to practice evidence-based, cost-effective medicine, it is necessary to be familiar with the methods and meanings of CEA. Thus, the purpose of this chapter is to review some essential concepts regarding cost-effectiveness studies and to provide some guidelines for reviewing and appraising CEAs of medical technologies. First, some general principles of CEA are provided, including the motivation for the analysis and the universe of possible outcomes. Second, key questions regarding the methodology and appropriateness of the analysis are presented. Like the process used to evaluate clinical studies, interested readers should be satisfied that these questions are addressed satisfactorily before accepting and possibly acting on the evidence. Finally, the chapter closes with some thoughts on why clinicians should care about economic evidence and how they might use this evidence in the course of clinical practice.

Principles of Cost-Effectiveness Analysis

CEA can be defined as a set of research methods to assess and quantify the costs and clinical consequences of medical care treatments to estimate the "economic value" of the treatment in relation to alternative treatments.[6] A CEA of competing medical treatments should incorporate evidence on the clinical consequences (i.e., efficacy and safety) and the costs and relative cost-effectiveness of treatment alternatives from a perspective designated by the analyst.[7] Guidelines for designing and reporting CEAs—including methods for incorporating evidence on costs and effects—are now available and should be read by those who are interested in conducting these types of studies.[4]

The "results" of CEAs are derived from a simple equation that integrates costs and outcomes:

$$\text{Incremental cost-effectiveness, therapy A} = \frac{\text{Cost}_A - \text{Cost}_B}{\text{Effectiveness}_A - \text{Effectiveness}_B}$$

Here, two therapies are compared: A (usually the new technology) and B (the established therapy). The incremental cost-effectiveness of A versus B is thus the attributable benefit per incremental level of expenditure for the new technology.

Given this equation, only four outcomes are possible from a CEA, as illustrated in Figure 11-1.[8] Quadrant B illustrates a treatment that is less efficacious or more harmful and costs more than the current treatment. Quadrant C depicts a dominant technology—one that improves health outcomes and achieves cost-savings. Outcomes B and C are unambiguous results, indicating that the new therapy should be rejected (B) or accepted (C) technologies adopted by clinicians and the health care system. Quadrant D represents a less expensive treatment with a reduced health outcome compared with standard therapy. Quadrant A shows the cost-outcome relationship of most new medical technology. Here, health benefits improve, but at an additional expense to the health care system. For outcomes in Quadrant D and A, clinicians, patients, and payers must decide whether the improvement or loss in health outcome is worth the additional costs or cost-saving of providing care with the new technology. Note that in a health care system with a fixed budget over time, additional expenditure on new treatments reduces the amount of resources that are available to treat other diseases. The second question, given that the results are valid, is whether the data applicable to the reader's setting are useful for his or her purpose(s).

Seven Essential Questions to Consider When Reading a Cost-Effectiveness Analysis

A well-done CEA integrates methods from clinical medicine, economics, epidemiology, and statistics. Few practicing clinicians have equally strong backgrounds in all of

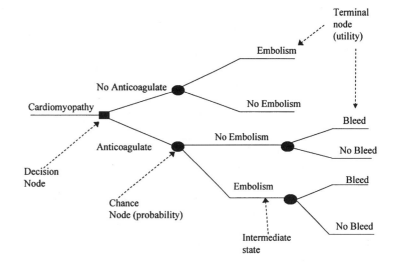

Figure 11-2. Decision pathway for choosing anticoagulation for patients with severe cardiomyopathy. (Reprinted with permission from WS Richardson, AS Detsky. Users' guide to the medical literature. VII: How to use a clinical decision analysis. A. Are the results of the study valid? JAMA 1995;273:1292–1295.)

these areas. This should not discourage potential readers from taking on these articles, however. At its core, CEA ultimately must attend to certain essential issues regarding study methods, presentation of results, and discussion of the implications of the results that will be quite familiar to anyone who reads the medical literature. The seven points listed below may be used as a guide to help the reader evaluate the economic analysis. They are taken in order below.

1. *Does the study accurately reflect a question that is an important issue in clinical practice?*
Often, a CEA is motivated by the development and introduction of a new drug, device, or procedure. An economic analysis of a new medical technology should start with an accurate description of the indications of the intervention as it is intended to be used in actual clinical practice, including a detailed description of the clinical indication, eligible patient population, path of diagnosis and therapy, and description of alternative intervention(s). The latter is particularly important because the choice of the comparison intervention has a great impact on the incremental cost-effectiveness of the intervention being evaluated (remember, from the equation above, incremental cost-effectiveness is the *difference* in cost divided by the *difference* in effectiveness for two alternatives). In most instances, the comparison intervention should represent what is accepted medical practice in the absence of the new intervention. Sometimes, this is a "do nothing" option (i.e., conservative care). In any event, the comparison should be justified among potential alternatives. For example, it would be inappropriate to test the cost-effectiveness of a new drug for congestive heart failure against "placebo," because angiotensin-converting enzyme inhibitors are considered the standard of care for this condition.

If the reader is satisfied that the clinical scenario and choice of interventions are appropriate, he or she can turn to the next issue: the description of the treatment pathway and services used when addressing the patient's problem.
2. *Does the analysis accurately describe the treatment pathway and identify all the medical and nonmedical services that one would expect to be incurred when the intervention is used in the course of addressing the patient's problem?*
The appropriate time horizon for a CEA is the duration of the clinical condition. In some cases, such as pneumonia, this duration is a matter of days or weeks. In others, such as emphysema or congestive heart failure, the duration is a lifetime. During the course of the illness, numerous diagnostic and treatment decisions are made, based on the results of tests and the patient's response to therapy. It is vitally important that all the relevant "downstream" consequences of a particular medical intervention are accounted for in the analysis. Thus, the CEA should include a detailed description of a treatment pathway, and this pathway should be an accurate representation of what happens in clinical practice. For example, if the CEA is evaluating whether to use warfarin for anticoagulation of patients with severe congestive heart failure, the pathway should reflect all the important decisions and events that can happen during the course of treatment (Figure 11-2). Along this pathway, patients consume medical and nonmedical resources. Medical resources include such items as office visits, laboratory tests, prescribed medications, and hospitalizations. Nonmedical resources can include such items as the cost incurred by the patient driving to and from the health care facility and the value of family members' time spent caring for patients whose ability to care for themselves is limited as a result of their illness. It is important that the CEA identifies all relevant resources because they must be valued and entered as costs in the

numerator of the equation. The reader should question whether any potentially important and costly resources were omitted from the analysis. For example, a study evaluating the value of CT scans versus plain films for screening patients with head trauma for cervical spine injury would be in error if it excluded the cost of the radiologist's reading of the films because the time and fee involved is different for the two types of films (the authors made such a mistake in this study).[9] In addition, *all* costs related to the therapy should be included, not just the costs of the therapy itself. In the example above, this would mean that the costs of "missing" a cervical spine fracture in the emergency department screening evaluation (patient suffers neurologic damage that requires lifelong care) is also included in the analysis.

If the reader is satisfied that all relevant diagnosis and treatment decisions and potential responses to therapy are included in the model, he or she should turn next to the important issue of evaluating the clinical end points and the strength of evidence regarding the effectiveness of the intervention at achieving those end points.

3. *Are the clinical end points meaningful? When describing the effectiveness of the intervention at reaching these end points, are credible sources cited?*
Patients and physicians are most interested in the end result of therapy, such as whether heart attacks or strokes were prevented, or if a cure was achieved using a given therapy. Likewise, in CEA, the clinical end points that are of interest are the final steps in the disease pathway: restoration of pre-illness health, chronic disability, or death. Unfortunately, many clinical studies are conducted over weeks or months and often focus on intermediate markers of illness rather than clinical outcomes that are important to patients and doctors. Readers of cost-effectiveness analyses should be alert for studies that extrapolate from intermediate end points to clinical end points because of the potential fallacies that can occur in this step. For example, a particular study of a chemotherapeutic regimen for lung cancer may list the percentage of patients with a "tumor response" as an end point. Of interest to patients and physicians, of course, are rates of long-term remission and survival among those who receive the therapy. Thus, tumor response would not be an appropriate end point for a CEA. When authors make a link between intermediate markers and clinical outcomes, the reader should be cautioned that the methods used to estimate associations should be subject to the same rigor as any other study design.

Interest is growing in including CEAs directly in randomized clinical trials.[10] Most cost-effectiveness studies, however, continue to base their estimates of the effectiveness of a particular health intervention on data from completed clinical trials. When this is done, the reader must ask whether the sources used to establish the efficacy of the intervention are credible evidence that the intervention actually works in clinical practice. The two dimensions to this credibility are the robustness of the original study design to test the efficacy of the intervention and the degree to which the original study reflects the style and level of care that occurs in actual clinical practice. The trial design methodologies that determine the robustness of a clinical efficacy study are core elements of evidence-based medicine.[11] These methodologies are not discussed here other than to say that randomized controlled trials provide the highest level of confidence that the intervention indeed is associated with the clinical outcome of interest. The degree to which the study reflects actual clinical practice is a more subtle issue for credibility, but reflects the difference between clinical *efficacy* (the success of the intervention for a narrowly defined patient population treated under the tightly controlled conditions of a clinical trial) and clinical *effectiveness* (how successful the intervention is when used on "real-world" patients in typical practice settings). Ironically, studies that have the highest validity for determining efficacy—randomized clinical trials—also present the greatest threat to validity for determining effectiveness. The reader should be sure to determine whether the study patients and clinical setting described in the CEA match the patients and setting described in the clinical trial. If they do not match (which is common), the authors must take steps to adjust for the dissimilarities between the trial and the clinical scenario that is the basis for the economic analysis.

4. *Were costs and outcomes valued credibly?*
Up to this point, this chapter has concentrated on identifying the health care resources and outcomes in the economic evaluation. Valuation of those resources and outcomes is another area for the reader's attention and critique.

Costs (the numerator of the equation) are the product of goods and services consumed and the valuation (prices) applied to those resources. When considering prices, it is important to distinguish between charges, reimbursement, and true costs.[12] *Charges* are the bills that patients and third-party payers are sent for the health care services. *Reimbursement* is the amount that is actually paid to the health care providers by patients and the insurer. *True costs* are what health care providers (i.e., hospitals, clinics, physicians) actually expend to provide the services, before markup or profit. In the managed care market, third-party payers often negotiate reimbursements that are less than what was charged by providers. In addition, when health care is covered under capitated insurance plans, reimbursement rates from payers to providers may actually fall below costs if patients suffer a higher than expected number of complications. True costs, charges, and reimbursement levels can differ substantially. Some disagreement exists among economists as to whether true costs or reimbursements are appropriate measures of value.[4] Nevertheless, all agree that using charges to value health resources are inappropriate, because charges almost always greatly overstate the value of the service relative to what it actually costs to provide the service and relative to what most parties in the market are willing to pay. The choice of which cost value to apply in a CEA depends entirely on the analytic perspective. For example, if the analyst is interested in evaluating a new inpatient diagnostic technology from the perspective of a hospital provider, then true hospital costs would be the variable chosen. On the other had, if the analyst is interested in assessing which of several technologies is most cost-effective for payment by health plans or managed care organizations, he or she would select reimbursement values as the appropriate metric.

One of the most difficult (and controversial) aspects of CEA lies in choosing the measure of effectiveness (the denominator in the equation). Effectiveness is measured a variety of ways in CEA. Nevertheless, it is most important to distinguish whether the measure of effectiveness is a natural unit (e.g., years of life or number of heart attacks avoided) or a measure that incorporates the quality of life that is associated with the clinical end points for the analysis. Some leaders in the field have stated that all CEAs should include quality of life in the measure of effectiveness.[4,13] Following this guideline, however, has proved to be impractical for many CEAs. Thus, interested readers should decide whether the clinical outcomes noted in the study can be reasonably measured in natural units or whether some type of adjustment to account for quality of life is necessary. The advantages and disadvantages of each approach are discussed later.

Most frequently, effectiveness in a CEA is measured in natural units, such as cases prevented, days free from symptoms, or years of life saved. Such ad hoc denominators have the advantage of being readily identifiable and unambiguous aspects of a disease that are clearly affected by the treatments in question. An important disadvantage is that important factors beyond the chosen measure of effectiveness that may also be affected by treatment are ignored. For example, focusing on life years gained as the measure of effectiveness ignores improvements in functional status and changes in quality of life, both of which may be affected by the therapies. In addition, it is difficult to compare multiple interventions in one disease area or across diseases when ad hoc measures are used. For example, how does one weigh two CEAs of cholesterol therapy for coronary artery disease when the measure of effectiveness for one is measured in milligrams of cholesterol reduction, and the other is measured in life years saved?

When quality of life is accounted for in CEAs, the most common measure of effectiveness is quality-adjusted life years (QALYs) gained. QALYs combine life expectancy in years adjusted for an individual's perceived quality of life, measured from 0 (death) to 1 (ideal health). The quality adjustment is derived from preference weights or health utilities. The advantages of cost-utility studies are that they (1) simultaneously capture changes in mortality and morbidity in the measure of effectiveness, (2) are applicable to all disease states and treatments, (3) consider patients' preferences for health outcomes, and (4) conform to normative theory of decision making under uncertainty.[14]

5. *Was an incremental analysis performed?*
CEA is a method for direct comparison of alternative health interventions. The comparison is most appropriately framed as the additional costs of one intervention over another intervention relative to the additional clinical benefit gained. This incremental analysis of costs and effectiveness allows readers to determine the additional health value realized for the expenditure on the intervention of interest.

The incremental analysis is performed using the equation described earlier. Total costs and effects are tallied for each intervention and the ratio of the difference in costs over the difference in effects yields the incremental cost-effectiveness of the intervention of interest. For example, Welch and Larson[15] performed a CEA of bone marrow transplantation versus chemotherapy for acute nonlymphocytic leukemia. They found that traditional chemotherapy cost an average of $136,000 per patient and yielded 2.24 years of life expectancy. Bone marrow transplantation cost an average of $193,000 per patient and yielded 3.32 years of life expectancy. Thus, the incremental cost-effectiveness of bone marrow transplantation versus chemotherapy for acute nonlymphocytic leukemia was $59,300 per life year gained.[15]

It is important to note that cost-effectiveness is a relative term—no generally agreed-on threshold value exists below which health care interventions are considered "cost-effective." Thus, it is ultimately a value judgement as to whether the additional health effect justifies the additional expenditure for a technology that is more expensive than an existing technology (the converse is whether the savings are justified for an intervention that has a worse health outcome but saves money compared with another intervention). In the case above, the authors suggest that spending an additional $59,300 per year of life gained for bone marrow transplantation does represent good health value for expenditure.

6. *Were confidence intervals or some measure of certainty provided around the estimate of cost-effectiveness?*
Clinical evaluations include statistical analyses to determine the level of certainty that the observed effect was due to the intervention itself rather than chance (e.g., the *P* value). Likewise, it is important for CEAs to include some measure of evaluation that conveys the degree of confidence that the incremental cost per incremental benefit is, in fact, accurate and precise. For example, suppose a paper describing a CEA of a new drug for myocardial infarctions reports a cost-effectiveness of $50,000 per life year gained for the new treatment. Although this result may seem reasonable, imagine that the true effectiveness of the drug was quite uncertain. As a result, depending on whether the best or worst level of effectiveness of the drug was entered into the CEA, the cost-effectiveness value that was derived varied between

$10,000 and $150,000 per life year gained. Readers of the CEA would want to know that a reasonable possibility existed that the drug may be extremely cost-effective or very cost-ineffective. Without providing some type of "confidence interval" around the original $50,000 per life year estimate, this important issue would not be apparent to the reader.

Measuring certainty is important in CEA because almost every study of this type makes assumptions about the relationship between the intervention and the outcome that are not derived directly from clinical trial data. For example, a particular CEA might link one study showing that a certain drug lowers serum cholesterol levels by a certain amount with another study showing that reducing serum cholesterol decreases the incidence of myocardial infarctions. Because assumptions are just that—hypotheses about cause and effect—it is important for the reader to understand how varying each assumption changes the outcome of the analysis.

Assessing levels of certainty in CEA is more complicated than evaluating certainty in clinical studies because the "outcome" in a CEA is a *ratio* of two different entities (costs and effects) rather than an estimate of a single outcome (e.g., a cholesterol level). Certainty is evaluated in CEA in two general ways. One method, known commonly as *sensitivity analysis*, involves varying the value of important parameters that were used in the CEA from "worst case" to "best case" values, then rerunning the analysis to determine how varying the input affects the ultimate cost-effectiveness value. For example, in a study of the cost-effectiveness of pneumococcal vaccine for older adults, Sisk and colleagues[16] varied the cost of the vaccine from $4 to $20 per injection. In the worst case ($20) the cost-effectiveness was $1,121 per QALY gained; in the best case ($4), giving the vaccine *saved* money and added QAL expectancy compared with withholding the vaccine (i.e., it was a "dominant" intervention in the language of CEA). It is possible to vary two or more values simultaneously and track the interaction of the variables as well as their impact on the ratio. If the cost-effectiveness ratio changes little despite wide variation in the input parameter, analysts say that the result is *robust* to changes in that parameter. If varying the input parameter has a great impact on the cost-effectiveness ratio, the result is said to be *sensitive* to changes in the value. Readers should scrutinize carefully those parameters to which the outcome is highly sensitive and decide, if they are based on assumptions, whether they are reasonably accurate estimates of the real world.

The second way certainty is assessed in CEA is through the use of confidence intervals. Although a discussion of the derivation of confidence intervals is beyond the scope of this chapter, it may suffice to say that they perform much like confidence intervals that are derived around estimates of effectiveness for clinical studies. As in clinical studies, narrow interval bands for the ratio of costs over effects are preferred to wider bands.

7. *Are the results discussed in context before economic evaluations and the realities of clinical practice?*
Cost-effectiveness studies are most useful for decision making at the population level rather than at the level of physician and patient. Nevertheless, the discussion and conclusion sections of a CEA have much in common with the discussion and conclusion sections of clinical studies. First, the results of the study should be compared with those of others who have investigated the same question. When making such comparisons, the discussion should address differences in study methodology between the current study and prior analyses. Second, the authors should discuss whether the results are generalizable to other settings and populations (as with clinical studies, generalizability is usually limited). Finally, the authors should discuss issues of implementation, such as the feasibility of adopting the preferred program. Because most programs, even cost-effective ones, consume additional resources compared with the status quo, it is important to discuss from where the additional funds might come (e.g., a new publicly funded program) and over what time period costs and benefits might accrue.

Finally, a word on the method of presentation of the results of a CEA. Although most analyses continue to be presented as a ratio of costs over consequences, a growing consensus states that cost-effectiveness results should also be presented in a "cost-consequence" format.[17] Here, all measures of resources used (and saved) and measures of effectiveness for the interventions are listed in tabular format, allowing the reader to review each separately. For example, the number (and cost) of all hospital days, emergency room visits, and key medications used might be listed for each treatment alongside measure of benefit, such as measures of quality of life and life expectancy. Because different readers may value the various outcomes differently, this format allows readers to draw conclusions on the study based on their own perspective and needs as decision makers.

Why Bother? Further Motivation for Reading Cost-Effectiveness Analyses

In general, cost-effectiveness studies are not designed for decision making at the physician-patient level because they take the perspective of populations rather than individuals. This does not mean that such studies are not of interest to clinicians, however. Physicians should familiarize themselves with the cost-effectiveness literature for three important reasons. First, cost-effectiveness studies may someday determine the practice boundaries around which clinicians operate and sometimes can influence national practice recommendations. For example, Medicare's decisions to cover pneumococcal and influenza vaccines were based in part on the economic analyses of these interventions. Because physicians can be directly affected by the outcomes of these studies, their effectiveness in contributing to discussions regarding appropriate use of new technologies is a function of their sophistication in understanding their methods and implications.

The second issue relates to the general concept around which cost-effectiveness is grounded: Given that health care budgets are limited, for each medical intervention it is important to know what health effect is realized for the expenditure (compared with no care or an alternative intervention). We would argue that, of all stakeholders in the health care system, physicians are in the best position to determine health value for expenditure for new and existing interventions. The other interested parties— patients, product manufacturers, and managed care organizations—usually have limited information or particular perspectives on the intervention of interest. Doctors see most clearly how patients are affected by new medical interventions and can observe the downstream implications of a particular therapy on patients' use of health resources throughout the medical care system.

Finally, physicians can take their time-honored position of serving as patient advocates when the inevitable ethical dilemmas arise when economic arguments are used to limit access to expensive technologies. Because CEA focuses broadly on the cost impact of therapies and takes a long-term perspective on outcomes, it can be valuable evidence to counter narrower views that may lead to inappropriate restriction or overuse of those therapies. For example, varicella vaccine has been shown to be effective in reducing rate of chickenpox among U.S. children.[18] The vaccine is expensive and may not be attractive to managed care organizations because chickenpox is usually self-limited and rarely requires costly medical therapy. From the perspective of society, however, the cost of varicella includes work-loss costs for the parents (indirect costs) and medical care costs. From this perspective, varicella vaccine may be *cost-saving* because both children and their parents benefit from the intervention.[19] The clinician who understands the implications of well-designed CEAs may be able to advocate for using medical interventions in ways that most benefit society than those with narrower perspectives and shorter time horizons.

Conclusion

CEA is a standardized methodology designed to help decision makers choose health care interventions that maximize the health of their populations, given the conflicts generated by constrained health budgets and rising demand for medical care. Physicians can and should be a part of the process of critically evaluating economic evidence for new medical interventions, just as they now evaluate clinical evidence. The task of becoming an effec-

tive evaluator of CEAs is not as daunting as it may first seem because these studies have more similarities than differences with the clinical literature. The knowledgeable clinician can play a role in ensuring that only high quality cost-effectiveness studies are used for decision making in their organizations. In addition, enlarging the audience of sophisticated, critical readers of CEAs will ultimately improve the quality of studies that are published in the medical literature. As economic evidence becomes more important in medical decision making, it is essential that clinicians can effectively participate in the process of translating this evidence into practice.

References

1. Sackett DL, Richardson WS, Rosenberg W, Haynes RB. Evidence-Based Medicine: How to Practice and Teach EBM. New York: Churchill Livingstone, 1997.
2. American Medical Association. Counsel on Ethical and Judicial Affairs. Ethical issues in managed care. JAMA 1995;273:330.
3. Drummond MF, O'Brien B, Stoddart GL, Torrance GW. Methods for the Economic Evaluation of Health Care Programmes (2nd ed). New York: Oxford University Press, 1997.
4. Gold MR, Siegal JE, Russell LB, Weinstein MC (eds). Cost-Effectiveness in Health and Medicine. New York: Oxford University Press, 1996.
5. Haddix AC (ed). Prevention Effectiveness: A Guide to Decision Analysis and Economic Evaluation. New York: Oxford University Press, 1996.
6. Drummond MF, Stoddart GL, Torrance GW. Methods for the Economic Evaluation of Health Care Programmes. New York: Oxford University Press, 1987.
7. Banta HD, Luce BR. Health Care Technology and Its Assessment. New York: Oxford University Press, 1993.
8. Ellwood P. Outcomes management: a technology of patient experience. N Engl J Med 1988;318:1549–1556.
9. Blackmore CC, Ramsey SD, Frederick AM, Deyo RA. Cervical spine screening with computed tomography in trauma patients: a cost-effectiveness analysis. Radiology 1999 (in press).
10. Drummond M, Davies L. Economic analysis alongside clinical trials. Revisiting the methodological issues. Int J Technol Assess Health Care 1991;7:561–573.
11. Muir Gray JA. Evidence-Based Healthcare. New York: Churchill Livingstone, 1997.
12. Evans RW. Organ Transplantation Costs, Insurance Coverage, and Reimbursement. In PI Terasaki (ed), Clinical Transplants. Los Angeles: UCLA Tissue Typing Laboratory, 1990;343–355.
13. Detsky A. Guideline for economic analysis of pharmaceutical products: a draft document for Ontario and Canada. Pharmacoeconomics 1993;3:354–361.
14. von Neumann J, Morgenstern O. Theory of Games and Economic Behaviour. Princeton, NJ: Princeton University Press, 1994.

15. Welch HG, Larson EB. Cost-effectiveness of bone marrow transplantation in acute nonlymphoblastic leukemia. N Engl J Med 1989;321:807–812.

16. Sisk JE, Moskowitz AJ, Whang W, et al. Cost-effectiveness of vaccination against pneumococcal bacteremia among elderly people. JAMA 1997;278: 1333–1339.

17. Stergachis A. Overview of cost-consequence modeling in outcomes research. Pharmacotherapy 1995;15:40S–42S.

18. White CJ. Varicella-zoster virus vaccine. Clin Infect Dis 1998;24:753–761.

19. Lieu TA, Cochi SL, Black SB, et al. Cost-effectiveness of a routine varicella vaccination program for U.S. children. JAMA 1994;271:375–381.

Chapter 12
Cost-Effectiveness of Primary Care*

Richard A. Deyo

Case 1

The resident described a new patient in clinic today, a 40-year-old woman with a cholesterol of 240 but no other coronary risk factors. She asked if it would be cost-effective to begin therapy with "statin" drugs to lower the patient's cholesterol. The attending physician, always skeptical of high technology and eager to promote preventive care, said, "Sure it is. Some of the statin drugs now cost approximately $50 per month. Compare that with $50,000 for a coronary bypass later on if she is not treated now."

This chapter follows up on the overview in Chapter 11 of cost-effectiveness analysis (CEA) with the intent to provide further clinical perspective on this subject. The goals are to provide a clear understanding of the difference between the cost of a treatment and its cost-effectiveness, to consider what is generally a socially acceptable range for cost-effectiveness, to give some examples of the cost-effectiveness of various treatments in primary care, and to provide for comparison some examples of cost-effectiveness in the world of specialty care. For readers interested in more details on this topic, excellent books and reviews are available, including the report of a U.S. Public Health Service–appointed expert panel.[1]

Cost-effective care is care that is judged to provide good health value for expenditure. *Health value* refers to the benefits of a particular medical intervention, which may include longer life, better quality of life, or both. Expenditures should include not only the costs of a test or treatment itself, but the subsequent costs it may cause, including additional medical interventions, work disability, costs of long-term care, and the like.

"Cost-effective" does not necessarily mean "cheap." The attending physician described in Case 1 made a common mistake—equating cost with cost-effectiveness and assuming that "low-tech" care is more cost-effective than "high-tech" care. Cost-effectiveness is always a ratio between cost and effectiveness and, therefore, some cheap interventions might not be cost-effective. Regardless of how inexpensive it is, if the effectiveness of an intervention is very low, the cost-effectiveness will be poor. On the other hand, expensive interventions do not necessarily have poor cost-effectiveness. If they are also very effective, then the cost-to-effectiveness ratio may be favorable. Cost-effective does not necessarily mean cost-saving; at a logical extreme, no care at all would be cost-saving but not cost-effective. Some introductory examples may illustrate these points.

We may all agree that a guaiac card for fecal occult blood is an inexpensive test. In a study published in the 1970s, the authors estimated the cost of guaiac cards to be $4 for the first test and $1 for each subsequent test. At the time, performing six stool guaiacs was the norm, comprising the regular screening test. Neuhaeuser and Lewicki[2] undertook a CEA to determine if performing all six screening tests was a reasonable strategy. Their analysis assumed that, for the first guaiac card, some

*Reprinted with permission from RA Deyo. Cost-effectiveness of primary care. J Am Board Fam Pract 2000;13:(in press).

cancer was picked up, and with this inexpensive test, the cost per case of cancer detected proved to be approximately $1,200. With the second guaiac card, less cancer is left to be detected. The effectiveness of the second guaiac card is therefore a little bit lower than the first, although the price is also lower. With the third guaiac card, some additional cases of cancer are detected, but now the yield is even lower. Most malignancies have been picked up with the first two cards, and not many more are discovered with the third guaiac. The cost of the third stool guaiac was estimated to be $49,000 per additional case of cancer detected (in 1975 dollars). By the time the sixth guaiac is obtained, although it costs $1 for that guaiac card, the cost-effectiveness is about $47 million dollars for each additional case of cancer detected. Why so dismal? Because not much additional cancer is detected after those first five guaiac cards have already been done. So the test is cheap, but the cost per case detected is enormous, even at $1 per card. This example illustrates the importance of examining the incremental value of additional expenditures.

On the other hand, consider coronary artery bypass surgery. This intervention costs approximately $30,000 per operation. For the highest-risk patients, who gain the most in terms of life expectancy, the cost per year of life saved can be quite good. Although it is a very expensive intervention, if we consider left main coronary bypass versus medical management, we have a cost-effectiveness ratio of approximately $2,300–$5,600 per year of life saved, a ratio that most people would find quite acceptable.[3]

If we examine three-vessel disease, as opposed to left main coronary disease, then the cost-effectiveness is not quite as good ($12,000 per year of life saved), but it is still in a generally acceptable range. This finding illustrates that it is important to consider exactly to whom we offer the intervention under consideration. If we look at two-vessel disease, a still milder form, the cost-effectiveness is somewhat worse again, not because the operation is more expensive, but because it does not have as big a "bang for the buck" in terms of lives saved or years of life added. The cost-effectiveness now is in the range of $28,000–$75,000 per year of life saved, and we are approaching a threshold at which many people begin to ask, "Is it worth it?"[4]

What Is Acceptable Cost-Effectiveness?

No hard-and-fast rules exist about what level of cost-effectiveness is acceptable, and any suggestions in this regard are debated. As a rough guide, however, society generally accepts treatments as appropriate if they cost less than approximately $50,000 for a quality-adjusted life year (QALY) gained (a conclusion from Laupacis and colleagues[4] roughly updated and converted by the author from Canadian to U.S. dollars). Such treatments are almost always accepted as part of our routine clinical repertoire. For interventions in the range of $50,000–$120,000 per QALY (defined later), we generally acknowledge that this is a high cost, and it is not clear in some cases whether the bang is worth the buck. We often provide services in that range, but access is sometimes limited. Interventions that cost more than $120,000 per QALY gained are often challenged and are infrequently implemented on a large scale. These figures are not rules, but rather they describe how we behave about cost-effectiveness, for better or worse.

When Is Cost-Effectiveness Analysis Important?

CEA does not need to be applied to everything that we do. In some situations, it makes no sense to bother with a formal analysis; for example, when a new test or a treatment is both cheaper and more effective (or even equally effective) than the older standard intervention, although some analysis is necessary to determine that this is the case. Also, it is usually pointless to do a CEA if the effectiveness of a treatment has not been demonstrated, because this is part of the cost-effectiveness ratio. If the treatment is of unknown effectiveness, then we cannot know its cost-effectiveness. In some circumstances, we might perform a CEA and decide that treatment effectiveness would have to be implausibly great to make the therapy cost-effective; therefore, it is not worth pursuing the intervention at all. When we are uncertain about the effectiveness of a treatment or a test, however, we should wait before attempting the CEA. Generally, the situation in which we want to do a CEA is when we have a new test or treatment that is both more expensive and more effective than the old treatments that were available. If a test or treatment is both less expensive and less effective, we may also ask whether the savings are worth what we are giving up in health benefits.

How Do We Describe the "Effectiveness" Part of the Ratio?

One of the problems in CEA is quantifying effectiveness—providing a number to be used in the cost-effectiveness ratio. One conceptually simple measure of effectiveness is years of life saved, a concept we all understand and about which we have some shared agreement. QALYs is a more complex notion. Most of us would agree that differences exist in quality of life, and we do not want to give the same credit to a lifesaving treatment that leaves somebody blind for the next 10 years as we would to a treatment that results in perfect vision for the next 10 years. Those are not equally effective treatments, so we "penalize" the treatment that reduces quality of life and give it less credit for effectiveness. How to make these quality adjustments remains very controversial. How do we quantify the value of being able to see? Techniques for approaching this quantification are described in detail elsewhere in this book.

One might think about effectiveness in terms of diagnoses made for a diagnostic test. For example, we looked at the cost per case of cancer detected for the stool guaiac test. Some analyses examine cost per hospitalization prevented or some other problem prevented. Of course, not all hospital days prevented or cancers found are the same in terms of health impact, introducing ambiguity even for these measures.

But many benefits of treatment are hard to measure and are poorly accounted for in these kinds of analyses. An example is the use of ultrasound during pregnancy. For some patients, ultrasound has an emotional benefit and a reassurance value, and it provides the thrill of "seeing" the baby. Some women are willing to pay for this benefit. But such effects typically are hard to account for in CEAs, because they have little bearing on years of life or more than momentary quality of life.

How Do We Measure the Cost Part of the Ratio?

The costs of a medical service seem deceptively easy to measure. The easiest thing to capture is the charge for direct medical care. It may be difficult, however, to actually figure out the total care costs for an illness, and we often substitute charges for costs. What we charge for a service, however, is not the same as the real resource cost—the real value of that service. Also, other costs exist that we all recognize as important and that might be affected by a treatment. An example is the cost of home care for a frail elderly person who cannot care for him- or herself. Someone bears that cost, and if it is not a family member, then society must pay for someone to provide that service. The cost of work

absenteeism or reduced productivity is another example: This is a real cost that somebody has to bear. For most purposes, cost-effectiveness analysts recommend this broad societal perspective in performing CEAs. If costs to the family or costs to the employer are substantially improved by a treatment, they may offset the direct medical cost, but it is more difficult to get a handle on the value of such nonmedical services.

Finally, economists are concerned about the *opportunity costs* of providing tests and treatments. This term refers to the fact that if we spend our money doing one thing, we cannot spend it for doing something else. If we spend an extra $500 million doing coronary bypass surgery, $500 million less is available for prenatal care, cancer screening, or other services, unless we agree to raise the overall cost (i.e., insurance premiums and taxes) of medical care. Thus, the clinical decisions we make are important for resource allocation, and may influence other day-to-day clinical decisions.

Examples from Primary Care

The precise methodology is not discussed in detail, but for purposes of comparison, the examples discussed here present only direct medical costs, not societal costs per year of life saved. Indirect costs are not considered, nor is there "quality adjustment" for years of life. Thus, these are the simplest, but perhaps least controversial, types of analyses. The studies have been adjusted to present data in 1993 dollars by previous analysts. These are at least theoretically lifesaving treatments; thus, the cost-effectiveness is expressed as cost per year of life saved. Although one may object to using these terms for the analyses, they at least offer illustrative examples for which costs and effectiveness are expressed in the same metric. The figures present graphs called *league tables* by economists, comparing the cost-effectiveness of different interventions. This makes some economists and policy makers very uncomfortable, because they may imply greater precision of these measures than is justified and the direct

---

Case 2

You are a member of the formulary committee for your health maintenance organization, which decides whether to add and financially cover new drugs as part of the health plan. Today's agenda includes a discussion of nicotine gum and nicotine patches, as well as misoprostol for preventing nonsteroidal anti-inflammatory drug–induced gastrointestinal bleeding. The chief of pulmonary medicine makes an impassioned plea for adding nicotine gum to the formulary, whereas the head of rheumatology wants to be sure misoprostol is added. The pharmacy director opposes both, saying they would be too expensive for the plan to cover. You ask what the cost-effectiveness of these treatments is, get only shrugs in response, and head off to the library after the meeting.

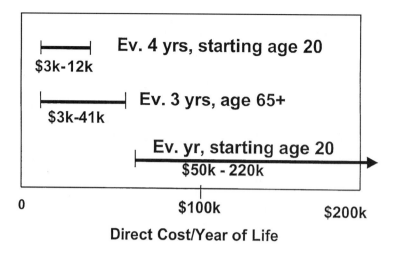

Figure 12-1. Published values for the cost-effectiveness of cervical cancer screening.

comparisons may be taken too literally. However, such comparisons seem essential if CEA is to have any practical value for resource allocation decisions.

Figure 12-1 presents published values for the cost-effectiveness of cervical cancer screening and makes several important points. First, cost-effectiveness here is expressed in ranges, reflecting various published values, rather than a single number. For many interventions, a fairly substantial range of published values exists. Second, the importance of patient targeting and precise definition of the intervention are illustrated here. Cancer screening for young women every 4 years has better cost-effectiveness than cancer screening every year, because every 4-year screening reduces the cost and retains most of the effectiveness. Cost-effectiveness is a little worse for women aged 65 years and older because the benefits are somewhat less. Cost-effectiveness of cervical cancer screening every year starting at age 20 years looks like a relatively poor value. This strategy adds costs but pro-

vides only modest added benefit in terms of additional cancer detected, resulting in a range of cost-effectiveness estimates for which many people would raise eyebrows and ask if we can really afford this on a large scale.

Figure 12-2 shows data for breast cancer screening. Again, a range of published values is presented, depending in part on which populations are considered. Mammography every 3 years for women aged 50–65 enjoys well-demonstrated efficacy, and cost-effectiveness is fairly good. For annual mammography and examinations starting at a younger age, cost-effectiveness estimates vary from $17,000–$100,000 per year of life saved. If one considers annual mammography and breast examination only for women aged 40–49, effectiveness is lower because fewer cases of cancer are present to detect and cost-effectiveness starts at a more daunting range.

Preventive care for cervical and breast cancer relies on early detection, a form of secondary prevention. What

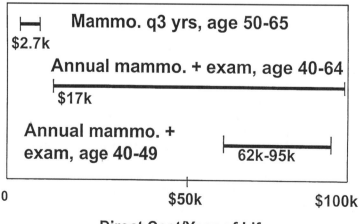

Figure 12-2. Published values for the cost-effectiveness of breast cancer screening. (mammo. = mammogram.)

Figure 12-3. Published values for the cost-effectiveness of some preventive treatments. (GI = gastrointestinal.)

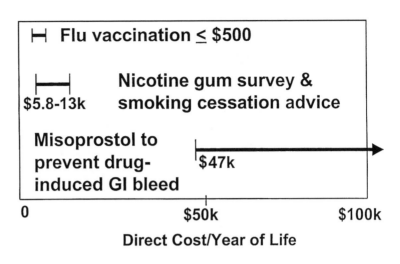

Direct Cost/Year of Life

about primary prevention strategies? Preventing influenza, for example, is very cost-effective. Some CEAs suggest that it may actually be cost-saving for certain patient groups, costing less to perform influenza vaccinations than not to perform them when taking into account all the costs of influenza and its complications. The estimate in Figure 12-3 is less than $500 per year of life saved, also very favorable.

Returning to Case 2, our member of the formulary committee discovers that nicotine gum and smoking cessation advice are also quite cost-effective (see Figure 12-3). These interventions are in the favorable range of $6,000–$12,000 per year of life saved. Comparing that with misoprostol to prevent drug-induced gastrointestinal bleeding, we find that the latter is very expensive per year of life saved, partly because a life is rarely saved with this type of treatment. We might prevent a gastrointestinal bleed, but that does not necessarily mean a life saved or a year of life saved, because most

bleeding episodes are not life-threatening. Estimates range as high as $200,000 per year of life saved. Our formulary committee member returns to the next meeting with a well-articulated argument in favor of adding nicotine gum, but not misoprostol.

Figure 12-4 illustrates the cost-effectiveness of some cardiovascular disease interventions. The cost per year of life saved for treating 40-year-old patients with a diastolic blood pressure higher than 105 is very good. For milder hypertension, cost-effectiveness is still acceptable but not as good as treating the more severe cases. This is not because the costs are higher but because the impact is less. For beta blockers after a heart attack, cost-effectiveness is very good because lives are saved in fairly short order.

The use of statin drugs for cholesterol lowering has produced a fairly wide range of published values, but again a dose-response is apparent in terms of coronary disease probability. If young men who already have

Figure 12-4. Published values for the cost-effectiveness of treating hypertension and providing beta blockers post–myocardial infarction. (BP = blood pressure.)

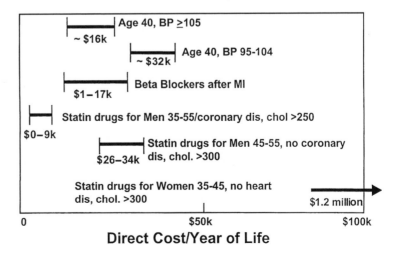

Direct Cost/Year of Life

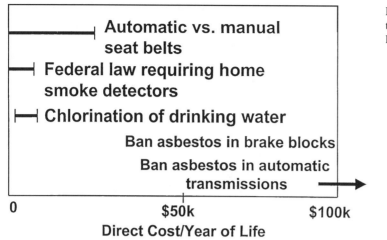

Figure 12-5. Published values for the cost-effectiveness of some public health and safety interventions.

coronary disease and high cholesterol levels are targeted, cost-effectiveness is very good. For middle-aged men with no coronary disease, even with high cholesterol, cost-effectiveness is not quite so good. For a lower-risk group, young women with no heart disease, even with high cholesterol, the cost-effectiveness value is approximately $1 million per year of life saved. This unattractive situation is the one presented in Case 1.

Examples of Public Health Interventions

For contrast, we may consider some public health interventions that have little to do with the field of medicine. As suggested in Figure 12-5, mandating automatic versus manual seat belts in cars has favorable cost-effectiveness, somewhere between $0 and $25,000 per year of life saved. Federal laws requiring smoke detectors in the home and chlorination of drinking water also appear highly cost-effective. Banning asbestos in automobile brake blocks costs up to $30,000–$40,000 per year of life—perhaps worth doing, but more expensive. The cost-effectiveness of banning asbestos in automatic transmissions is approximately millions of dollars per year of life saved, which might be a public health intervention that is not worth the cost.

Examples from Specialty Care

At the opposite extreme from public health, we might consider highly specialized forms of medical care. The beginning of this chapter presented the example of surgery for coronary artery disease, and Figure 12-6 shows some examples from nephrology for home dialysis, hospital dialysis, and kidney transplantation. Although kidney transplantation may be relatively expensive, it is also fairly effective. Thus, its cost-effectiveness is within a reasonable range. Home dialysis is

more expensive per year of life saved, and hospital dialysis is more expensive still. This figure illustrates the importance of defining treatments precisely, because the cost-effectiveness of all dialysis is not the same.

Common Flaws in Published Studies

The published literature on CEA has many flaws, emphasizing the need for a critical eye. For example, Table 12-1 lists some problems identified in 46 published CEAs.[5] Most studies did not explicitly identify whose perspective they were taking. Only 13% explicitly indicated whether the perspective was that of the payer, the patient, society, or some other stakeholder. The costs of treatment of side effects were often missing from published analyses. Induced costs (e.g., necessary additional tests or monitoring) and averted costs (e.g., costs of complications) were often omitted from these analyses. Sensitivity analysis was performed in only a minority of the studies reviewed. Thus, many of the published studies are seriously flawed, and a critical appraisal is very important. A detailed list of criteria for performing and reporting CEAs was published in a prominent medical journal in 1996.[6]

An important problem that is often ignored in CEAs is the opportunity costs of providing certain treatments, even if they appear to be relatively cost-effective. This raises the problem of making good resource allocation decisions, and CEA is only one component of such decision making. As an example, one CEA demonstrated that the additional costs of tissue plasminogen activator as opposed to streptokinase for thrombolysis in the event of acute myocardial infarction were relatively cost-effective.[7] The incremental cost-effectiveness over streptokinase was $33,000 per life year saved. This treatment would increase the survival rate of acute myocardial infarction by approximately 1.1%. If this strategy were

Figure 12-6. Published values for the cost-effectiveness of specialty care: treatment for end-stage renal disease.

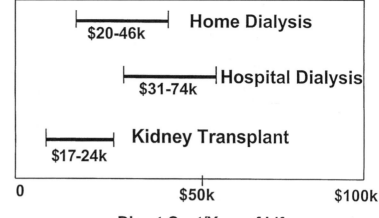

implemented nationally, however, the additional cost of health care overall would be $500 million. Where would this money come from? Would it come from other medical treatments that would be made unavailable? Would a reluctant public be willing to increase their taxes or their insurance premiums to reduce the risk of death by 1.1% after a myocardial infarction? This problem illustrates that CEA is not the only relevant factor in making resource allocation decisions and that value-laden judgements cannot be avoided or precluded by performing CEAs.[8,9]

Conclusions about Cost-Effectiveness Analysis in Primary Care

Cost-effectiveness may be one aspect of clinical decision making if physicians accept that they have responsibility to patients other than the individual facing them in the examining room. However, many would argue that its role in individual patient care is modest and that simple treatment effectiveness should be the first priority.[10] Identifying effective treatment is the first step in practicing evidence-based medicine, and cost-effectiveness simply

adds a refinement to this consideration. However, clinicians are likely to find CEAs very useful in their common roles in helping to set clinical policies. Many physicians are involved in developing drug formularies, clinical guidelines, or decisions about allocating resources within an organization. All of these roles for the physician may benefit from including CEA as one component of the decision making. Furthermore, for physician executives, cost-effectiveness often may be an important component of decision making.

In summary, cost and cost-effectiveness are very different. We should insist on good evidence of effectiveness before accepting speculative estimates of cost-effectiveness. It is important to remember that low-tech interventions are not necessarily cost-effective, nor are high-tech interventions necessarily characterized by poor cost-effectiveness. Finally, it is important to remember that patient targeting is critical and that applying interventions where they offer the most benefit is a key to maximizing the cost-effectiveness of our care.

Acknowledgments

Thanks to Pamela J. Hillman for preparation of the manuscript and to Scott D. Ramsey, Sean D. Sullivan, and Hanan S. Bell for many useful conversations. Supported in part by grant No. HS-08194 from the Agency for Health Care Policy and Research.

Table 12-1. Common Problems in Cost-Effectiveness Analyses*

Perspective explicitly stated:	13%
Costs of side effects included:	35%
Induced costs included:	4%
Averted costs included:	24%
Sensitivity analysis done:	35%

*Information taken from 46 articles published in 1985–1987. Source: Reprinted with permission from IS Udvarhelyi, GA Colditz, A Rai, AM Epstein. Cost-effectiveness and cost-benefit analyses in the medical literature: are the methods being used correctly? Ann Intern Med 1992;116:238.

References

1. Gold ME, Siegel JE, Russell LB, Weinstein MC (eds). Cost-Effectiveness in Health and Medicine. New York: Oxford University Press, 1996.
2. Neuhauser D, Lewicki AM. What do we gain from the sixth stool guaiac? N Engl J Med 1975;293:226–228.
3. Tengs TO, Adams ME, Pliskin JS. Five hundred life-saving interventions and their cost-effectiveness. Risk Anal 1995;15:369–390.

4. Laupacis A, Feeny D, Detsky AS, Tugwell PX. How attractive does a new technology have to be to warrant adoption and utilization? Tentative guidelines for using clinical and economic evaluations. CMAJ 1992;146:473–481.

5. Udvarhelyi IS, Colditz GA, Rai A, Epstein AM. Cost-effectiveness and cost-benefit analyses in the medical literature: are the methods being used correctly? Ann Intern Med 1992;116:238–244.

6. Siegel JE, Weinstein MC, Russell LB, Gold MR. For the Panel on Cost-Effectiveness in Health and Medicine. Recommendations for reporting cost-effectiveness analyses. JAMA 1996;276:1339–1342.

7. Mark DB, Hlatky MA, Califf RM. Cost effectiveness of thrombolytic therapy with tissue plasminogen activator as compared with streptokinase for acute myocardial infarction. N Engl J Med 1995;332:1418–1424.

8. Singer PA. Resource allocation: beyond evidence-based medicine and cost-effectiveness analysis. ACP Journal Club 1997;Nov/Dec:A16–A18.

9. Gafni A. Economic evaluation of health care interventions: an economist's perspective. ACP Journal Club 1996;Mar/Apr:A12–A14.

10. Detsky AS, Naglie IG. A clinician's guide to cost-effectiveness analysis. Ann Intern Med 1990;113:147–154.

Chapter 13
Clinical Guidelines: A Strategy for Translating Evidence into Practice

Linda E. Pinsky and Richard A. Deyo

Guidelines are constructed to improve clinical practice and, primarily, patient outcomes. Physicians, when surveyed, support the idea of practice guidelines in theory but are hesitant about using them in their actual practices.[1] Many reasons exist for this incongruence. Some physicians are suspicious of a financial motivation, believing health care institutions guidelines are implemented primarily to decrease expenses.[2] Alternatively, guidelines may be seen by some as a threat to their autonomy or their self-image. As one physician expressed, "We [physicians] like to understand pathophysiology. We like to understand the logic of our patient's disease; we like to bring that logic to how we treat them."[3] Although a scientific shift is occurring in medicine's underlying paradigms from one based on pathophysiological inferences to one based on clinical evidence, the cultural transformation is much slower. We have not reached the stage at which most doctors view themselves as being sophisticated, scientific physicians who can understand the epidemiology of a disease, can apply clinical guidelines to individual patients, and can discuss the risk-benefit probability with these patients.

Physicians have always used informal practice guidelines, whether they be self-formulated, local or national expert opinions, textbooks, standards of care, or medical traditions ("Because we have always done it that way"). The move, first to more formalized guidelines and subsequently to explicit evidence-based guidelines, is the result of many factors. In a simplified sense, these guidelines result from a rapid increase in the amount of information available (harder to process), the availability of more effective treatments (more at stake), and the increasing numbers of intriguing technologies of often unproved efficacy (potentially unnecessary costs). The frequent disparity between results of studies assessing surrogate or intermediate markers (e.g., lowering cholesterol) and subsequent studies of morbidity and mortality outcome (e.g., lowering cardiovascular events or deaths) reinforces the concern that personal observation, pathophysiological reasoning, and expert opinion—although necessary—are not sufficient to provide the best care for patients. Wide variations in practice habits among physicians and physician specialties[4] and by geographic areas[5] highlight the need for determining what works best and most efficiently.

Physicians are faced with a staggering quantity of information to apply to increasingly busy clinical practices. For example, between 1990 and 1995, more than 14,000 articles in the field of hypertension were published on calcium-channel blockers alone. Physicians often are forced to interpret contradictory data and incorporate emerging studies without having time to review the existing literature that it joins. Thus, physicians can benefit from guidelines developed with the same process used by the individual physician, if that process is transparent and described sufficiently so as to permit critical evaluation.

Physicians contemplating using a guideline must ask themselves the following questions: Will this guideline help me give better care to my patients? Will following it result in my patients living longer and/or being healthier while they are alive? Is it clear for which patients the guideline is helpful and for which patients it is not? Will it help me choose the most effective and cost-efficient approach and avoid harmful or unnecessarily expensive treatments? Does it represent the best evidence available on the subject and will it be updated when better evidence is available? Guidelines represent a "wide spectrum of intellectual properties."[6] To assess their validity, applicability, and usability, it is helpful to go through the process of analysis discussed in the next section.

Deconstructing Guidelines

The overall themes for critiquing a guideline relate to its stated purpose, the perspectives and agendas of the people

Table 13-1. Comparison of Medical Paradigms

Principles of Clinical Observation Medicine	Principles of Evidence-Based Medicine
Practice derived from personal observation	Practice explicitly derived from the best external clinical evidence available
Reasoning based on pathophysiology	Reasoning based on clinical studies
Guidelines based on expert opinion	Guidelines based on evaluation of medical literature

who construct it, the principles under which it was developed and the degree of adherence to those principles, the transparency of the process as reflected in the final product, and the applicability of the guidelines to the patient population for whom you are caring.

Why Was This Guideline Developed?

One of the first questions to consider in analyzing guidelines is, "Why does this guideline exist?" Is the subject of the guideline a clinically relevant problem? Was the guideline developed to improve patient care, decrease variation in care, save money, or all of these? Whose perspective does it reflect: that of the patient; the physician or other health care provider, the health care institution (clinic, hospital, health maintenance organization), or an outside entity with a financial stake in that institution, such as an insurance company? Although there is no one "right" perspective to have, it is helpful to know what the underlying viewpoint is when considering the guideline.

What Is the Composition of the Panel Who Developed the Guideline?

The composition of the panel should be explicitly stated. Panels may comprise participants with different experiences—patients, primary care providers, specialists, nonphysician providers (e.g., nurses, physical therapists, vocational counselors, alternative therapists), research experts, and health care policy makers. Such multifaceted panels may be more likely to produce balanced guidelines than a panel comprising only physicians of a single specialty. Panel members with varied backgrounds have outlooks that vary with their experience and underlying philosophy of health care. Patients, in considering quality care, often place greater emphasis on doctor-patient communication and patient preference issues than do others at the table. Primary care providers may bring a population-based perspective along with knowledge of the realities and challenges of day-to-day care, including time limitations and competing demands of other health problems. Specialists may have a greater depth of experience and knowledge of a particular problem, but the limited population they see, often weighted towards unusual or severe cases, influences their perspective.

Potential financial or proprietary interests in a particular guideline outcome must be considered. For example, consider the possible bias of a radiologist versus a gastroenterologist on the recommendation of using barium enema versus endoscopy for colon cancer screening. Content experts and researchers may have an advocacy bias towards approaches with which they are familiar and confident.

The underlying philosophy of the members also influences the panel's conclusions. For example, a group whose approach to cancer screening is, "Find all cancer that is out there" might recommend a screening test with high sensitivity and low specificity whether or not a treatment was available with proven benefit, whereas a group who advocates for screening only if a proven net benefit exists might recommend against such testing.

What Decision Making Process Was Used in Developing the Guidelines?

As the evidence-based framework has informed more of medical decision making, a shift away from expert opinion guidelines and towards evidence-based guidelines has occurred, as suggested in Table 13-1. Inherent in this shift is a change in the process by which guidelines are formed. Previously, decisions often were made by a "global subjective" process, based on an informal or formal consensus of expert opinion.[7] The evidence and processes by which the individual experts reached their opinion would not be apparent to the readers of the guideline. With evidence-based guidelines, in contrast, the attempt is to make the process explicit, or as some call it, *transparent*. The criteria for reaching recommendations assume that decisions should be based on the best possible evidence. This involves a multistep process of identifying, evaluating, and applying the literature as described here:

1. *Stating the clinical question.* In reporting its recommendations, the guideline framers should begin with a concise description of the clinical question the guideline addresses, including the population it covers and the type of intervention (screening, diagnostic procedure, therapy) it involves. Because high quality studies that address the overarching question rarely, if ever, exist, an "analytic framework" often is constructed, delineating the chain of

questions that combine to address the overall question.[8] The evidence for each step along the framework is then sought.

2. *Gathering the evidence.* Varying degrees of thoroughness are used in identifying the appropriate medical literature for a guideline. The most thorough approach entails fanning out from an initial computer-based search for articles, searching citations noted in these articles, and querying experts about key articles. Searching, sometimes by hand, of non-English publications expands the scope. Contacting researchers in the area provides access to articles that might not have been published, sometimes because they had negative results or were redundant (publication bias). Such contacts also can provide updates of the existing studies, if available.

3. *Evaluating the evidence.* Authors of evidence-based guidelines acknowledge that a hierarchy exists in the quality of evidence, and they create evidence tables with explicit grading of the quality of each study. The level depends on the inherent strength of different types of studies (e.g., randomized clinical trial versus cohort study versus case control). Rigor is also typically evaluated with regards to the following:

The application of single or double blinding
The use and results of an intention-to-treat analysis
The length of follow-up and the dropout rate
Comparability of treatment and control groups (if applicable) with respect to baseline measures
The type and scope of outcomes considered, including 95% confidence intervals surrounding the results
The generalizability of the results

Chapter 5 has an expanded discussion of such critical appraisal criteria.

4. *Linking the evidence to the recommendations.* An explicit statement of the line of reasoning used in developing recommendations should be present that links data interpretation to the recommendations that are made.

5. *Grading the recommendations.* It is important to explicitly label the strength of the recommendation. A grading system is a shortcut means of making explicit both the strength of the evidence used and that of the extrapolation from the evidence to the recommendation. Different groups have used slightly different systems, but they basically resemble that of the U.S. Preventive Services Task Force (Table 13-2):

A: Good evidence to support recommendation for use of intervention
B: Fair evidence to support recommendation for use of intervention
C: Insufficient evidence to support recommendation for use of intervention
D: Fair evidence to support recommendation against use of intervention

Table 13-2. Quality of Evidence

I.	Properly randomized controlled trial
II.1.	Well-designed controlled trial without randomization
II.2.	Well-designed cohort or case-control analytic study
II.3.	Time series with or without the intervention or dramatic results in an uncontrolled experiment
III.	Opinion of respected authority, descriptive study or case report, or report of expert committee

Source: Adapted from U.S. Preventive Services Task Force. Guide to Clinical Preventive Services (2nd ed). Baltimore: Williams & Wilkins, 1996.

E: Good evidence to support recommendation against use of intervention

6. *Explicit labeling of the use of lower quality evidence, including expert opinion.* In some cases, clear, high quality evidence exists of benefit or harm that argues for or against an intervention. In other cases, extrapolation is necessary from less than optimal evidence. In the latter cases, an explicit discussion of the gaps in the evidence and how new evidence might alter the recommendations should be present. Some extrapolations are made on stronger grounds than others. Consider, for example, the extrapolation needed to recommend colon cancer screening at an early age for patients at high genetic risk compared with that needed to recommend early ovarian cancer screening for patients with a similarly high genetic risk. For colon cancer screening, the screening test (colonoscopy) is known to be effective in the general population, and a treatment intervention (polypectomy or colectomy) that has known efficacy in high-risk patients exists. In ovarian cancer screening, the tests (CA-125 or ultrasounds) are of uncertain effectiveness in the general population, no evidence exists that their performance is better in a high-risk population, and treatment (prophylactic oophorectomy) efficacy is uncertain.

Guidelines extrapolated from related data, or lower quality data (including expert opinion) should indicate the reason for making recommendations in the absence of high quality data. For example, Table 13-3 lists "other grounds" on which decisions are made that were extracted from the 1996 U.S. Preventive Services Task Force report. The guidelines should explicitly label expert opinion and the strength of extrapolations used in forming the opinion and should provide a discussion of alternative conclusions that could be reached from the data.

7. *Incorporating patient preferences.* Means should be provided for clinicians to incorporate patient preferences into the application of the guidelines. To facilitate this, guidelines should discuss the benefits and harms considered in arriving at a recommendation and indicate the relative weight placed on specific benefits and harms in

Table 13-3. Factors Used to Argue For or
Against Intervention

Availability of an alternative high-quality intervention
Burden of suffering on an individual or population level
Comorbidity
Compliance
Costs
Decision analysis results
Degree of practicality or convenience
Easy treatment when symptoms appear
Expert opinion
Legal requirements
Likelihood of recurrence
Patient preferences
Potential benefit to others (e.g., communicable disease)
Potential harm or improvement
Test limitations (e.g., inaccuracy, imprecision)

Source: Adapted from A Berg. Review of other grounds for
recommendations from U.S. Preventive Services Task Force.
Guide to clinical preventive services, 1996. Personal communication, 1998.

Table 13-4. Assessing the Quality of Guidelines

Explicit disclosure of panel's members, their expertise and
  perspective (e.g., primary care, population-based, high-
  risk case finding, group with potential advocacy bias or
  self-interest)
Financial sponsors of the guidelines clearly stated
Construction of analytic framework
Description of how evidence was found and filtered and
  how the references were used
Critical review of literature informing the pathway and
  explicit grading of the quality of evidence
Explicit labeling of gaps in evidence
Explicit discussion of other reasonable conclusions that
  could be reached from this data
Explicit discussion of the evidence, when available, that
  would override opinion
Explicit labeling of expert opinion, reasons for its inclusion, line of reasoning, and strength of extrapolation
  from other data used in formation of the expert opinion
Explicit discussion of benefits and harms considered in
  arriving at the opinion and relative weight placed on specific benefits and harms in different scenarios to provide
  means of incorporating patient preference
Discussion of cost-effectiveness
Proposed plan and explicit date for upgrading the
  guidelines

different scenarios. The patient's own values and system of weighting these factors can then help direct the appropriate decision in individual cases. Chapter 8 has an expanded discussion of methods for assessing patient preferences.

8. *Discussing cost-effectiveness.* Cost is an important but secondary consideration in making clinical decisions. A discussion of the cost-effectiveness of interventions, supported by the literature, can help make policy deci-sions. Knowledge of a less expensive treatment that is clinically equivalent to a more expensive choice can direct the choice of treatment.

9. *Planning for updates.* Evidence in the field of med-icine is constantly changing. If guidelines are to be based on the best possible evidence available, it is necessary to have a mechanism and time schedule for updating the guidelines so that they incorporate the evidence that has been gathered in the interim.

Assessing the Quality of the Guideline

The quality of the guideline can be assessed by the adher-ence to the principles discussed earlier, summarized in Table 13-4. Clinicians have greater confidence in guide-lines that have been tested on actual patient populations than in guidelines that are the results of a decision analy-sis or theoretical construct.

Of great importance is the applicability of the guide-lines to your own population. Are the patient(s) you see similar to those the guidelines address? If not, are the differences significant? Do factors about your popula-tion exist that would make the intervention less effec-tive or the treatment course different? Will the

intervention be acceptable to your patient(s)? Are other barriers present, such as access to care or financial fac-tors, that would adversely affect patient compliance? A guideline is most helpful when it provides a range of acceptable options, allowing built-in flexibility to accommodate differences in patient populations and patient preferences.

Incorporating Guidelines into Clinical Practice

Finally, it is important to consider whether the guideline can be incorporated into your practice situation. Barriers to implementation include not only the practicality of the guidelines, but also the presence of office systems to expedite them. For example, if you are planning to fol-low a guideline about screening, you need a reminder sys-tem (e.g., flags on patients' charts, written or electronic health maintenance lists) that states the desired frequency of the screening, records the last time it was performed, and provides prompts when it is due. In addition, it should include a permanent means for you to indicate if the screening intervention is not appropriate for a specific patient (e.g., Papanicolaou smears in a patient after hys-terectomy for nonmalignant causes).

To incorporate guideline-based changes in your prac-tice, a mechanism for retrieval of information is needed, rather than trying to remember it all. For example, for guidelines that you accept but that may represent problems that are seen infrequently in your patient populations (e.g., the Ottawa ankle rules guiding the appropriate x-ray in some practices), it is helpful to have a system, often electronic, that prompts you as to what the guidelines suggest. Using guidelines that have been constructed according to the principles discussed earlier helps manage the plethora of information physicians face, but these require thoughtful implementation.

References

1. Tunis SR, Hayward RS, Wilson MC, et al. Internists' attitudes about clinical practice guidelines. Ann Intern Med 1994;120:956–963.

2. Inouye J, Kristopopatis R, Stone E, et al. Physicians' changing attitudes towards guidelines. J Gen Intern Med 1998;13:324–326.

3. Weber M. National ACP meeting, oral presentation.

4. Cherkin DC, Deyo RA, Wheeler K, Ciol MA. Physician variation in diagnostic testing for low back pain. Who you see is what you get. Arthritis Rheum 1994;19:1329–1334.

5. Wennberg JE, McPherson K, Caper P. Will payment based on diagnosis-related groups control hospital costs? N Engl J Med 1984;311:295–300.

6. McDonald CJ, Overhage JM. Guidelines you can follow and can trust. JAMA 1994;271:872–873.

7. Berg A, Atkins D, Tierney W. Clinical practice guidelines in practice and education. J Gen Intern Med 1997;12(Suppl):25–33.

8. Battista RN, Fletcher SW. Making recommendations on preventive practices: methodologic isssues. Am J Prev Med 1998;4(Suppl):53–67.

Chapter 14

Use of Balance Sheets in Developing Clinical Guidelines*

Mick Braddick, Michael E. Stuart, and Jennifer Hrachovec

Improving quality while containing costs is arguably the highest priority in health care today. Problems with the quality and cost of care in the United States include wide variations in clinical practice,[1–3] medical practices with marginal benefit to patients with considerably increased costs, ineffective practices, and clinical practices initially expected to improve care but that may actually cause harm.[4–8] Managed care organizations (MCOs) must provide the best available care to their populations under cost constraints, and clinical guidelines may help in achieving this goal. Useful clinical guidelines should contain more than clear recommendations. The evidence and reasoning on which the recommendations are based should be explicit, and the expected outcomes of implementing the guideline should be stated.

Group Health Cooperative of Puget Sound is a large MCO in the Pacific Northwest with an enrollment of approximately 600,000 patients and more than 900 staff physicians and 2,500 nonstaff physicians. Within this MCO, teams of providers with administrative and epidemiologic support developed 30 evidence-based clinical practice guidelines using an explicit approach to systematically analyze evidence and to project the impacts of each guideline on health care outcomes.[9–11] These guidelines are used by providers and patients as an aid to shared decision making, and key outcomes are monitored to check that the guidelines have been successfully implemented. Before completion of each

guideline, the impacts on all pertinent outcomes (i.e., health status, patient satisfaction, provider satisfaction, cost and utilization, and capital needs) are determined by developing a balance sheet.[10,11]

The balance sheet in clinical guideline development work has been described by Eddy[12] as a tool to

Estimate the health and economic outcomes from clinical research and clinical experience

Assist decision makers in developing an accurate understanding of the important consequences of adopting the different options

Condense important information into a space that can be grasped visually and mentally at one time

Assist in planning organizational change (e.g., organize thinking, structure the analysis of evidence, and focus debates)

A balance sheet is used to ensure that the effects of various clinical practice changes being contemplated by guideline developers have been formally considered before finalizing and implementing the clinical guideline. Balance sheets have been especially useful in assisting teams in developing clinical guidelines at Group Health Cooperative of Puget Sound, to simultaneously consider cost, quality, and satisfaction (Table 14-1). In this chapter, we provide examples of balance sheets of varying complexity that have assisted our health care providers and administrators in understanding the full range of consequences of adopting different diagnostic or treatment options before guideline implementation. Although patients are not members of our guideline development teams, we have endeavored to represent their perspective when developing guidelines.

---

*Reprinted with permission from M Braddick, M Stuart, J Hrachovec. The use of balance sheets in developing clinical guidelines. J Am Board Fam Pract 1999;12:48–54.

Table 14-1. Functions of the Balance Sheet in Clinical Guideline Development

Organizes benefits, harms, and costs of various clinical practice changes in one chart
Benefits can be compared with harms in a quantifiable way (e.g., the number of post-operative pulmonary emboli prevented by subcutaneous heparin and the number of major bleeds caused)
Health outcomes (both benefits and harms) are displayed in natural units (e.g., deaths avoided)
Patient and provider satisfaction are projected
Costs and utilization, including start-up costs and marginal costs, are estimated
Can be used to assist decision making regarding individual patients or populations
Shows all the projected impacts of any clinical practice change (e.g., guideline implementation)
Balance sheet information can be used to create decision support for providers and patients (e.g., baseline risk, absolute risk reduction with various treatments, information regarding number of patients needed to treat [NNT] to benefit one patient)

Case 1

A 23-year-old man presented after he twisted his ankle playing soccer. Your nurse had arranged for foot and ankle x-rays before his visit with you. The x-ray showed no fracture, and you advised the standard treatment of rest, ice, compression, and elevation.

Clinical Examples of Balance Sheet Use

Eliminating Unnecessary Investigations and Recognizing Barriers to Changing Clinical Practice

Wondering how best to determine whether a patient with an ankle injury really needs to have an x-ray (Case 1), you search MEDLINE. You find a multicenter study of the Ottawa ankle rules (i.e., a set of prospectively validated decision rules).[13] When introduced to emergency departments at eight hospitals, these rules reduced the use of ankle radiography with no increase in the rate of missed fractures. This guideline would save time for the patient and reduce costs. You wonder if it would be worth encouraging other providers in your MCO to use these decision rules. You obtain the number of patients presenting with ankle injuries within your organization and

assume that you could achieve a similar change in radiography as experienced in the study (i.e., reduction from 83% to 61%). After discussing the potential reduction in radiography with a colleague, you decide to broaden your analysis to include other factors, such as patient satisfaction, provider satisfaction, and health outcomes. Information about waiting times was available in the paper; however, patient and provider satisfaction were not discussed in detail. In the absence of information on provider satisfaction, you assume that your colleagues and their patients may, at times, find it hard to accept the implications of the decision rules (Table 14-2).

In view of the substantial savings that the Ottawa ankle rules could generate for your organization, you decide to try to develop an acute ankle injury guideline, while recognizing that patient and provider satisfaction issues constitute barriers that need to be addressed.

Table 14-2. Acute Ankle Injury X-Ray

	Current				Projected		
	Number per Year	Unit Cost ($)	Total Annual Costs ($)	Change (%)	Number per Year	Total Annual Costs ($)	Annual Savings (Costs) ($)
Ankle and foot x-ray series	12,450	50	622,500	−26	9,213	460,650	161,850

Other outcomes of implementing an ankle injury guideline include the following:
    Reduction in radiation exposure
    Length of office visit reduced by 33 minutes in those not requiring an x-ray
    Satisfaction among patients and providers may be reduced as a result of disagreement with the decision rules

---

Case 2

At the end of a busy morning, a pharmaceutical representative visited you to describe the benefits of potassium-sparing diuretics for the treatment of hypertension. He explained that case-control studies of hypertensive patients on thiazide diuretics demonstrate that the rate of sudden death is lowest in those on low doses of thiazides combined with a potassium-sparing diuretic.[14] You wonder whether you should switch all your patients currently on a thiazide alone to a potassium-sparing diuretic.

Making Uncertainty Explicit

Recalling your colleague's advice to include all outcomes, you construct a simple balance sheet for Case 2.

Health outcomes: The only definite improvement in health outcomes is an estimated 50% reduction in the number of sudden cardiac deaths. However, sudden cardiac death is not the only outcome related to hypertension. Low-dose thiazides have been shown to reduce the risk of stroke, heart failure, coronary artery disease, total mortality, and cardiovascular mortality, but the effect of the combination of a thiazide and potassium-sparing diuretics on these outcomes has not been studied.

Cost: The combination of a thiazide and potassium-sparing diuretics costs approximately six times as much as a thiazide alone. Although neither drug is expensive, you are aware that little-ticket items, such as these drugs, lead to considerable expense for the organization as a whole. The cost of testing for hypokalemia was not included because there is uncertainty regarding both the need to test for hypokalemia in patients on low-dose thiazides alone and the need to test patients on a thiazide and a potassium-sparing diuretic.

Satisfaction: Advertising by the pharmaceutical industry to both providers and patients stimulates interest in potassium-sparing diuretics. Any attempt to restrict their use may encounter resistance and needs to be addressed sensitively.

In summary, there are known significant costs, uncertain overall health benefits, and commercial forces that are likely to increase the use of potassium-sparing diuretics. You decide against substituting a combination of a thiazide and a potassium-sparing diuretic for a low-dose thiazide alone as standard treatment of hypertension.

Making Decisions about New, More Effective but More Costly Interventions

In Case 3, the first study included women with low bone density but without a previous symptomatic osteoporotic vertebral fracture. The main outcome in this study was a 48% reduction in the relative risk of radiologically detected vertebral fractures.[15] You regard this as an intermediate marker rather than an outcome of clear clinical significance and discard the paper.

The second study was of women with low bone density and a previous osteoporotic vertebral fracture. After 2.9 years of follow-up, the hip fracture rate was 1.1% in those randomized to alendronate, compared with 2.2% in the placebo group. You calculate that the absolute risk reduction is 1.1% over 2.9 years and that you would have to treat 90 patients (111/1.1) for 2.9 years to prevent a single hip fracture (this is the number needed to treat [NNT]). Using the cost of the medication, the NNT, and the duration of treatment, you calculate that the cost to prevent one hip fracture is $172,000. In addition, there would be 1.7 fewer wrist fractures and 2.5 fewer symptomatic vertebral fractures.[16]

The difficulty in establishing how many women within your MCO would be candidates for alendronate therapy precludes the construction of a formal balance sheet, so you briefly document your conclusions. Although this approach does not give a complete picture of the impact of using alendronate at a population level, it is helpful when estimates are considered to be unreliable.

Case 3

While scanning advertisements in a medical journal, you noted that alendronate reduces the risk of hip fracture by approximately 50%. Knowing that the lifetime risk of hip fracture in women is approximately 15% and that this event frequently is followed by reduced mobility and a substantial increase in mortality, you wonder whether you should actively encourage older patients to take this drug. You select two randomized controlled trials for critical appraisal.

Table 14-3. Balance Sheet Showing the Benefits, Harms, and Costs of a Range of Strategies for Preventing Deep Vein Thrombosis (DVT) and Pulmonary Embolism (PE) Applied to 1,000 Elective Hip Surgery Patients Receiving Prophylaxis for 4 Days

	Intervention Cost per Patient ($)	Relative Risk Reduction (%)	Number of Patients with PE	Number of Patients with Clinical DVT	Major Bleeds Caused	Total Costs Related to DVTs, DVT Prevention, and Bleeding ($)
No prophylaxis	0	0	40	120	0	380,000
FIT	97	86	6	17	0	150,000
IPC stockings	122	38	25	74	0	357,000
Aspirin	4	26	30	89	3	290,000
Warfarin	73	73	11	32	13	199,000
Fixed dose unfractionated heparin	8	45	22	66	29	269,000
LMW heparin	128	79	8	25	18	240,000
FIT + aspirin*	101	90	4	12	3	145,000
FIT + warfarin*	170	96	2	5	13	207,000
FIT + fixed dose unfractionated heparin	170	92	3	9	29	251,000
FIT + LMW heparin*	225	97	1	4	18	268,000
IPC + aspirin*	126	54	18	55	3	305,000
IPC + warfarin*	195	83	7	20	13	282,000
IPC + fixed dose unfractionated heparin*	130	66	14	41	29	311,000
IPC + LMW heparin*	250	87	5	16	18	331,000

FIT = foot impulse technology; IPC = intermittent pneumatic compression; LMW = low molecular weight.
Notes: Total costs are rounded to the nearest $1,000. This balance sheet was developed as part of Group Health Cooperative's DVT prevention guideline. Although the estimates of effectiveness and harms associated with individual preventive strategies are based on a literature review, space constraints preclude us from describing the review in detail. Costs are likely to vary between organizations.
*Unproved benefit of combining these strategies.

Health outcomes: Alendronate is effective in reducing the risk of osteoporotic fractures. Of some concern is potential for esophagitis and the absence of long-term safety data on a drug that is permanently fixed to bone. In addition, it is unclear how much advantage alendronate provides to patients taking hormone replacement therapy and higher doses of vitamin D (in this study, women received only 250 IU).

Cost: Even if alendronate is restricted to patients with low bone density and a previous osteoporotic vertebral fracture, paying $172,000 to prevent a hip fracture is not highly cost-effective.

Patient and provider satisfaction: There is likely to be interest among both patients and providers in another therapeutic option for osteoporosis, although this interest may be reduced on learning of the requirement to take the medication on an empty stomach and to remain upright for half an hour afterwards to reduce the risk of esophagitis.

You are reluctant to abandon the use of an effective medication and consider that this drug would be cost-effective if used in patients at high risk of osteoporotic fracture. A MEDLINE search reveals a prospective study of more than 8,000 community living women that developed a model for predicting hip fracture risk based on risk factor scoring and bone density.[17] You calculate that if alendronate were offered to women with an annual risk of hip fracture of 3% or more, then it would only cost $44,000 to prevent a hip fracture. At this point you decide to (1) use the well-established therapies, such as calcium, vitamin D, and hormone replacement therapy, as first-line therapy; (2) stimulate a discussion within your organization as to how much it is willing to pay to prevent a hip

Table 14-4. Balance Sheet for Diabetic Glycemic Control Guideline

	Current				Projected		
	Number per Year	**Unit Cost ($)**	**Total Annual Costs ($)**	**Change (%)**	**Number per Year**	**Total Annual Costs ($)**	**Annual Savings (Costs) ($)**
Primary care visits	100,000	100	10,000,000	+15	115,000	11,500,000	(1,500,000)
HbA$_{1c}$ tests	40,000	10	400,000	+25	50,000	500,000	(100,000)
Diabetic medication	10,000	200	20,000,000	No change	10,000	20,000,000	0
Total			30,400,000			32,000,000	(1,600,000)

HbA$_{1c}$ = component of hemoglobin used to monitor control of diabetes.

Health outcomes: The mean HbA$_{1c}$ is expected to decrease by 0.5%. Over 15–20 years, the annual incidence of major complications is expected to decrease by approximately 40 (14 fewer diabetics will become blind, 18 fewer patients will develop end-stage renal failure, and nine fewer lower extremity amputations will be performed). These projections must be balanced against an additional 163 severe hypoglycemic episodes per year. Whereas the reduction in incidence of major complications is expected to occur in both type 1 and type 2 diabetes, the risk of severe hypoglycemia will principally be borne by patients with type 1 diabetes (the absolute annual risk of severe hypoglycemia is expected to increase by 8% in type 1 diabetes).

Provider Satisfaction: The guideline's concise approach to diabetes control should help to clarify uncertainties and increase satisfaction. The guideline will increase workload, however, which may create some resistance.

Patient Satisfaction: Overall, this guideline should increase patient satisfaction. Patients are likely to have different views about intensive glycemic control with the associated increase in risk of hypoglycemia, together with a heightened awareness that their own behavior will have a direct impact on the future risk of complications. Nonetheless, patients are expected to appreciate increased information and the fact that a consistent approach is applied throughout the managed care organization, even if they change primary care providers.

fracture and to develop a hip fracture risk scoring tool to identify those patients for whom alendronate would be considered cost-effective; and (3) discuss cost and benefit information with patients interested in beginning alendronate therapy who also pay for their own medications.

Choosing between Many Options and Weighing Benefits, Harms, and Costs

So far we have considered three examples in which there was a choice between a new approach and an old one. By explicitly setting out benefits, harms, and costs, a balance sheet can be particularly helpful when there are multiple interventions and several outcomes to consider. Prevention of deep vein thrombosis (DVT) and pulmonary embolism after total hip replacement is a good example. Several possible preventive strategies exist, including mechanical approaches (foot impulse technology and intermittent pneumatic compression stockings) and medications (aspirin, warfarin, heparin). These interventions vary in their effectiveness, are associated with different rates of bleeding, and have different costs. Keeping all of these factors in one's head is very difficult. Indeed, some review articles and meta-analyses have concentrated on DVT prevention and paid less attention to the impact of bleeding.[18,19]

The balance sheet shows that no one correct approach exists (Table 14-3). If you wished to minimize costs, you

would opt for warfarin alone. For every 1,000 patients treated, an average of 11 would have a pulmonary embolus, 13 would have major bleeds, and 32 would develop clinical DVT. In contrast, if you wished to minimize the risk of pulmonary embolus, you would combine foot impulse technology with low molecular weight heparin, giving a 1 in 1,000 risk of pulmonary embolus. This strategy, however, is associated with more major bleeds and higher costs. A pragmatic approach combines foot impulse technology with aspirin, thereby reducing the risk of pulmonary embolus to 4 in 1,000. This strategy would cause only three major bleeds per 1,000 patients treated and appears to be the most cost-effective strategy. Given that costs vary from one organization to another, it is possible that two organizations with similar values could adopt different strategies.

Making All the Implications of a Clinical Change Explicit

The previous case studies illustrate the role of balance sheets in helping providers and planners to use evidence from the literature combined with local costs and values before choosing between different strategies. Balance sheets are also helpful when considering a new program in its entirety. Consider implementation of a guideline on diabetic glycemic control. Table 14-4 shows the

Table 14-5. Common Types of Economic Analyses

Cost-effectiveness analysis	Health outcomes are reported in natural units, such as deaths avoided, life years gained, cases successfully treated. The cost-effectiveness ratio is a measure of the amount of benefit provided by an activity for a specified amount of cost.
Cost-utility analysis	Health outcomes are valued or weighted. For example, the quality-adjusted life year allows for the valuation of time spent in less than full health. Valuing health outcomes makes it possible to compare various types of outcomes.
Cost-benefit analysis	All outcomes are valued in the same units (usually dollars), making it possible to determine what consumers will pay for various interventions or services.
Balance sheet	Health, satisfaction, cost, and utilization outcomes of current practice and various alternatives are listed. Components are not combined, and relative importance of outcomes are not indicated. Users are expected to make judgments based on their values and local conditions.

costs, health outcomes, and patient and provider satisfaction associated with this guideline. It is important to acknowledge that many of the figures in this balance sheet are estimates and that it includes an assumption that patients with type 2 diabetes benefit from glycemic control. Whenever uncertainty exists, we take a conservative approach, using high-range cost estimates and low-range estimates of benefit. In the absence of easily available local data regarding rates of major complications of diabetes, we relied on estimates from the medical literature.[20] In view of the difficulties of assigning a financial cost to these outcomes and the difficulties of discounting benefits that are expected many years in the future, we simply state these facts in a footnote.

Discussion

Balance sheets display estimates of benefits, harms, and costs and are best thought of as a type of practical and useful economic analysis. Table 14-5 summarizes the most common types of economic analysis and their uses in health care.[12,21,22] *Economic analyses* can be defined as approaches used to compare alternative strategies in health care using formal, quantitative methods to estimate outcomes and resource utilization.[22] Underlying the increasing interest in economic analysis is the understanding that an astounding and ever-increasing number of health care activities exists, each associated with different benefits, harms, and costs. A key concept in economic analysis is the notion that interventions can be prioritized beyond benefit to an individual patient or population. Through economic analysis, interventions can be ranked by the total benefit they provide to a population for a given cost. Economic analyses have been distinguished from decision analyses and clinical practice guidelines by their explicit measurement and valuation of resource consumption or cost.[22] We believe that balance sheets are a critically important part of an explicit, evidence-based guideline process. They require

the collection, interpretation, and integration of valid and clinically important evidence from the medical literature and costs from internally derived organizational data. Information is frequently missing, and estimates are often necessary to complete a balance sheet. For example, how likely is it that the benefits observed in a randomized controlled trial will be achieved in routine clinical practice (this is the difference between efficacy and effectiveness [Table 14-6]) and, realistically, what proportion of patients will be treated according to a newly implemented guideline?

Balance sheets display both health outcomes and cost outcomes, but they leave the health outcomes in natural units, such as number of myocardial infarctions prevented or number of hospitalizations avoided. Balance sheets, in contrast to some types of economic analysis, do not place an economic value on health states. Dollar valuing of health states, for example, is the distinguishing feature of cost-benefit analyses. Because balance sheets leave economic and health outcomes in their natural units, users of balance sheets are required to use their own values and local conditions to guide their recommendations. The balance sheet is thus a tool to assist in the planning of clinical improvement activities. It facilitates decision making by setting out alternatives, and it shows all expected impacts of a guideline or other clinical improvement project. An additional step is required to compare various guidelines. To rank diagnostic or treatment interventions of different types (e.g., a cervical cancer screening program compared with a coronary artery bypass program), a cost-utility analysis is required in which health outcomes are weighted or valued, for example, in quality-adjusted life years, or *QALYs*.

Summary

Balance sheets are designed to assist decision makers regarding outcomes in their practice setting. For this reason, they must include data generated in that practice

Table 14-6. Comparison of Efficacy and Effectiveness

Efficacy	Effectiveness
Best represented by randomized controlled trials in which *ideal conditions* for interventions can be created because of steps taken to assure full cooperation with medical advice Study population may exclude 　Complex cases (patients with comorbidities)[a] 　Older patients[b] 　Women[c] Frequently, there is optimal support for 　Personnel to deliver care 　Necessary facilities and equipment 　Implementation methods 　Attention to patients in the form of follow-up, 　　reminders, and the like to keep drop-out rates low	The "reality" of practice settings in which conditions usually are not ideal—conditions differ from those in randomized controlled trials. Effectiveness is established if more good than harm results from interventions offered to patients: 　Patients are more likely to be older, female, taking 　　multiple medications, or to have multiple 　　medical problems 　Usually, fewer personnel are available 　　to deliver care 　Usually, less support is available for encouraging 　　compliance with treatment and follow-up

[a]Greenhalgh T. Is my practice evidence-based? Should be answered in qualitative, as well as quantitative terms. BMJ 1996;313:957–958.

[b]Gurwitz JH, Col NF, Avorn J. The exclusion of the elderly and women from clinical trials in acute myocardial infarction. JAMA 1992;268:1417–1422.

[c]Fletcher RH, Fletcher SW, Wagner EH. Clinical Epidemiology: The Essentials. Baltimore: Williams & Wilkins, 1988.

setting and project the impact of a change in clinical practice on health outcomes, cost, and patient and provider satisfaction. To complete a balance sheet, it is often necessary to make assumptions that should be both conservative and realistic. Balance sheets are particularly useful for presenting all the expected outcomes of implementing a clinical guideline or other change in clinical practice and frequently lead to insights and improvements.

Acknowledgments

We gratefully acknowledge David Eddy, whose lucid writings have inspired our guideline development work at Group Health Cooperative. We also acknowledge our clinical and administrative colleagues with whom we have discussed and refined these ideas over the years.

References

1. Wennberg J, Gittelsohn A. Small area variations in health care delivery. Science 1973;182:1102–1108.
2. Perrin JM, Homer CJ, Berwick DM, et al. Variations in rates of hospitalization of children in three urban communities. N Engl J Med 1989;320:1183–1187.
3. Chassin MR, Brook RH, Park RE, et al. Variations in the use of medical and surgical services by the Medicare population. N Engl J Med 1986;314:285–290.
4. Schroeder SA. Strategies for reducing medical costs by changing physicians' behavior. Int J Technol Assess Health Care 1987;3:39–50.
5. Grimes DA. Technology follies; the uncritical accep-
tance of medical innovation. JAMA 1993;269:3030–3033.
6. Epstein AE, Hallstrom AP, Rogers WJ, et al. Mortality following ventricular arrhythmia suppression by encainide, flecainide, and moricizine after myocardial infarction. JAMA 1993;270:2451–2455.
7. Franks P, Clancy CM, Nutting PA. Sounding board: gate keeping revisited—protecting patients from over treatment. N Engl J Med 1992;327:426–429.
8. Eddy DM. Medicine, money, and mathematics. Am Coll Surg Bull 1992;77:36–49.
9. Stuart ME, Macuiba JM, Heidrich F, et al. Successful implementation of an evidence-based clinical practice guideline: acute dysuria/urgency in adult women. HMO Practice 1997;11:150–157.
10. Handley MR, Stuart ME. An evidence-based approach to evaluation and improving clinical practice: guideline development. HMO Practice 1994;8:10–19.
11. Handley MR, Stuart ME. An evidence-based approach to evaluating and improving clinical practice: implementing practice guidelines. HMO Practice 1994;8:75–83.
12. Eddy DM. Comparing benefits and harms; the balance sheet. JAMA 1990;263:2493–2505.
13. Stiell I, Wells G, Laupacis A, et al. Multicentre trial to introduce the Ottawa ankle rules for use of radiography in acute ankle injuries. BMJ 1995:311:594–597.
14. Siscovick DS, Raghunathan TE, Psaty BM, et al. Diuretic therapy for hypertension and the risk of primary cardiac arrest. N Engl J Med 1994;330:1852–1857.
15. Liberman UA, Weiss SR, Broll J, et al. Effect of oral alendronate on bone mineral density and the incidence of fractures in postmenopausal osteoporosis. N Engl J Med 1995;333:1437–1443.

16. Black DM, Cummings SR, Karpf DB, et al. Randomised trial of effect of alendronate on risk of fracture in women with existing vertebral fractures. Lancet 1996;348:1535–1541.
17. Cummings SR, Nevitt MC, Browner WS, et al. Risk factors for hip fracture in white women. N Engl J Med 1995;332:767–773.
18. Clagett GP, Anderson FA Jr, Heit J, et al. Prevention of thromboembolism. Chest 1995;108(Suppl):312–334.
19. Imperiale TF, Speroff T. A meta-analysis of methods to prevent venous thromboembolism following total hip replacement. JAMA 1994;271:1780–1785.
20. Eastman RC, Javitt JC, Herman WH, et al. Model of complications of NIDDM. II: Analysis of the health benefits and cost-effectiveness of treating NIDDM with the goal of normoglycemia. Diabetes Care 1997; 20:735–744.
21. Gold MR, Seigal JE, Russell LB, Weinstein MC (eds), Cost-Effectiveness in Health and Medicine. New York: Oxford University Press, 1996;27–29.
22. Drummond MF, Richardson WS, O'Brien BJ, et al., for the Evidence-Based Medicine Working Group. Users' guides to the medical literature. XIII: How to use an article on economic analysis of clinical practice. A. Are the results of the study valid? JAMA 1997;277: 1552–1557.

Chapter 15
Summarizing Evidence for Clinical Use

Fredric M. Wolf

Medicine is a science of uncertainty and an art of probability.

—*Sir William Osler*

Case 1

Suppose a proposal is made to offer a cardiac rehabilitation program of uncertain effectiveness to people who have experienced a heart attack. Following are five statements derived from five randomized trials published in medical journals. On the basis of each, please take a moment to indicate how likely you are to agree to the implementation of a cardiac rehabilitation program based on this information. For the sake of the example, assume that the costs of each program are the same and that each result was deemed to be statistically significant. Please rate from 0 (would not) to 10 (would) the degree of support you would be willing to recommend each of the following programs if during a 10-year follow-up

1. **Program A reduced the death rate by 13%.**
2. **Program B produced an absolute reduction in deaths of 4%.**
3. **Program C increased the rate of patient survival from 70% to 74%.**
4. **Program D prevented one death for every 25 people who entered a rehabilitation program.**
5. **Program E reduced the odds of death by 18%.**

The results of the five programs in Case 1 are typical of how the results of new research studies are reported in professional medical journals and subsequently quoted in the popular press. In fact, these are actual results taken from the published medical literature. The translation of research findings into improved quality and efficiency of care is critical for research to be of ultimate practical value. How findings like those in Case 1 are interpreted are critical when physicians and patients make health care decisions. The underlying assumption is to provide the highest quality, most effective health care given a particular patient's situation.

What may not be evident is that all five results presented in Case 1 are derived from exactly the same underlying data. This case is described further after stating the purpose of this chapter and providing some background for this discussion. Specifically, the purpose of this chapter is to discuss the following topics:

The general context of health care reform and the role of evidence;

What distinguishes evidence from information and the difficulty in identifying high quality evidence;

The potential use of decision support tools to assist us in weaving through the maze of information;

Some specific, high quality sources of information, including electronic resources such as the Cochrane

Database of Systematic Reviews, Best Evidence, Scientific American Medicine Online, and a variety of Internet-based resources, including the National Guideline Clearinghouse;

The impact language and communication about the effects of health care interventions have on physician and patient decision making; and

How language might be used to communicate evidence more meaningfully and understandably for it to enhance patient care.

Health Care Reform, Information Overload, and the Role of Effectiveness Evidence

No one would doubt that the health care system in the United States is in the process of significant change because now the majority of Americans are being served by some form of managed care organization. It can be argued that this change is being largely, if not exclusively, driven by efforts to hold down the costs of care and, some might add, to bolster the bottom line of for-profit health care systems. Issues of quality of care are currently coming to the forefront of the debate. An appropriate question is, "What role does effectiveness evidence play in third-party reimbursement decisions for approved, covered, and reimbursed services?" If rational decision making were indeed based on evidence, then a serious problem would be identifying the best evidence and distinguishing information from evidence. Dictionaries define *information* as news, whereas *evidence* is something that tends to *prove* or provide grounds for holding a certain belief. A higher standard exists for something to be called *evidence* rather than simply *information*—yet this distinction is often lost.

A recent editorial in the *British Medical Journal* bemoaned, "We have much too much information of poor quality, too little that's good, and no effective way of sorting it out."[1] Advances in medical science and information technology are combining to create ever-increasing amounts of information, resulting in what has been commonly termed *information explosion* at a systems level, creating the challenge of *information overload* at the individual level. This phenomenon is evidenced by a more than 10-fold increase in the number of professional journals across all disciplines.[2] For example, the number of journals in the biomedical sciences increased from 2,300 in 1940 to more than 23,000 in 1993! If you multiply 23,000 by the number of issues per year in each journal and the number of articles per issue, clearly it is increasingly difficult to stay abreast of new advances reported in the literature. The problem is exacerbated for primary care providers, generalists who are expected to know an increasing amount of information about an increasing number of topics. Mulrow estimates that approximately 2 million medically related articles are published annually.[3] If you also use electronic mail and access the Internet regularly, you may feel like the patient suffering from information overload and burnout illustrated in the editorial cartoon in Figure 15-1.

To make matters worse, research studies designed to answer the same question do not always reach consistent conclusions. In some cases, studies reach conflicting conclusions, leaving people confused as to what the "right" course of action is, as illustrated in the editorial cartoon in Figure 15-2. This leads to a general skepticism about the worth and credibility of the scientific enterprise. As one editorial cartoonist mocked, the "random medical news from the New England Journal of Panic Inducing Gobbledygook" randomly assigns cause, effect (i.e., resulting medical condition or outcome), and population (e.g., adults, children, men, women) to studies.

Finding High Quality Evidence in the Information Age

So what is one to do? A possible solution is to turn to one of the available decision support systems. These include (1) literature databases like MEDLINE or its European counterpart, EMBASE, (2) computer-based textbooks that offer enhanced (Boolean) searching capabilities for identifying relevant information, (3) drug databases that alert users to potential side effects and drug interactions, (4) clinical practice guidelines, (5) reminder or alert systems, (6) diagnostic or treatment decision support systems that provide consultations once the characteristics of a patient's problem are entered in the system, and (7) systematic reviews of the effectiveness of health care interventions. I try to make the case that this latter tool, systematic reviews of the effectiveness of health care interventions, offers some unique advantages or "added value" over the others, and I describe one particular database of systematic reviews (the Cochrane Database of Systematic Reviews) that may be particularly useful for the physician, patient, and for policy-oriented decision making.

Searching MEDLINE, EMBASE, or other health-related databases for articles that are relevant to a particular patient's problem often results in many references. These references typically describe studies whose research designs, patient groups, methods, and even results often differ. It is not easy to make sense of and synthesize these varied findings into a concrete summary of the evidence. This is exactly the goal of a good systematic review (or meta-analysis), which can also inform us about the consistency and replicability of the findings across studies.

Electronic textbooks, such as *Harrison's Textbook of Medicine* or *Scientific American Medicine*, both of which are available on CD-ROM, offer the advantage of being easier to search than standard, printed texts. Electronic drug databases also can be useful reference and

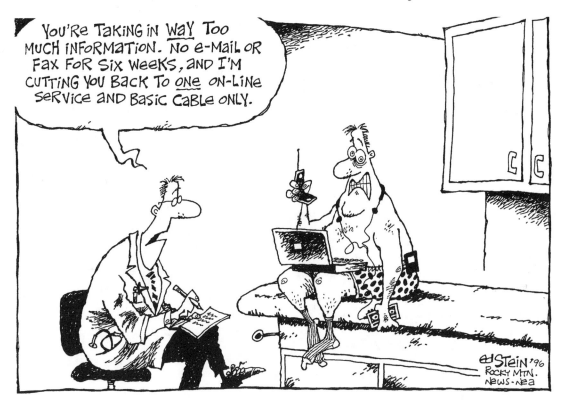

Figure 15-1. The effects of information overload. (Reprinted with permission from Rocky Mountain News Service.)

decision support tools. Information in textbooks and drug databases, however, must be based on good evidence, which a well-done, systematic review or meta-analysis can provide.

Systematic reviews also can provide good sources of evidence required to construct practice guidelines, which typically rely on the best available evidence and/or expert opinion as the basis for making recommendations. Some of the best guideline sources can be found in the Canadian and U.S. Prevention Task Force Guidelines, as well as in the National Guideline Clearinghouse. The National Guideline Clearinghouse is a "public resource for evidence-based clinical practice guidelines . . . sponsored by the Agency for Health Care Policy and Research in partnership with the American Medical Association and the American Association of Health Plans." It is readily accessible on the Internet (http://www.guideline.gov/index.asp).

Systematic reviews also can be good sources of the evidence that is necessary to develop decision rules for treatment or diagnostic computer consultation programs (e.g., DXplain, ILIAD, or QMR). These decision support tools allow clinicians to enter their patients' findings into the system to receive a differential diagnosis or treatment plans ranked on the basis of likelihood of accuracy or effectiveness, respectively. What is a systematic review, then?

Elements of High Quality Systematic Reviews of Effectiveness Evidence

According to the Cochrane Collaboration,[4] a good systematic review has at least eight key elements, as summarized in Table 15-1. The first is to state the objectives of the review and outline the eligibility criteria for including and excluding studies in the review. This is typically not done in more traditional narrative reviews and is a key element in trying to elevate the quality of a review by enhancing its "objectivity." Explicit criteria for inclusion and exclusion of studies in the review should specify the population, intervention, outcome, and methodologic criteria for the studies included in the review. The next steps are to search for all the studies, both published and unpublished, that seem to meet eligibility criteria and tabulate the relevant characteristics of each study. Comprehensive search methods are used to locate relevant studies by examining reference lists of key articles (often referred to as the *ancestry* approach) and conference proceedings, directly contacting experts in the field, and searching a wide range of computerized databases using a combination of appropriate key words and free text searching strategies. Coding the characteristics of each study typically includes an assessment of the methodologic quality of the study using predefined criteria.[5,6] Coding should

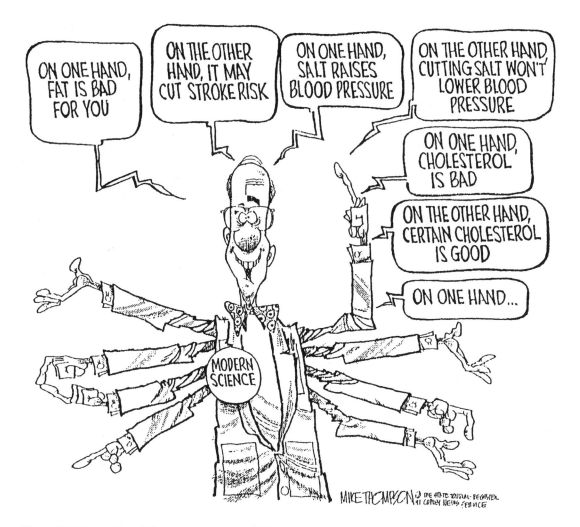

Figure 15-2. Perceptions of disarray and lack of credibility can result from conflicting study results in medical research. (Reprinted with permission from Copley News Service.)

attempt to avoid bias and be reproducible, which typically requires each study to be coded independently by at least two "judges." Exploration of variation between the findings of the studies enables the authors and readers to determine the degree to which characteristics of the study design itself may be accounting for some of the findings. Even differences in the design of randomized controlled trials have been shown to account for differences in the effect of therapy. [6] This is particularly true for the precise manner in which patients are assigned to the various treatment groups. The coding of study quality essentially serves as an assessment of the validity of the primary studies.

The next step is to apply the eligibility criteria to each study and to justify the exclusion of each study. A table listing the excluded studies, with reasons justifying their exclusion, are typically included as part of a systematic

review, along with a table summarizing the characteristics of the studies included in the review. This should result in the most complete data set feasible, often including information to supplement published data that is requested and obtained directly from the authors of the primary studies.

The results from the eligible studies are then synthesized and summarized. If appropriate and possible, results from each of the primary studies are pooled quantitatively using statistical synthesis methods (i.e., meta-analysis). Regardless of whether results are pooled quantitatively, it is important to adhere to the other elements of a systematic review to maintain as much objectivity and minimize as much bias in the review as possible. It is important to recognize that a systematic review is not a meta-analysis if it does not quantitatively pool results across studies. Conversely, a meta-analysis is not a systematic review if it does not explicitly state (1) the eligibility criteria for including studies in the review, (2) what databases have been searched, and (3) what search terms were used to identify relevant studies for the review.

Once the synthesis of the overall findings is reported, sensitivity and/or subgroup analyses typically follow. For example, it is important to know whether the treatment is equally effective for men and women, younger and older people, people with varying degrees of disease severity, and so forth, and whether particular characteristics of the intervention, such as duration, dose, and study design, affect outcomes. Finally, a structured report of the review—stating aims, describing materials and methods, and reporting results—is prepared.

The growth of meta-analysis since the late 1980s has been quite remarkable, with more than 3,000 meta-analyses or articles about meta-analyses indexed in MEDLINE since the term *meta-analysis* was first coined by Gene Glass in 1976.[7] This growth has been exponential, with more than 400 articles a year referenced in MEDLINE since 1994,[8] as shown in Figure 15-3. An increasing number of print and electronic resources are evidence-based, many of which rely on evidence from systematic reviews and meta-analyses. These include the Agency for Health Care Policy and Research's Internet-based National Guideline Clearinghouse and *Best Evidence*, a CD-ROM published by the American College of Physicians. *Best Evidence* contains the full text of all articles and clinical commentaries published in the journal *Evidence-Based Medicine* and the *ACP Journal Club*, a supplement to the *Annals of Internal Medicine*. The *Journal of Family Practice*'s Journal Club has evolved into *POEMs* (*Patient-Oriented Evidence that Matters*). Eight articles are identified each month from more than 80 journals "with patient-oriented outcomes that have the greatest potential to change the way primary care clinicians practice. These articles are then critically appraised by expert family physicians, educators, and/or pharmacologists" (see *Journal of Family Practice*'s Internet site for details at http://www.infopoems.com). The validity of systematic reviews is typically determined by the quality of (1) the clinical question that is asked (Is it well focused?), (2) the criteria for including articles in the review (Are they appropriate?), (3) the completeness of the studies included (How likely is it that relevant studies were missed?), and (4) the consistency of findings across studies (Are the results similar from study to study?).

Jordon Cohen, president of the Association of American Medical Colleges, observed, "The practice of medicine is about to be revolutionized by the convergence of two immensely powerful developments: information technology and evidence-based decision-making. . . . [T]he academic community need not wait for more evidence . . . to lead the fundamental reorientation toward evidence-based medicine that is needed throughout the

Table 15-1. Elements of a High Quality Systematic Review

State objectives of the review and outline eligibility (inclusion/exclusion) criteria for studies

Exhaustively search for studies that seem to meet eligibility criteria

Tabulate characteristics of each study identified and assess its methodologic quality

Apply eligibility criteria and justify any exclusions

Assemble the most complete data feasible, with involvement of investigators

Analyze results of eligible studies; use statistical synthesis of data (meta-analysis) if appropriate and possible

Perform sensitivity analyses, if appropriate and possible (including subgroup analyses)

Prepare a structured report of the review, stating aims, describing materials and methods, and reporting results

Source: Adapted from Chalmers I. The Cochrane Collaboration: preparing, maintaining, and disseminating systematic reviews of the effects of health care [review]. Ann N Y Acad Sci 1993;703:156–163.

health care delivery system."[9] A 1998 editorial in *Lancet*[10] stated, "The most important effort to gather evidence that might change practice has come from the Cochrane Collaboration." The Cochrane Collaboration also has been called "an enterprise that rivals the Human Genome Project in its implications for modern science."[11] The Cochrane Collaboration is an international effort to prepare, update, and disseminate systematic reviews of the effects of health care.[4,12]

Cochrane Collaboration and Cochrane Database of Systematic Reviews

Evidence obtained from at least one good, properly designed randomized clinical trial traditionally has been considered the highest quality evidence available (e.g., see the U.S. Preventive Services Task Force). Evidence from a properly designed systematic review of all the available properly designed randomized trials has been deemed to be evidence of the highest quality for use in decision making, and it is superior to the results from any one randomized clinical trial. The Cochrane Database of Systematic Reviews is an electronic journal published quarterly that first appeared in 1995. It is distributed as part of the Cochrane Library by British Medical Journal Publishing in the United Kingdom and the American College of Physicians in the United States and is available worldwide on CD-ROM and now on the Internet.[13] The Cochrane Database of Systematic Reviews is one of four components of what has evolved into the Cochrane Library.[13,14] The other three components are (1) the Database of Abstracts of Reviews of Effectiveness (DARE),

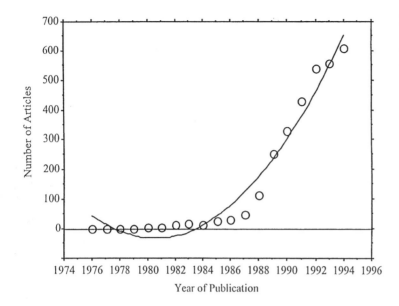

Figure 15-3. Illustration of the growing trend in the appearance of citations for "meta-analysis" available in MEDLINE from 1976–1994. (Adapted from FM Wolf, C Lefebvre, WC McGaghie. Identification of meta-analyses in MEDLINE: all that glitters is not gold, or is it [abstract]? Prof Educ Res Q 1996;17:13.)

which includes more than 1,600 critical assessments and structured abstracts of good systematic reviews not published by the Cochrane Collaboration, (2) the Cochrane Controlled Trials Register, which contains bibliographic information on more than 175,000 controlled trials, and (3) the Cochrane Review Methodology Database, a bibliography of articles and books on the science of research synthesis. Unlike articles appearing in medical journals,

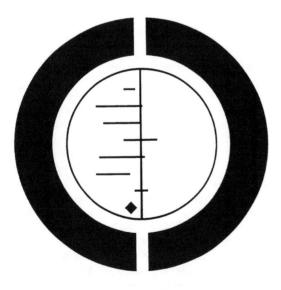

Figure 15-4. The logo of the International Cochrane Collaboration. Understanding how to interpret the logo allows the reader to interpret any research finding reported in the Cochrane Database of Systematic Reviews. (Reprinted with permission from the International Cochrane Collaboration.)

for example the *New England Journal of Medicine* or *Journal of the American Medical Association*, one can interpret any review in the Cochrane Database of Systematic Reviews regardless of subject matter or area of medicine if one is able to interpret the logo of the Cochrane Collaboration, illustrated in Figure 15-4.

Each of the seven horizontal lines represents the 95% confidence interval for the results of one randomized trial comparing the effectiveness of an intervention with standard care or placebo (in this case an inexpensive course of a corticosteroid given to pregnant women at risk of preterm delivery). More certain results are represented by shorter lines, with horizontal lines crossing the vertical line indicating no difference between the two treatments. A horizontal line to the left of the vertical line indicates that the study result favored the intervention, whereas a horizontal line to the right of the vertical line indicates that the study result favors standard therapy or placebo. For example, the top trial favors the intervention, whereas the two below it suggest an advantage in favor of the intervention, but seem to border on "no difference," whereas the fourth trial from the top clearly indicates that the two treatments have similar effects. The pooled result across all seven trials is summarized by the diamond, which indicates that the weight of all the evidence favors a significant reduction in infant mortality as a result of corticosteroid use. Results from any systematic review in the Cochrane Database of Systematic Reviews are interpreted in an analogous fashion, regardless of the topic of the review—for example, diabetes, asthma, cardiovascular disease, cancer, depression, and so forth. One example can be seen in Figure 15-5, a screen from a Cochrane Database of Systematic Reviews review of the effects of family psychosocial interventions

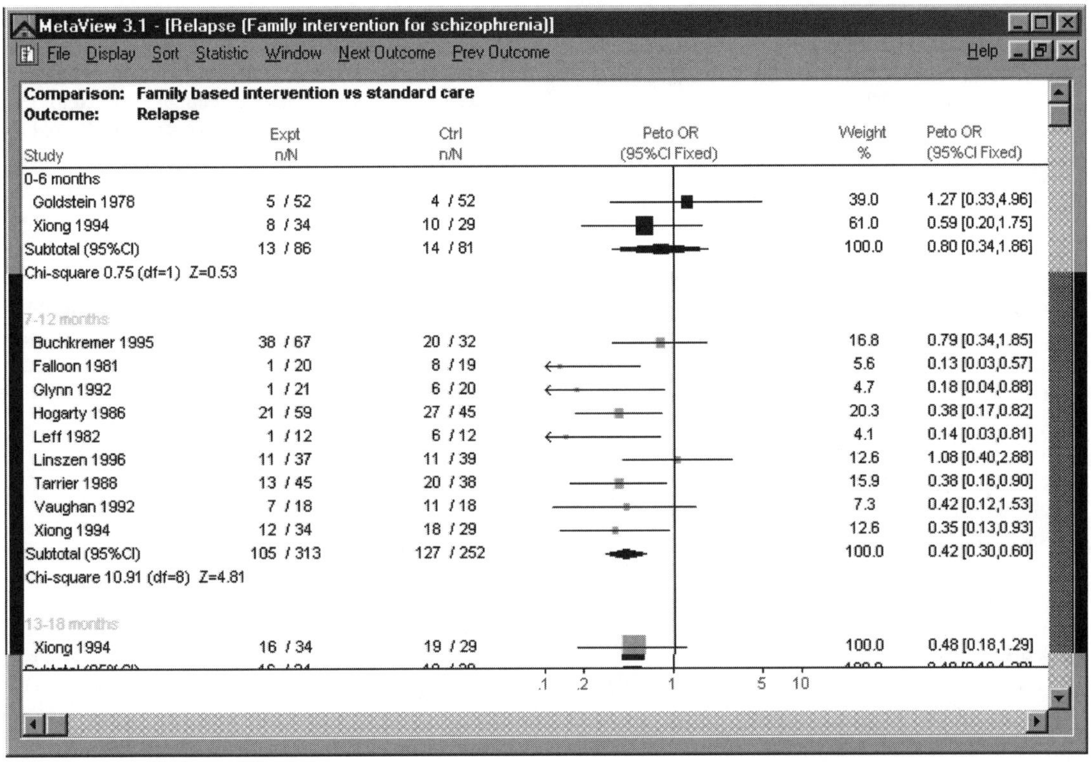

Figure 15-5. Example of results from a Cochrane review. (CI = confidence interval; Ctrl = control group; df = degrees of freedom; Expt = experimental group; Peto OR = Peto-modified Mantel-Haenszel odds ratio.) (Reprinted with permission from JJ Mari, D Streiner. Family Interventions for Schizophrenia. [Cochrane Review]. The Cochrane Library, Issue 2. Oxford: Update Software, 1998.)

versus standard care in community settings for the care of individuals with schizophrenia.[15]

Figure 15-5 summarizes an interesting subgroup analysis based on the length of time of the intervention. The authors of this review were able to locate only two randomized trials in which the interventions lasted no more than 6 months. These two trials involved a total of 167 patients (86 randomized to the family intervention groups and 81 randomized to the standard care) and showed the interventions to be equally effective in preventing relapse (i.e., no difference between them). Thirteen of 86 patients in the intervention group experienced relapse, whereas 14 of 81 patients receiving standard care experienced relapse. On the other hand, for interventions lasting between 7 months and 1 year, the results for all patients pooled across all seven trials showed a significant reduction in relapse for patients in the family intervention groups (105 of 313 patients relapsed) compared with standard care (127 of 252 patients relapsed). This resulted in an average reduction of 58% in the odds of relapse—that is, 1 minus 0.42 under the column labeled *Peto OR*. At this point, it is important to review the language used to report and discuss the results of research, including such terms as *odds*, *risk*, and *survival*.

Language of Medical Research: Communication among and between Providers and Patients

Let us now focus on Case 1 and Case 2, presented next. The results of both cases are based on actual results reported in the published medical literature.[16,17] Although Case 1 focuses on intervention and Case 2 deals with screening (prevention), the issues of interpretation and communication of research findings are the same.

The two problems introduced in Cases 1 and 2 typify the language used to report new clinical research findings and were modified from those presented by Fahey and colleagues.[18] What may not be so readily apparent is that the five results for each case are actually alternative representations of the same research findings. This fact implies that your preference for each intervention, whether therapy or screening, should be the same regardless of how the information is presented or framed.

Table 15-2. Example of 2 × 2 Table Summarizing Breast Cancer–Specific Survival at 7-Year Follow-Up for Women at Least 50 Years of Age with and without Breast Cancer Screening

Group	Dead	Alive	Total
Mammography	71	58,077	58,148
Controls	76	41,028	41,104
Total	147	99,105	99,252

Source: Data from L Tabar, A Gad, LH Holmberg, et al. Reduction in mortality from breast cancer after mass screening with mammography. Lancet 1985;1:829–832.

Results of studies using problems like these and others suggest that the manner in which information is framed can affect the decisions people make and that preference reversals do occur when the same "evidence" is presented in different ways.[18–20] These studies suggest that people are significantly more supportive of treatments when outcomes are expressed in terms of relative risk reduction but less supportive when outcomes are expressed as the absolute risk difference or the number of patients needed to treat to prevent one patient from experiencing an adverse event. We address how these preference reversals might occur after explaining how the various representations of the same results are derived.

The study results reporting various measures of effect in Cases 1 and 2 are derived from 2 × 2 tables that can be constructed from data provided in the original articles.[16,17] For illustration purposes, the 2 × 2 table for Case 2 is provided in Table 15-2. The table is based on results reported in the original Scandinavian multinational randomized trial conducted by Tabar et al.[16] that was designed to examine the effectiveness of mammog-

raphy screening in reducing breast cancer–specific deaths after 7 years of follow-up. These effect size measures are (1) relative risk reduction, (2) risk difference, (3) survival rates, (4) number of patients needed to treat (or screen) to prevent one adverse event, and (5) reduction in odds.

Program A reduced the death rate by 34%. This is the common language used to describe what is more technically referred to as the *relative risk reduction*. To determine the relative risk, simply divide (or take the ratio of) the risk of an adverse outcome for people randomized to one group by the risk of an adverse event for people randomized to the other group and then subtract this from one to estimate the reduction in relative risk:

Risk (mammography) = 71/58,148 = 0.00122
Risk (controls) = 76/41,104 = 0.00185
Relative risk = 0.00122/0.00185 = 0.659
Relative risk reduction = 1 − 0.659 = 0.341 = 34%

Program B produced an absolute reduction in deaths from breast cancer of 0.06%. Rather than take the ratio of the risks for the two groups, simply subtract the risk of one group from that of the other to estimate the risk difference, which is sometimes referred to as the *absolute risk reduction*.

Risk (mammography) = 71/58,148 = 0.00122
Risk (controls) = 76/41,104 = 0.00185
Risk difference = 0.00122 − 0.00185 = −0.00063 = −0.06%

Program C increased the patient survival rate of breast cancer from 99.82% to 99.88%. Divide the number of patients *not* experiencing the adverse event by the total number of people in that group and take the difference between the two groups:

Case 2

Suppose a proposal is made to offer a breast screening program of uncertain effectiveness to women older than 50 years. Following are five statements derived from five randomized trials published in medical journals. On the basis of each, indicate how likely you are to agree to the implementation of a breast screening program. Assume that the costs of each program are the same and each result was deemed to be statistically significant. Rate from 0 (would not) to 10 (would) the degree of support you would be willing to give the screening program if during a 7-year follow-up:

1. Program A reduced the death rate by 34%.
2. Program B produced an absolute reduction in deaths from breast cancer of 0.06%.
3. Program C increased patient survival rate of breast cancer from 99.82% to 99.88%.
4. Program D prevented one death for every 1,588 individuals screened.
5. Program E reduced the odds of death by 34%.

Survival rate (mammography) = 58,077/58,148 = 0.9988 = 99.88%

Survival rate (controls) = 41,028/41,104 = 0.9982 = 99.82%

Program D prevented one death for every 1,588 individuals screened. The number of patients needed to be treated or screened to prevent one adverse outcome is simply the inverse of the absolute risk difference.

Risk difference = 0.00122 − 0.00185 = −0.00063 (0.06%)

Risk difference = absolute risk reduction

Number needed to treat = 1/(absolute risk reduction)

Number needed to treat = 1/0.00063 = 1,588

The number needed to treat can be adjusted for the underlying risk group that is most representative of a particular patient's characteristics and risk if the patient were to go untreated (or receive standard care).

Program E reduced the odds of death by 34%. Estimate the odds of an adverse event for each group by dividing the number of adverse events for each group by the number of people not experiencing that adverse event in that group and then take the ratio of these odds to estimate the odds ratio. The reduction in odds is simply one minus the odds ratio.

Odds (mammography) = 71/58,077 = 0.00122

Odds (controls) = 76/41,028 = 0.00185

Odds ratio = 0.00122/0.00185 = 0.659

Odds reduction = 1 − 0.659 = 0.341 = 34%

This breast cancer screening problem illustrates the special case in which the risk and odds are identical. This only occurs when the number of events is small and the sample sizes are large for both groups, because it does not matter whether the number of events (e.g., deaths) in patients randomized to one group or another (e.g., mammography group) is divided by the total number of people in that group (to calculate relative risk) or by the total number of people who did not experience the event (i.e., were still living), because these numbers are both large and tend to approximate each other.

So why does this matter? People, including physicians, generally tend to confuse odds with risks. It is argued that the concept of *risk* is more easily understood than *odds* and therefore is a more desirable indicator to use to communicate the degree of effectiveness of an intervention.[21] Odds, however, have certain statistical properties that make their calculation and use easier (e.g., in multivariate prediction modeling), whereas calculating "risks" may not be appropriate in some circumstances— for example, in the estimation of effects based on results from case-control studies. Estimates of risk should not be based on results from case-control studies because it is possible to obtain "any value we like for the risk by vary-

ing the number of cases and controls that we choose to study."[22] That is, the investigators choose the number of patients to include in each group and can inflate or deflate the denominator, which does not allow us to calculate an unbiased estimate of risk. All this is made even more problematic because of the well-known difficulty people (both lay and professional) have in understanding statistical and probabilistic concepts.[23]

Applying Evidence to Individual Patients

So the question remains, what is the best way to communicate the results of research studies to make the most informed decisions? Decisions based on a reduction in risk of 34% tend to vary from decisions based on an absolute reduction of risk of less than 1%, although both measures are derived from the same evidence. Empirical data examining the impact of communicating information on actual behavior are lacking, as research in this area is in the early stages of development. Perhaps one way of dealing with this problem when discussing options with patients, particularly those who desire to be more involved in decisions regarding their own care, would be to take the time to walk them through the various representations of the evidence so that they may be fully informed, particularly when the consequences of the decisions are greater.

It is not easy to apply evidence-based medicine in everyday clinical practice. Haynes[24] has identified at least four major barriers. These include (1) the difficulty in finding sound evidence, (2) the lack of clarity of standards of evidence and interpretation, and (3) the mismatch between existing evidence and the clinical situation at hand. All three of these barriers are affected by a huge fourth barrier that underlies the first three: the increasing time pressures and constraints on clinicians that make it difficult, if not almost impossible, to find, synthesize, and interpret evidence in real time that is relevant to a patient's problem. Many experiments, both planned and naturally occurring, are under way to try to overcome these barriers. Just as pharmacists, physician assistants, social workers, and other health professionals are becoming part of group physician practices, so too might information specialists, to whom physicians may turn for identifying evidence. Just as patient care and management plans are reaffirmed or modified when the results of laboratory tests arrive after the patient goes home, so too might they be reaffirmed or modified after the evidence becomes available.

We should keep in mind that evidence-based medicine is not a panacea whose practice will lead to the best solution to each patient's problem. "Evidence-based medicine involves integrating clinical expertise with the best available clinical evidence derived from systematic research," along with patient preferences and

Table 15-3. Five Steps Needed to Practice Evidence-Based Medicine

1. Convert the need for information about a patient's problem into clinically relevant, answerable questions.
2. Find, in the most efficient way, the best evidence with which to answer these questions (whether this evidence comes from clinical examination, laboratory tests, published research, or other sources).
3. Critically appraise the evidence for its validity (i.e., closeness to the truth) and usefulness (i.e., clinical applicability).
4. Integrate the appraisal with your clinical expertise and apply the results to your patient.
5. Evaluate your decision, particularly in light of how well the patient responds.

Source: Reprinted with permission from SE Straus, DL Sackett. Using research findings in clinical practice. BMJ 1998;317:339–342.

choice.[25,26] It is not intended to replace clinical experience and judgment but rather inform and enhance it. "The practice of evidence-based medicine is a process of lifelong, self-directed learning in which caring for patients creates a need for clinically important information about diagnoses, prognoses, treatment, and other health care issues." Straus and Sackett[23] assert that practicing evidence-based medicine is a way for clinicians to keep up with the rapidly growing body of medical literature and to sharpen their skills in asking answerable questions and finding the best evidence to answer these questions by providing a framework for critically appraising evidence.[27–33] The goal is to integrate valid and useful evidence with clinical expertise and each patient's unique features to provide the best care possible. The steps that are considered necessary to effectively practice evidence-based medicine are

Table 15-4. Factors to Consider When Applying Evidence to Individual Patients

Is the relative risk reduction that is attributed to the intervention likely to be different in this case because of the patient's physiologic or clinical characteristics?

What is the patient's absolute risk of an adverse event without the intervention?

Is there significant comorbidity or a contraindication that might reduce the benefit?

Are social or cultural factors present that might affect the suitability of treatment or its acceptability?

What do the patient and the patient's family want?

Source: Reprinted with permission from TA Sheldon, GH Guyatt, A Haines. Getting research findings into practice: when to act on the evidence. BMJ 1998;317:139–142.

summarized in Table 15-3. It is critical always to evaluate how well your decisions and actions based on the evidence actually work when applied to the patient and to modify future decisions and actions accordingly in what may be a very "trial and error" iterative process for some patients.

Some of the factors that are helpful to consider when applying evidence to individual patients have been described by Sheldon et al.[34] and are summarized in Table 15-4. These include (1) whether the relative risk reduction that is attributed to an intervention is likely to be different in your particular patient because of the patient's demographic, physiologic, or clinical characteristics, which may differ from those of the research patients; (2) what the absolute risk of an adverse event without the intervention for this patient would be; (3) whether a significant comorbidity or contraindication exists that might reduce the benefit for your patient; (4) whether social or cultural factors exist that might affect the suitability of treatment or its acceptability; and (5) what the patient and the patient's family prefer to do. Sheldon et al.[34] summarize these steps well when they state, "The decision whether to implement research evidence depends on the quality of the research, the degree of uncertainty of the findings, relevance to the clinical setting, whether the benefits to the patient outweigh any adverse effects, and whether the overall benefits justify the costs when competing priorities and available resources are taken into account." They emphasize that "systematic reviews that show consistent results are likely to provide more reliable research evidence than nonsystematic reviews or single studies." Many social, organizational, or institutional barriers exist that inhibit the incorporation of research-based evidence into clinical practice. The fact that it is often difficult to locate and access patient-relevant information at the point of care should not stop us from using the best evidence that does exist in our decision making. The efforts of individuals working within the Cochrane Collaboration and elsewhere, combined with the ongoing remarkable advances in information technology,[35–37] virtually ensure that the amount and accessibility of valid, reliable evidence to use for informed decision making continues to grow and become increasingly available in real (patient care) time. It is incumbent on us that we begin to make the best use of the best evidence that we can.

Acknowledgments

This work was supported in part by a Fogerty Senior International Fellowship awarded to the author by the National Institutes of Health Fogerty International Center, grant No. NIH 1 F06 TW 02123. The author thanks Jennifer Hoock, M.D., for the many discussions that have helped clarify points raised in this chapter; however, the author assumes sole responsibility for the opinions expressed.

References

1. Doctors' information: excessive, crummy, and bent [editor's choice]. BMJ 1997;315(13 September).

2. Olkin I. Statistical and theoretical considerations in meta-analysis. J Clin Epidemiol 1995;48:133–146.

3. Mulrow CD. Rationale for systematic reviews. BMJ 1994;309:597–599.

4. Chalmers I. The Cochrane Collaboration: preparing, maintaining, and disseminating systematic reviews of the effects of health care [review]. Ann N Y Acad Sci 1993;703:156–163.

5. Chalmers I, Altman DG (eds). Systematic Reviews. London: BMJ Publishing, 1995.

6. Schultz K, Chalmers I, Haynes RJ, Altman DG. Empirical evidence of bias: dimensions of methodological quality associated with estimates of treatment effects in controlled clinical trials. JAMA 1995;273:408–412.

7. Glass GV. Primary, secondary, and meta-analysis of research. Educ Res 1976;5:3–8.

8. Wolf FM, Lefebvre C, McGaghie WC. Identification of meta-analyses in MEDLINE: all that glitters is not gold, or is it [abstract]? Prof Educ Res Q 1996;17:13.

9. Cohen JJ. Higher quality at lower cost: maybe there is a way. Acad Med 1998;73:414.

10. Changing, from top to bottom [editorial]. Lancet 1998;351:997.

11. Naylor CD. Grey zones of clinical practice: some limits to evidence-based medicine. Lancet 1995;345:840–842.

12. Bero L, Rennie D. The Cochrane Collaboration: preparing, maintaining, and disseminating systematic reviews of the effects of health care. JAMA 1995;274:1935–1938.

13. Update Software Home Page. Available at: http://www.update-software.com. Accessed March 31, 1998.

14. Cochrane Collaboration Home Page. Available at: http://www.cochrane.org. Accessed April 6, 1998.

15. Mari JJ, Streiner D. Family Intervention for Schizophrenia. (Cochrane Review). The Cochrane Library, Issue 2. Oxford: Update Software, 1998.

16. Tabar L, Gad A, Holmberg LH, et al. Reduction in mortality from breast cancer after mass screening with mammography. Lancet 1985;1:829–832.

17. Yusef S, Zucker D, Peduzzi P, et al. Effect of coronary artery bypass graft surgery on survival: overview of 10-year results from randomised trials by the Coronary Artery Bypass Graft Surgery Trialists Collaboration. Lancet 1994;344:563–570.

18. Fahey T, Griffiths S, Peters TJ. Evidence based purchasing: understanding results of clinical trials and systematic reviews. BMJ 1995;311:1056–1060.

19. Wolf FM. Using evidence of effectiveness from randomized trials and meta-analyses to make health care decisions: how information is framed may affect judgments [abstract]. Med Decis Making 1996;16:464.

20. Wolf FM. Interpreting Results of RCTs and Meta-Analyses: Implications for Providers, Consumers, and Policy Makers [abstract]. In 2nd International Conference on the Scientific Basis of Health Servies and the 5th Annual International Cochrane Colloquium. Amsterdam, The Netherlands: Dutch Cochrane Centre, 1997;240.

21. Sinclair JC, Bracken MB. Clinically useful measures of effect in binary analyses of randomized trials. J Clin Epidemiol 1994;47:881–889.

22. Altman DG. Practical Statistics for Medical Research. London: Chapman & Hall, 1991;268.

23. Tversky A, Kahneman D. Judgment under uncertainty: heuristics and biases. Science 1974;185:1124–1131.

24. Haynes RB. Some problems in applying evidence in clinical practice [review]. Ann N Y Acad Sci 1993;703:210–224.

25. Straus SE, Sackett DL. Using research findings in clinical practice. BMJ 1998;317:339–342.

26. Sackett DL, Richardson SR, Rosenberg W, Haynes RB. Evidence-based medicine: how to practice and teach EBM. London: Churchill Livingstone, 1997.

27. Guyatt G, Sackett DL, Cook DJ. Users' guides to the medical literature. II: How to use an article about therapy. A. Are the results of the study valid? JAMA 1994;270:2598–2601; B. What were the results and will they help me in caring for my patients? JAMA 1994;271:59–63.

28. Hayward RSA, Wilson MC, Tunis SR, et al. Users' guides to the medical literature. VIII: How to use clinical practice guidelines. A. Are the recommendations valid? JAMA 1995;274:570–574; B. What are the recommendations and will they help you in caring for your patients? JAMA 1995;274:1630–1632.

29. Jaeschke R, Guyatt G, Sackett DL. Users' guides to the medical literature. III: How to use an article about a diagnostic test. A. Are the results of the study valid? JAMA 1994;271:389–391; B. What are the results and will they help me in caring for my patients? JAMA 1994;271:703–707.

30. Levine M, Walter S, Lee H, et al. Users' guides to the medical literature. IV: How to use an article about harm. JAMA 1994;271:1615–1619.

31. Evidence-Based Medicine Working Group. Evidence-based medicine: a new approach to teaching the practice of medicine. JAMA 1992;268:2420–2425.

32. Oxman AD, Cook DJ, Guyatt G. Users' guides to the medical literature. VI: How to use an overview. JAMA 1994;272:1367–1371.

33. Oxman AD, Sackett DL, Guyatt G. Users' guides to the medical literature. I: How to get started. JAMA 1993;270:2093–2095.

34. Sheldon TA, Guyatt GH, Haines A. Getting research findings into practice: when to act on the evidence. BMJ 1998;317:139–142.

35. Kassirer JP. The next transformation in the delivery of health care. N Engl J Med 1995:332:52–54.

36. Glowniak JV. Medical resources on the Internet. Ann Intern Med 1995;123:123–131.

37. Goldwein JW, Benjamin I. Internet-based medical information: time to take charge. Ann Intern Med 1995;123:152–153.

Chapter 16
Computer Aids to Clinical Practice

Thomas H. Payne

Use of computers in clinical care has increased dramatically during the 1990s. Many clinicians and health care organizations have made substantial investments in information technology in efforts to speed access to patient information, sort through data that is relevant to patients, and meet other information needs inherent in clinical practice. In many cases, this effort is justified by evidence, but like the use of other new technologies, use of computing systems in the clinical setting has exceeded what is firmly supported by evidence. An increasing number of well-conducted clinical trials, however, demonstrate that computing systems can be beneficial to patient care. While more research is conducted on the benefits of computers in patient care, we must decide whether to purchase new equipment or modify our practice style, and we must make these decisions without as much evidence as we would like.

Information needs of clinicians are discussed in more detail in Chapter 17, but to summarize, clinicians need information gathered from a variety of sources. Most critical is evidence gathered directly from patients through the history and physical examination, from prior medical records, and from the results of laboratory and radiology tests. Several questions typically arise after clinicians assimilate these data: Could these findings be explained by a well-described clinical syndrome? What confirmatory tests are needed, and how can these be arranged in an efficient sequence? Of available therapies, which is best suited to the patient at hand, and what initial dose might be selected? Is what I have discovered today relevant to others within my practice or patient population? How can I quickly identify those patients?

A classic article on the information needs of physicians revealed that the source physicians turned to most frequently for answers was not a computer, a textbook, or the medical literature but a nearby colleague.[1] Why is this? The colleague is easily accessible, responds to questions in a form that is familiar to all of us (i.e., spoken

English), can provide judgments on available literature and, in many cases, will be accountable for the advice given.

For computers to be useful, they must simplify the process of answering questions clinicians face when making the right decisions. Access to those answers must be rapid and simple or, despite the potential value of computer systems, the answers are unlikely to be used.

In this chapter, we review how computing systems help physicians to gather information on individual patients and patient populations, make better decisions, deliver and document care electronically, and communicate with other professionals and with patients.

These capabilities come with a cost. We begin with an overview of the investment required and end with some cautions to consider when balancing these costs with the advantages discussed.

Investment Required

In the 1990s, any use of computers requires an investment of time to learn to use operating systems and computer programs (called *applications*). Most computers use one of only a few operating systems. Although computers are easier to use than they were in the 1970s, computer use is not intuitive. It takes time to learn to use a mouse and to learn the metaphors of the graphic user interface, such as using windows to find and read text on a screen. Typing skills are needed for many applications; learning to type can reduce anxiety associated with using computer applications.[2]

Purchasing and maintaining computing equipment is expensive. It is encouraging that the cost of powerful computers drops annually, but because newer, more sophisticated software requires more powerful machines, the cost for computing equipment used in an office does not drop as rapidly. To be convenient in practice, com-

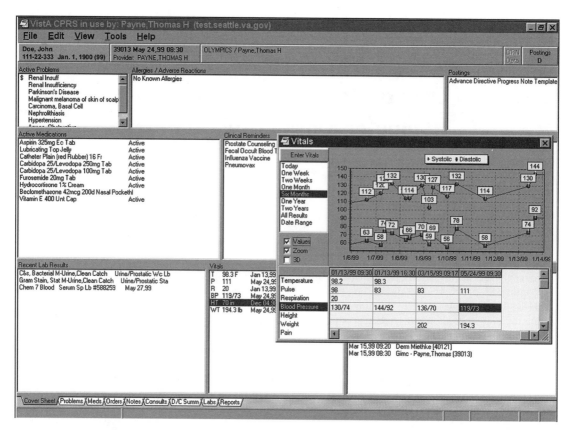

Figure 16-1. Results-reporting screen from the Veterans Administration's Computerized Patient Record System (CPRS).

puters must be available where patient care takes place. Sturdy, portable computers or multiple desktop machines can be used but, with either choice, the computers must be connected by cables and software (a *network*) to access local and Internet information sources. This adds to cost and complexity.

Many of the applications that are most useful to clinicians depend on a substantial infrastructure: databases containing patient data, the ability to send orders from a desktop machine to a laboratory system, or a World Wide Web database that can display patient information from another organization. Individual physicians usually cannot develop or purchase this infrastructure but can advise and lobby organizations where they practice to do so. They can also work to assure that the clinical computing system purchased meets their needs.

How Computing Systems Can Aid Clinical Practice

There are six general ways that computing systems help us take better care of our patients. They can help us gather information about individual patients, manage patient

populations, make clinical decisions, deliver and document care, and communicate with colleagues and patients.

Gathering Information about Individual Patients

Because a large proportion of medical record content is created electronically, display and retrieval of patient information—referred to as *results review*—is one of the most common and useful functions of computers in most physician practices (Figure 16-1). Results review applications are popular because they are a highly convenient means of gathering important data but require little or no practitioner data entry. Results review applications are easier for information systems staff to implement because the data they display—dictated narrative text notes, laboratory and radiology results—are nearly always available from their source system in electronic form. Results review is the "'low-hanging fruit" of clinical computing.

Automated results review is most useful if it includes the patient information from all health care organizations where the patient has received care. Electronic transfer of data from one organization to the next is far less common than collection of laboratory and other data from within the multitude of sources inside a single organization. An increasingly popular method for allowing authorized users to view records of patients from another organization is to use a World Wide Web browser to access a patient data repository,[3] which requires only that the physician have access to the Internet or dial-up access to the sending organization's Intranet and a World Wide Web browser.

Computing systems make possible the storage and review of far more information than numeric and textual information. Radiologic and endoscopy images, electroencephalogram tracings, video clips, and other multimedia data gathered during patient care can be stored and reviewed in computing systems. Adding image review capability to results review applications can increase costs; whether these costs are justified by better decision making, better resource use, and improved patient outcomes is the subject of current research.

Population Management

Searching for literature and guidelines relevant to your practice will be more effective if you are familiar with your patient population. This means understanding the prevalence of health problems in your population, identity of individuals with those problems, medications being used, disease risk factors, and other information derived from records of many patients. Although population-level information of this type can be gathered by reviewing paper charts, this is time consuming and expensive. Automated records make it possible to report clinical characteristics and current therapeutic and patient outcome information on a regular basis. One should not assume, however, that commercially available clinical computing systems allow population-level views of patient information—most focus on viewing data from one patient at a time.

Once a practitioner has an understanding of the demographic and clinical characteristics of the practice population, the next logical step is to use this information to design population-level interventions—to manage the population. With the proper automated tools, for example, it is possible to regularly review data of all patients with diabetes mellitus for whom a practice is responsible. The health care team can then order hemoglobin A_{1c} tests for patients who need them, refer patients for retinoscopy, and arrange foot examinations or a review of cardiovascular risk factors. The combination of a well-organized health care team in which each member knows what role they play and the right population management computing tools can result in better utilization of interventions proved to be effective.[4] The following section details how such tools can be used to increase compliance with health maintenance organization recommendations and clinical practice guidelines.

Aids to Clinical Decision Making

After obtaining a history, conducting a physical examination, and reviewing test results, physicians should consider competing diagnoses and develop a plan for distinguishing between them. Since the 1970s, many computing programs have been created to assist in this task. Because they exhibit characteristics we associate with human intelligence—posing questions and considering a large number of possible or even coexisting conditions—they are referred to as examples of *artificial intelligence*. To be most useful, these programs require substantial amounts of data on the case to be entered, which is time consuming if done by hand. Many of the programs are best suited for relatively limited domains within medicine, such as management of cancer treatment. For these reasons, artificial intelligence applications have not been as broadly adopted in medicine as was predicted.[5,6] The extensive disease databases on which these programs rely, however, have been used for other purposes.[7,8] Commercially available differential diagnostic programs can be very useful for individual complex cases and for educational purposes.

The strongest evidence that computing systems improve care quality comes from applications in which decision aids are embedded in computing systems clinicians are already using. It takes very little effort, for example, for a clinician to place an order for a needed medication if he or she is already using a workstation for order entry. An excellent example of the effectiveness of reminders that are interwoven into the daily routine comes from Boston's Beth Israel Hospital.[9] When clinicians were prompted to order prophylactic antibiotics to prevent *Pneumocystis* pneumonia in patients with low CD4 counts, it required only an additional keystroke to begin the order for the medication. The time between the availability of two CD4 counts of less than 200 cells/mm^3 and the prescription of prophylactic medication was 11 days for patients whose providers received these reminders; for the control patients, the interval was 122 days—a statistically and clinically important difference. Similar results were seen for reminders used to implement other human immunodeficiency virus guidelines.

One of the best examples of the effectiveness of decision aids when they are embedded in clinical computing applications in daily use by clinicians comes from a system used to prescribe antimicrobials at LDS Hospital in Salt Lake City.[10,11] A clinician usually orders antimicrobials after considering patient allergies, likely pathogens, local patterns of antimicrobial resistance, the antimicrobials on the formulary, hepatic and renal function, the results of cultures, and other factors. Even using a results review application, gathering these data can take as long as 25 minutes. In a trial conducted in the critical care unit, the LDS Hospital group studied outcomes for patients for whom antimicrobials were ordered using a program that considers all of these data and makes recommendations for therapy. Patients treated using this computer-assisted management program for antibiotics received fewer doses of antibiotics, had fewer days of excessive drug dosage, fewer prescriptions for drugs to which the patient was allergic, shorter lengths of hospital stay, and lower hospital costs compared with patients treated without this program. Several other improvements were apparent beyond these, leaving little question of the advantage of such an application over the traditional methods for ordering antimicrobials.

The greatest advances in assisting clinician decision making have been in resources available through the Internet and in published data collections on CD-ROM. Bibliographic citation databases; reference texts; and newly released information on therapy, new conditions, and guidelines are now routinely accessible via the World Wide Web from credible organizations. The challenge for the clinician is to distinguish what is valuable for the question at hand from what is preliminary or inaccurate.[12] Numerous reviews are available to direct clinicians to the best available information on the Internet; these guides are available over the World Wide Web.[13] The Uniform Resource Locator (commonly referred to as the *URL*) is the Internet address cited in publications and elsewhere to direct the reader to the resource. The challenge is to make access to all of these resources rapid enough to be practical for clinicians to use during a busy clinic or hospital day. Several excellent examples exist of how a clinical computing system can be designed to simplify access to external (CD-ROM or other) resources during the process of reviewing patient data.[14,15]

Deliver and Document Care: Computer-Based Medical Record Systems

Because a large proportion of patient-specific information needed in day-to-day care is stored in the medical record, computer-based medical record systems have the potential to meet many of clinicians' information needs. Computer-based medical record systems allow review of results, review and creation of notes, order entry, and a view of the longitudinal patient record.[16] Computer-based records have the potential advantages of allowing simultaneous access to the record from many geographically distinct locations, improved legibility, and automatic summarization.[17] The ability to display graphs of laboratory results over time and to list notes sorted by author, topic, or encounter can give the viewer a rapid overview of a patient's history and present condition (Figure 16-2). The paper record can only be arranged one way; information in the electronic record can be organized according to the present need.

Automated reminders for needed care can be generated based on specified algorithms if data on which the algorithm is based are stored in a processible form

rather than solely in narrative text documents (Figure 16-3). This caveat is important: if one wishes to remind a provider to examine the feet of a patient with diabetes who has not recently had this done, then the algorithm to generate the reminder requires data to determine whether a foot examination has been recently performed. For this algorithm to operate, some encoded value must be entered when the foot examination is done—it is not sufficient for a narrative text note to contain that information in an unstructured way. Capturing physical examination findings or other procedures usually means imposing some structure on the way providers enter data into the automated record, but an important benefit of this structure is the ability of automated reminder systems to improve performance of effective preventive and chronic care maneuvers.[18-20]

Some computer-based medical record systems allow practitioner order entry. Those systems that do allow this function have the additional potential to bring data needed to create an order to the attention of the clinician at the time the order is being created. Examples of intelligently designed order entry systems are those from Beth Israel Hospital and LDS Hospital, described above. Other advantages to direct clinician entry of orders are the potential to speed transmission of the order to the filling service, to reduce order transcription errors, and to improve legibility. Costs also can be reduced as was demonstrated when Tierney and colleagues showed that simply displaying past test results in the ordering screen used to order new tests reduces the laboratory test charges by 13%[21] because it is often simpler to order a new test than it is to search for prior results.

An advantage of computer-based record systems that is not as obvious as a listing of individual features is the synergy that can occur when clinicians begin to use the automated medical record for a large number of purposes. For example, if clinicians in an organization regularly turn to the computer-based record to view results, enter orders, and create notes, then they are more likely to see and act on reminders for needed care. It may be easier for the user to learn one new feature of an application with which he or she is already familiar than to learn and regularly use an entirely new application.

The advantages of improved organization and access to the medical record and the ability to modify clinician ordering and patient management behavior have led to growth in the use of computer-based record systems in the United States and internationally.

Introducing a computer-based medical record system has potential disadvantages as well. Clinic and hospital workflow is changed substantially when time-tested paper record and ordering systems are replaced with automated versions.[22] Roles of physicians, nurses, pharmacists, other health professionals, and clerical staff change. Of great concern to clinicians is the additional time that order and note entry can take. It is very quick to write a

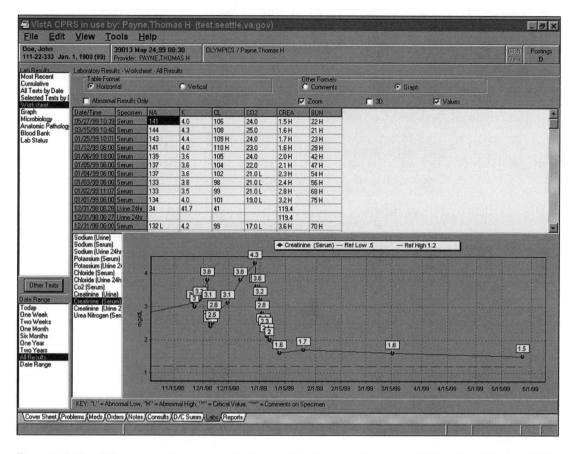

Figure 16-2. Plot of laboratory results created by the Veterans Administration's Computerized Patient Record System (CPRS).

relatively unstructured, marginally legible order on paper but potentially more time consuming to enter required fields for a prescription so that pharmacists can quickly dispense the medication. Even if a net reduction occurs in the time it takes the patient to receive the medication, if it takes more time for the clinician to enter the prescription, the tight clinic schedule is disrupted. If computing applications save physicians time and are viewed as helpful, they are far more likely to be embraced than if they do not. Additionally, potential for error arises when clinicians enter automated orders into the system. Clinicians who are learning to use order entry applications or to enter automated notes may be more prone to error than those with more experience. The potential to detect order entry errors at the time they are entered and to reduce errors due to illegibility are among the strongest incentives for the development of automated order entry applications.[23,24] Whether orders entered directly by clinicians result in fewer errors should be examined with each new order entry application developed.

All computing systems malfunction or "crash" eventually. When clinicians depend on a computer-based record system, the availability of that system is critical.

Contingency plans describing the use of manual or automated backup computing systems must be developed to assure that patient care proceeds when the automated record is not available.

Change of any kind is difficult to introduce into complex organizations such as clinics and hospitals. Computer-based medical record systems are no exception.

How Much Information Is Enough?

As the potential to compile patient information grows, we should recognize that very little research exists to tell us how much information clinicians need to make patient care decisions. Is review of a record summary, including the problem list, medication list, and pertinent recent laboratory results adequate? Should the entire content of the medical record, including scanned versions of outside records, be available? If the entire record is available, can clinicians assimilate and use all of it to make decisions necessary at the time? Is a rudimentary results review application adequate, or is a sophisticated results review system that costs the organization 10 times more worth the cost? Not enough well-designed studies exist to definitively answer these questions.[25]

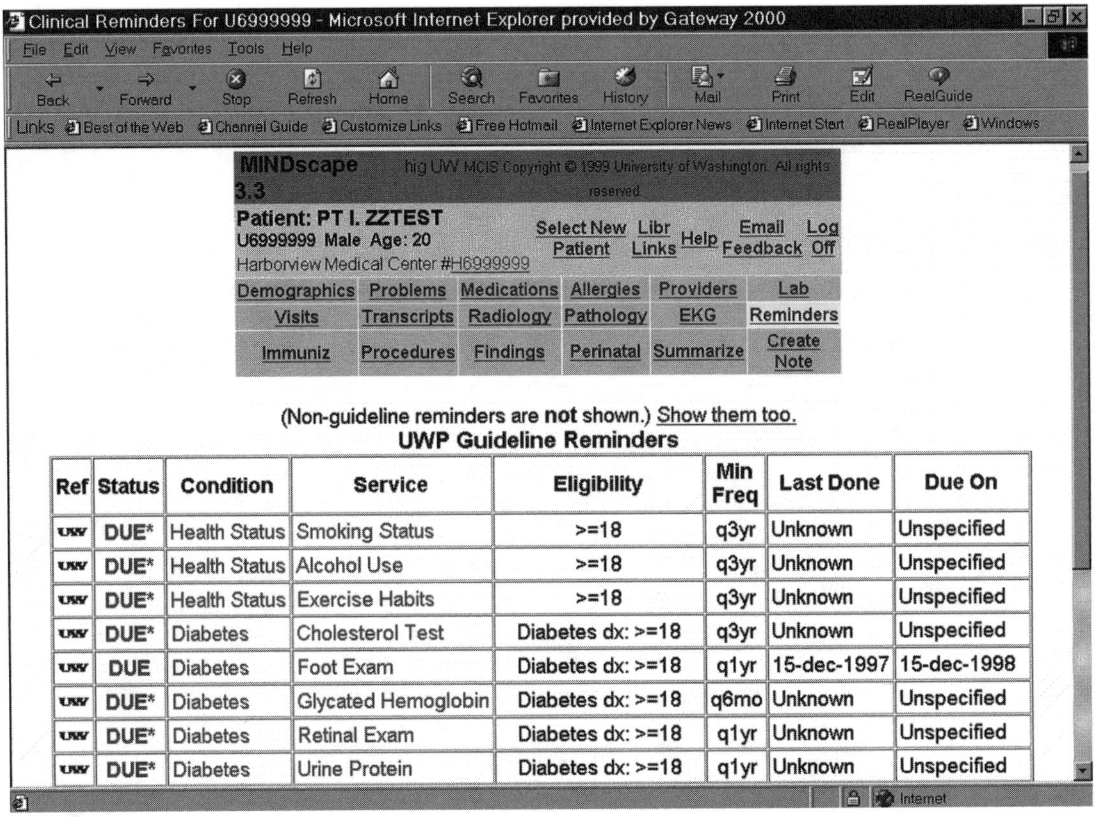

Ref	Status	Condition	Service	Eligibility	Min Freq	Last Done	Due On
UW	DUE*	Health Status	Smoking Status	>=18	q3yr	Unknown	Unspecified
UW	DUE*	Health Status	Alcohol Use	>=18	q3yr	Unknown	Unspecified
UW	DUE*	Health Status	Exercise Habits	>=18	q3yr	Unknown	Unspecified
UW	DUE*	Diabetes	Cholesterol Test	Diabetes dx: >=18	q3yr	Unknown	Unspecified
UW	DUE	Diabetes	Foot Exam	Diabetes dx: >=18	q1yr	15-dec-1997	15-dec-1998
UW	DUE*	Diabetes	Glycated Hemoglobin	Diabetes dx: >=18	q6mo	Unknown	Unspecified
UW	DUE*	Diabetes	Retinal Exam	Diabetes dx: >=18	q1yr	Unknown	Unspecified
UW	DUE*	Diabetes	Urine Protein	Diabetes dx: >=18	q1yr	Unknown	Unspecified

Figure 16-3. Reminders for preventive and chronic care as displayed on a Web-based clinical computing system used at the University of Washington. (Courtesy of Harold Goldberg, M.D.)

Confidentiality of Computer-Based Medical Records

Patients and practitioners are appropriately concerned that electronic health records remain confidential. This concern is growing as computer-based records become more common and contain more health information. Many organizations with computer-based records use a combination of policies and technical measures to prevent unauthorized access to patient information. User agreements, for example, describe appropriate and inappropriate use of computer-based records, policies determine how passwords are issued and what levels of access users have, and firewalls are used to reduce the risk of unauthorized break-ins from the Internet. There are myriad other policy and technical measures that can be adopted to protect electronic health records, as outlined in an excellent review of this topic.[26]

An approach to confidentiality adopted by many computer-based record developers is to audit record access rather than try to anticipate who will need access to each record. It is difficult, for example, to anticipate when one physician will cover for another or when a physician previously uninvolved in a particular patient's care will need record access during an emergency. Knowing that an audit trail exists and providing patients who request it with a list of individuals who have viewed their records may serve as potent deterrents to inappropriate viewing of confidential records.

Two important points must be kept in mind in any discussion of the confidentiality of health records, whether electronic or paper: (1) The risk of inappropriate viewing of electronic patient records may be greater with users who have access to the computing system than with those breaking in from the outside,[27] and (2) measures to protect the confidentiality of health information should extend beyond the bounds of individual health care organizations. Identified health data may be transmitted to health and life insurance companies, pharmacy benefit managers, attorneys, and possibly employers.

Communication with Colleagues

A computer-based medical record system can help with communication concerning a particular patient if all parties have access to such a system—if not, electronic mail may be a very efficient communication tool. Clinical questions, informal consultations, and administrative issues all can be sent via electronic mail to health professionals involved in a patient's care. Because electronic mail systems often are not covered by the security and confidentiality envelope of a well-designed computer-based medical record system and may be connected to the Internet, however, precautions must be taken to protect patient confidentiality.

An important example of the need for communication between all members of a health care team is the presence of an advance directive in the patient's medical record. Evidence suggests that, in the transition between outpatient and inpatient care, inpatient clinicians are often unaware of the presence of advance directives.[28] Many automated medical record systems have provisions for electronic alerts to make the existence of an advance directive known to clinicians wherever the patient is seen. This feature alone can make computing systems worthwhile to clinicians.

Communication with Patients

The proportion of the U.S. population with access to electronic mail is increasing.[29] It is not surprising that patients and their providers find that the advantages of electronic mail also apply to patient-provider communication. The ability to avoid "telephone tag" and to communicate information that would need to be committed to writing (e.g., instructions or directions) make electronic mail well-suited to solving communication problems in health care settings. A growing literature describes how such communication can be organized and efficiently used. Because electronic mail is a relatively new medium for clinical care delivery, it is important to be careful when using it and to make patients aware of its limitations. Published guidelines can help providers understand how electronic mail can be most safely used to communicate with patients.[29]

Other Uses

Clinical computing systems that have been installed and integrated into practice will eventually contain data both on the content and process of care. If health records are computer based, clinical research projects may be conducted without the expense of a paper-chart review. If automated order entry and results review applications are used, enormous potential exists to use the automated record for continuous quality improvement projects.[30] Finally, automating the financial aspects of care is possible using practice management software.

Caveat Emptor

When seeking to capitalize on the potential advantages of computing in clinical care, clinicians should remember several principles. First, the difference between efficacy and effectiveness—well-known in trials of pharmacologic

interventions[31]—applies to this newer technology also. What works well when used by clinicians who are facile with computing and who may have developed the program may not be successful when used by the general physician population. Second, advancements in clinical computing must be tested and proved effective just as with other new technologies. Only through critical testing can problems be identified and solved.[32] Finally, physicians should be open minded in appraising computing technology. Although it often requires substantial and painful change to our practice patterns, irrefutable evidence exists that well-designed clinical computing systems can complement our humanistic abilities and allow us to provide the best possible care to our patients.

References

1. Covell DG, Uman GC, Manning PR. Information needs in office practice:are they being met? Ann Intern Med 1985;103:596–599.
2. Brown SH, Coney RD. Changes in physicians' computer anxiety and attitudes related to clinical information system use. J Am Med Inform Assoc 1994;1:381–394.
3. van Wingerde FJ, Schindler J, Kilbridge P, et al. Using HL7 and the World Wide Web for unifying patient data from remote databases. Proc AMIA Annu Fall Symp 1996;643–647.
4. Taplin S, Galvin MS, Payne T, et al. Putting population-based care into practice: real option or rhetoric. J Am Board Fam Prac 1998;11:116–126.
5. Schwartz WB, Patil RS, Szolovits P. Artificial intelligence in medicine. Where do we stand? N Engl J Med 1987;316:685–688.
6. Miller RA, Masarie FE Jr. The demise of the "Greek Oracle" model for medical diagnostic systems. Methods Inf Med 1990;291:1–2.
7. Miller RA. Medical diagnostic decision support systems—past, present, and future. J Am Med Inform Assoc 1994;1:8–27.
8. Warner H Jr, Blue SR, Sorenson D, et al. New computer-based tools for empiric antibiotic decision support. Proc AMIA Annu Fall Symp 1997;238–42.
9. Safran C, Rind DM, Davis RB, et al. Guidelines for management of HIV infection with computer-based patient's record. Lancet 1995;346:341–346.
10. Pestotnik SL, Classen DC, Evans RS, Burke JP. Implementing antibiotic practice guidelines through computer-assisted decision support: clinical and financial outcomes. Ann Intern Med 1996;124:884–890.
11. Evans RS, Pestotnik SL, Classen DC. A computer-assisted management program for antibiotics and other antiinfective agents. N Engl J Med 1998;338:232–238.
12. Silberg WM, Lundberg GD, Musacchio RA. Assessing, controlling, and assuring the quality of medical information on the Internet. Caveant lector et viewor—let the reader and viewer beware. JAMA 1997;277:1244–1245.

13. Sikorski R, Peters R. Internet anatomy 101. Accessing information on the World Wide Web [directory]. JAMA 1997;277:171–172.

14. Nielson C, Smith CS, Lee D, Wang M. Implementation of a relational patient record with integration of educational and reference information. Proc Annu Symp Comput Appl Med Care 1994;125–129.

15. Tarczy-Hornoch P, Kwan-Gett TS, Fouche L, et al. Meeting clinician information needs by integrating access to the medical record and knowledge resources via the Web. Proc AMIA Annu Fall Symp 1997; 809–813.

16. Dick RS, Steen EB, Detmer DE (eds). The Computer-Based Patient Record: An Essential Technology for Health Care. Washington, DC: National Academy Press, 1997.

17. Barnett GO. The application of computer-based medical-record systems in ambulatory practice. N Engl J Med 1984;310:1643–1650.

18. McDonald CJ, Hui SL, Smith DM, et al. Reminders to physicians from an introspective computer medical record. A two-year randomized trial. Ann Intern Med 1984;100:130–138.

19. Johnston ME, Langton KB, Haynes RB, Mathieu A. Effects of computer-based clinical decision support systems on clinician performance and patient outcome. A critical appraisal of research. Ann Intern Med 1994; 120:135–142.

20. Shea S, DuMouchel W, Bahamonde L. A meta-analysis of 16 randomized controlled trials to evaluate computer-based clinical reminder systems for preventive care in the ambulatory setting. J Am Med Inform Assoc 1996;3:399–409.

21. Tierney WM, McDonald CJ, Martin DK, Rogers MF. Computerized display of past test results. Effect on outpatient testing. Ann Intern Med 1987;107:569–574.

22. Sittig DF, Stead WW. Computer-based physician order entry: the state of the art. J Am Med Inform Assoc 1994;1:108–123.

23. Schiff GD, Rucker TD. Computerized prescribing: building the electronic infrastructure for better medication usage. JAMA 1998;279:1024–1029.

24. Bates EW, Leape LL, Cullen DJ, et al. Effect of computerized physician order entry and a team intervention on prevention of serious medication errors. JAMA 1998;280:1311–1316.

25. Whiting-O'Keefe QE, Simborg DW, Epstein WV, Warger A. A computerized summary medical record system can provide more information than the standard medical record. JAMA 1985;254:1185–1192.

26. Committee on Maintaining Privacy and Security in Health Care Applications of the National Information Infrastructure. For The Record. Washington, DC: National Academy Press, 1997.

27. Rind DM, Kohane IS, Szolovits P, et al. Maintaining the confidentiality of medical records shared over the Internet and the World Wide Web. Ann Intern Med 1997;127:138–141.

28. Morrison RS, Olson E, Mertz KR, Meier DE. The inaccessibility of advance directives on transfer from ambulatory to acute care settings. JAMA 1995;274: 478–482.

29. Kane B, Sands DZ. Guidelines for the clinical use of electronic mail with patients. JAMA 1998;5:104–111.

30. Ornstein SM, Jenkins RG, Lee FW, et al. The computer-based patient record as a CQI tool in a family medicine center. Jt Comm J Qual Improv 1997;23:347–361.

31. Weinstein MC, Fineberg HV. Clinical Decision Analysis. Philadelphia: Saunders, 1980.

32. McDonald CJ, Overhage JM. Guidelines you can follow and trust. An ideal and an example. JAMA 1994;271:872–873.

Chapter 17
Information at the Point of Care: Answering Clinical Questions*

Mark Ebell

I have no particular talent. I am merely inquisitive.

—*Albert Einstein*

As physicians, we gather information from patients in the form of answers to questions, patient stories, physical examination maneuvers, and test results. We integrate that information with information about our patient, the patient's family and community, and information from original research, colleagues, textbooks, and a variety of other sources. We then develop a plan for evaluation and management and implement it by communicating it to the patient and other parts of the health system. This flow of information is expensive: Physicians spend more than one-third of their time recording and synthesizing information, and communications consume one-third of a typical hospital's budget.[1]

As we approach the twenty-first century, however, most of us are still using outdated tools to manage medical information. We scribble illegible notes in a chart, try to keep problem and medication lists up-to-date by hand, send letters to consultants, and call the laboratory for results. Questions arise at the point of care but go unanswered. Practice patterns ossify, and our textbooks become outdated. Several questions arise as we consider this dilemma:

1. What questions do clinicians ask at the point of care?
2. What is the relationship between clinical questions, lifelong learning, and evidence-based medicine (EBM)?

3. How can clinicians answer clinical questions at the point of care, when the answers are most likely to affect clinical practice?
4. As a primary care physician, how can I begin to answer my clinical questions more effectively?

This chapter addresses all of these questions. However, it is important first to define what is meant by a clinical question. Researchers often use the term *information need* to describe the broad range of questions asked by physicians during the care of patients. It can include patient-specific information needs such as "Does this patient have rales?", "What is the serum creatinine?", and "I wonder why he or she has back pain?" asked during the data-gathering phase of the encounter. It can also include logistic and administrative questions such as "Does this patient's insurance cover x-rays?" and "Does Dr. Hart accept patients with Medicaid?" asked during the implementation phase. For this discussion, we focus on generalizable questions about patient care that can potentially be answered by the medical literature. These questions are typically generated when patient data are being integrated with generalizable medical knowledge to develop a management plan. Some examples of such clinical questions include:

1. What is the appropriate regimen for treatment of herpes zoster infection with famciclovir?
2. How effective is famciclovir at preventing postherpetic neuralgia?

*Reprinted with permission from M Ebell. Information at the point of care: answering clinical questions. J Am Board Fam Pract 1999;12:225–235.

3. What test, if any, should I order for an otherwise well but worried dyspeptic patient whose brother was just diagnosed with pancreatic cancer?
4. What is the best test for a jaundiced, 50-year-old man who has lost 20 pounds and has a family history of pancreatic cancer?
5. Should I empirically treat this febrile child with sore throat for streptococcal pharyngitis or should I order a rapid antigen test?
6. What should I do for this 53-year-old male smoker who has a cholesterol of 260 mg/dl?
7. Does my patient with a corneal abrasion need a patch?
8. What is the most cost-effective approach to the management of a urinary tract infection?

Clinical questions are the result of critical reflection by a clinician on his or her practice. By better understanding their clinical questions generated at the point of care, family physicians can identify strategies for answering these questions using relevant and valid information and thereby improve the care of patients. We answer some of the above clinical questions in the rest of this chapter as we discuss the information needs of primary care physicians at the point of care.

What Questions Do Clinicians Ask at the Point of Care?

When asked at the end of a half-day of patient care to recall how many questions they had that related to patient care, physicians reported one question for every four patients.[2] Direct observation of primary care physicians, however, has shown that they generate an average of two questions for every three patient encounters.[3] For a physician seeing 25 patients per day, this represents approximately 15 questions.

These and similar studies have shown that a tremendous variety exists in the questions asked by physicians and that these questions are often complex and patient-specific. Approximately 33% relate to treatment, 25% to diagnosis, and 15% to pharmacotherapeutics.[3–5] When questions are pursued and answered, more than half of the answers come from textbooks and human sources, including both office partners and consultants.[5] The *Physicians' Desk Reference* is perhaps the most commonly identified source of answers. Electronic sources of information rarely are used.[3,4] Approximately two-thirds of the clinical questions generated at the point of care, however, go unanswered.[3] Are these questions important? In one study, researchers gave the unanswered questions to medical librarians. The authors of the study then gave the answers to the physicians who had asked the questions and found that approximately half of the answers would have had a direct impact on patient care.[6]

Why are more of these questions not answered? Limitations include a lack of convenient access to reference materials at the point of care, the time needed to search for information, and the challenge of formulating an "answerable" question.[4] Two characteristics that predict whether physicians seek and find an answer to a clinical question are the urgency of the problem and the physician's confidence that he or she will find an answer.[7] Consider the physician, for example, who wants to know how to prescribe famciclovir for herpes zoster virus. Although he or she can be confident of finding a dosage recommendation in the *Physicians' Desk Reference*, this reference does not answer questions about the medication's effectiveness. Information about the number of patients he or she would have to treat to prevent a case of postherpetic neuralgia might be found in a randomized trial, but the physician is unlikely to be able to access that information at the point of care, and the question remains unanswered. Thus, the information a patient and physician needs to decide whether it is worth paying for and taking the medication is not available.

A useful way to think about clinical questions is by the "type of information need."[8] A relatively large randomized controlled trial has shown, for example, that patching corneal abrasions only increases discomfort and healing time.[9] A family physician who is unaware of this continues to patch corneal abrasions and has an unrecognized information need because his or her patients would benefit from such a change in practice. When that family physician asks the clinical question, "I wonder whether any evidence exists that patching corneal abrasions improves outcomes that my patients and I care about?", he or she has recognized an information need and asked a clinical question. When the physician asks a colleague, he or she begins to pursue the information need. Searching the *Journal of Family Practice* POEMs (*patient-oriented evidence that matters*) Web site (http://www.infopoems.com) using the term *corneal abrasion* identifies an article that answers the clinical question, and the information need is now satisfied. Finally, the information must be implemented in the physician's practice to affect patient outcomes.

This pathway is not linear; rather, it is a cycle, because medical science is dynamic rather than static, and new information is constantly becoming available. Yesterday's satisfied and implemented information need is tomorrow's unrecognized need. A new study has convincingly shown, for example, that topical nonsteroidal anti-inflammatory drops reduce pain and speed healing in corneal abrasion.[10] If use of nonsteroidal anti-inflammatory drops was not the standard practice for this physician, he or she has an unrecognized need and begins the process anew. One way to illustrate this search for information is shown in Figure 17-1.

In addition to the type of need, several other ways exist to classify physician information needs. Woolf describes several other characteristics of an information need: the *type* of information (e.g., diagnostic, prognostic, therapeutic), the *organ system*, and the *source* of information used to answer the question.[5] Osheroff describes the generalizability of an

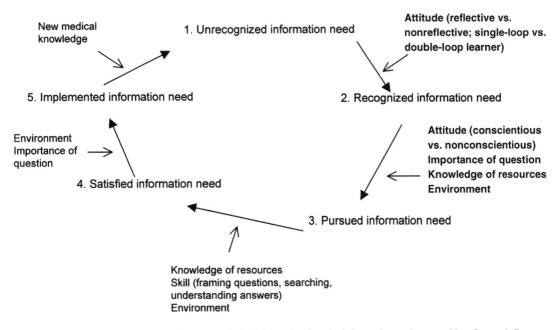

Figure 17-1. A model for the information needs of physicians, showing the information pathway and key factors influencing each step.

information need as whether it can be satisfied by generalizable sources of information, such as original research and the *Physicians' Desk Reference*, or whether the information need is specific to a particular patient.[8] These different ways of classifying information needs (including clinical questions) are summarized in Table 17-1.

Clinical Questions, Lifelong Learning, and Evidence-Based Medicine

Although physicians are encouraged to practice lifelong learning, and continuing medical education is required by many organizations, lifelong learning has not been successful at improving patient outcomes.[11] Physician practice changes in haphazard ways that are not often driven by the best available evidence. In fact, the best predictor of physicians' prescribing behavior regarding antihypertensives is their year of graduation from medical school![12] Adult learning theory suggests that physicians learn best when learning[13]

Is in the context of patient care
Answers their questions
Is directly applicable to their work
Does not take too much time

Physicians who want to be successful lifelong learners, therefore, need highly developed critical reflection skills. Applying these skills to their practice and generating clinical questions at the point of care is central to physician education and lifelong learning. To take an evidence-based approach to practice, these questions must be answered using the most valid, relevant information available.

Recall Figure 17-1, which diagrams a continuous process of identifying information deficits and meeting them. The ideal evidence-based practitioner critically reflects on his or her practice on a regular basis, asking whether a better way to do things exists. He or she then answers the questions generated by this process of critical reflection using relevant, valid information rather than anecdote or opinion whenever possible. Finally, answers to questions that change the physician's practice are implemented. Many potential barriers to this ideal model of reflective, evidence-based practice exist. These are summarized in Figure 17-1, along with the information pathway itself.

The first step in the information pathway is recognition that an information need exists. The willingness to recognize that one's knowledge may not be complete appears to be driven primarily by physician attitude and personality. Work by educators in the area of critical reflection suggests that this is a mature, high-level skill,[14] but that it may be undermined by an emphasis on what Argyris calls *single-loop* rather than *double-loop* learning.[15] Consider the example of a patient who presents with a cough, is diagnosed with bronchitis, and is given erythromycin. When he or she returns two days later with persistent symptoms, the physician changes the antibiotic.

Table 17-1. Ways to Classify Medical Information Needs

Axis	Components	Example
I. Type of need		
	Unrecognized	Should have looked for drug interaction.
	Recognized	Thought about drug interaction but did not pursue.
	Pursued	Looked for drug interaction information but did not find it.
	Satisfied	Found information about a drug interaction.
	Implemented	Does not prescribe a medication because of the interaction.
II. Type of information		
	Etiology	Can *Mycoplasma pneumoniae* cause a sore throat?
	Differential diagnosis	What diagnoses should I consider in this patient with sore throat?
	Clinical diagnosis	Is viral pharyngitis likely in a patient with exudate and adenopathy?
	Laboratory diagnosis	Is the rapid streptococcus screen accurate enough to rule out streptococcus if negative?
	Treatment	Is amoxicillin, 500 mg bid, for 6 days as effective as 250 mg tid for 10 days?
	Prognosis	If my patient is still symptomatic in 2 days, should I change therapy?
	Patient education	What should I tell my patient about communicability?
	Administrative	Does this patient's insurance cover the cost of antibiotics?
III. Organ system		
	Cardiovascular	What is the appropriate starting dose for enalapril in an 80 year old?
	Pulmonary	When should I start inhaled corticosteroids in an asthmatic patient?
	Gastrointestinal	Is there a role for *Helicobacter pylori* eradication in nonulcer dyspepsia?
IV. Source of information		
	Colleague	Asked one of my partners
	Textbook	Consulted *Harrison's Textbook of Internal Medicine*
	Original research	Referred to a recent *Journal of the American Medical Association* article
	Online database	Did a MEDLINE search
	Other	—
V. Generalizability		
	Generalizable knowledge	What is the likelihood ratio for a CAGE score of 3?
	Patient-specific question	What is this patient's most recent serum creatinine level?

CAGE = screening test for alcoholism (Have you ever felt the need to *c*ut down or tried to quit? Have others been *a*nnoyed at your use? Have you felt *g*uilty about your use or behavior when using? Have you taken a morning drink or pill [*e*ye opener] to feel better?).

This type of learning is *single-loop*, because the physician reacts to the situation without questioning his or her underlying assumptions. A more reflective practitioner practices *double-loop* learning: When the patient returns, both the underlying diagnosis and the treatment strategy are questioned. Perhaps the patient does not have bronchitis? Perhaps the patient has reflux or allergies? What if the patient's bronchitis is viral and the antibiotic is not going to help anyway? Do antibiotics help even if the bronchitis is bacterial? The reflective practitioner, even in this simple clinical situation, generates a host of important questions.

In addition to generating more clinical questions, the reflective practitioner is more likely to practice patient-centered medicine, tailoring their management strategy to the patient's clinical picture, needs, and situation. For example, taking a "one-size-fits-all" approach to the management of sore throat by ordering a rapid antigen test on everyone provides too much care for some and not enough for others. By reflecting on practice and asking whether a rapid antigen test is needed for this particular patient, care is individualized and, it is hoped, outcomes are improved.

Traditional medical education, however, values knowing the right answer more than asking the right question. Too often, the intern or medical student who asks a question is "punished" with the task of reporting the answer back to the group the next day! The traditional, paternalistic view of physicians as all-knowing may make them afraid to admit that they do not know everything and less likely to critically appraise their current practice. Phrases such as, "This is the Michigan State (or Harvard or Duke) way" and "We have always done it this way and my patients do fine," further undermine our willingness and ability to critically reflect on our practice. Argyris has described similar defensive strategies in the business setting and called them *learned incompetence*. Just as General Motors was slow to change its practices during the 1970s and 1980s, physicians find many reasons to justify the status quo and resist positive change.

The decision to pursue a clinical question is perhaps the most complex step in the information pathway, influenced by physician attitude, personality, and work ethic; the characteristics of the question; and the practice environment. Research has shown that the decision to pursue a clinical question is driven most strongly by the importance of the question and the perceived availability of an answer to the question.[7] The former may vary depending on physician characteristics, such as conscientiousness, work ethic, and sense of duty to their practice. One physician, for example, may feel that it is important to find out the best way to treat corneal abrasions because the wrong decision may adversely effect some patients. Another may be more complacent, however, and feel that using a patch has always worked well enough. The perceived availability of an answer to the question depends in part on the physician's knowledge of available resources. For example, a physician wondering about the efficacy of corticosteroids in preterm labor might continue to wonder because he or she feels that it would be too difficult to find the answer. Knowing, however, that the Cochrane Database of Systematic Reviews has many excellent systematic reviews on perinatal topics might stimulate the physician to look there for an answer, especially if he or she has the necessary computer skills. Finally, environmental factors, such as access to information sources and the time available between patients, affect the decision to pursue a clinical question. Having the Cochrane Database of Systematic Reviews abstracts on a handheld computer or CD-ROM in the clinical area would eliminate a trip to the library and reduce the time needed to access the review.

Physicians' abilities to satisfy an information need and answer clinical questions is determined by the their knowledge of available resources, their skill at framing a question and searching these resources, and their context or environment. Physicians tend to frame questions in relation to specific patients[4,8] rather than in a generalizable fashion as advocated by teachers of EBM.[16] For example, a family physician might ask, "I have a 38-year-old patient with dyspepsia whose father was diagnosed with pancreatic cancer. He is very worried that he has pancreatic cancer and I want to reassure him. What is the best test to rule out pancreatic cancer

for him? Should I order an ultrasound?" A clinical epidemiologist or EBM proponent might frame this question as, "What is the test with the best negative likelihood ratio for pancreatic cancer among outpatients like this with dyspepsia?" Finally, a research article might provide information in terms of sensitivity and specificity but not mention the term *likelihood ratio*. In addition, the researchers may present data as false-positive and false-negative rates rather than sensitivity or specificity, further confusing the naive reader.

Bridging these gaps between the language of physicians, clinical epidemiologists, and researchers will be a challenge for teachers and researchers as we try to link research findings to practice. Although physicians may have to learn to frame their questions in a more generalizable way, information sources should also avoid jargon and help us bridge this gap from clinical question to original research. For example, a software "Answer Wizard" could help physicians frame questions in a way that is most likely to get a useful answer from a medical database.

The practice environment also influences our ability to answer a clinical question in terms of time and availability of resources. A physician with rapid access to a handheld computer version of a clinical prediction rule for the diagnosis of streptococcal pharyngitis could determine that the likelihood of streptococcus in a child with fever, sore throat, adenopathy, exudate, and no cough exceeds 40% and that empiric treatment is appropriate. Without that clinical prediction rule in a rapidly available format, he or she might order a rapid antigen test and be misled by a false-negative test result.

Finally, the decision to implement the answer to a clinical question in practice depends on environmental factors, such as cost, health system constraints, patient acceptance, acceptance of colleagues, and local practice patterns. The amount of work needed to implement a change and the importance of the question are both important. It is easy to stop patching corneal abrasions, for example, but very difficult to establish a stroke unit in a local hospital. Nevertheless, if the outcomes are important enough in terms of reduced morbidity and mortality, then it should be worth the effort to establish such a unit.

An evidence-based approach to care is potentially very information intensive. It challenges physicians to not only know the *what* of care, but the *how much* as well. Taking an evidence-based approach to answering clinical questions challenges physicians to take their answers to the next level, using tools such as likelihood ratios and the number needed to treat to choose the right test or intervention for a particular patient. This approach should improve the care of patients by helping physicians select the right tests and the most effective therapies for their patients. Practicing in this way, however, may actually intensify the information needs of primary care physicians at the point of care.

Consider the diagnostic example of a worried patient with dyspepsia who is convinced that he or she has pancreatic cancer. When the likelihood of disease is low and a patient needs reassurance—a common situation in primary care practice—our job is more about ruling *out* disease than ruling *in* disease. Many physicians might order a serum amylase, thinking that a normal level reduces the likelihood of disease. Amylase has a negative likelihood ratio of close to 1 for the diagnosis of pancreatic cancer, however, meaning that a normal value does not appreciably reduce the likelihood of disease.[17] Ordering the test is wasteful and could even be harmful if the patient and physician are falsely reassured. Ultrasound is a better test because it is noninvasive and does a better job of ruling out disease.

When discussing therapeutics, it is common to think in terms of risk reduction. For example, how much does pravastatin (Pravachol) reduce the risk of death in men at high risk of developing heart disease? One study[18] showed that over a 5-year period use of pravastatin decreased the all-cause mortality rate from 4.1% to 3.2%, a 22% *relative* risk reduction ($[4.1 - 3.2]/4.1 = 22\%$). However, the *absolute* risk reduction is only 0.9% ($4.1 - 3.2 = 0.9\%$). This is a less impressive number than the 22% relative risk reduction, even though the underlying data have not changed! An even more clinically meaningful way of describing the benefits of treatment uses the number needed to treat (commonly referred to as *NNT*). Dividing the absolute risk reduction of 0.9% into 100, one finds that 110 adults at high risk of developing heart disease would have to take pravastatin for 5 years to prevent one death. This information can help physicians and patients put the costs, risks, and benefits of cholesterol-lowering therapy into perspective.

In conclusion, for physicians to become reflective, evidence-based practitioners, it is important that they

Critically reflect on their practice, using double-loop learning that questions underlying assumptions about care

Value the questions

Have the skills, time, and resources to answer questions using evidence-based sources of information

Implement the answers to questions in the care of patients

How Can We Answer Clinical Questions at the Point of Care?

Information Mastery Instead of Evidence-Based Medicine

Richard Smith, editor of the *British Medical Journal*, states, "New information tools are needed: they are likely to be electronic, portable, fast, easy to use, connected to both a large valid database of medical knowledge and the patient record, and a servant of the patient as well as doctors."[4] David Slawson and Allen Shaughnessy have described the usefulness of medical information as follows:[19]

$$\text{Usefulness of information} = \frac{\text{relevance} \times \text{validity}}{\text{work}}$$

Thus, the most useful information is relevant to your practice, highly valid, and takes very little work to acquire. This insight can guide us in identifying and even designing resources for answering clinical questions at the point of care.

The traditional approach to EBM involves a five-step approach: question, search, appraise, apply, and evaluate. This approach emphasizes validity assessment more than relevance, advocates formal MEDLINE searches, and encourages physicians to read the original research literature and do their own critical appraisal.[20] This is a time-consuming process, however, that is impractical for the busy clinician. Slawson and Shaughnessy have advocated an approach that they call *information mastery*. Information mastery takes a more balanced approach and emphasizes an initial assessment of outcomes and relevance before proceeding to the assessment of validity. Central to information mastery is the concept of POEMs.[19] A POEM has several key characteristics:

1. The article asks a question that is relevant to primary care practice.
2. It uses patient-oriented outcomes such as symptoms, mortality, cost, or quality of life.
3. If they are valid, the results have the potential to change your practice.

Articles that meet these criteria are POEMs, and physicians are obligated to know about them because they can help patients live better or longer lives. Slawson and Shaughnessy argue that they should be the focus of efforts to both stay up-to-date and answer clinical questions.[19] They also apply their criteria for validity and relevance to information sources other than the original literature and emphasize use of secondary sources of literature such as *Evidence-Based Practice, Evidence-Based Medicine, Journal of Family Practice* POEMs, and the *ACP Journal Club*.

The difference between traditional EBM and information mastery is shown graphically in Figure 17-2. Although the traditional approach remains the basis for those who perform meta-analyses, systematic reviews, and critical appraisals for secondary literature journals, information mastery provides a much more accessible and efficient way for physicians to be up-to-date and to answer their clinical questions rapidly at the point of care. For example, it is much easier to search the Cochrane

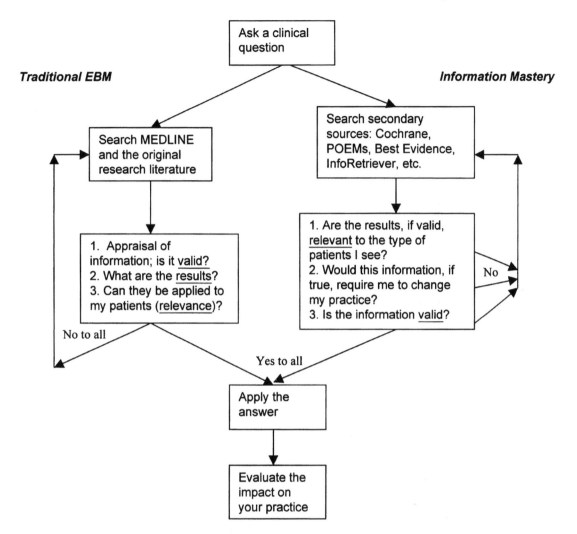

Figure 17-2. Traditional evidence-based medicine (*left path*) and information mastery (*right path*). Note that information mastery offers a more efficient approach to implementing an evidence-based approach to patient care because it emphasizes the use of "predigested" sources of information and a brief relevance screen before the more lengthy validity evaluation. (EBM = evidence-based medicine; POEMs = *p*atient-*o*riented *e*vidence that *m*atters.)

Database of Systematic Reviews, Best Evidence, or InfoRetriever CD-ROMs than to search all of MEDLINE. Also, rather than beginning with a time-consuming validity assessment, Slawson and Shaughnessy advocate reading the abstract to see whether the outcomes are patient-oriented and whether the conclusion recommends a change to your current practice. If either answer is no, you can stop and move on to the next article.

Using Computers at the Point of Care

One way to reduce the work of answering clinical questions is to make information easily available on a computer. Two studies have looked at physician expectations and desires for computer-based information. Woolf found that the places

where information was most needed (i.e., clinic and ward) were not considered the most convenient for a terminal-based solution, suggesting that a mobile, handheld solution would be especially useful to physicians.[5] This is particularly true for family physicians, whose clinical questions may arise in the office, the hospital, the nursing home or extended care facility, or at home while on call.

In a survey of Michigan family physicians, Ebell and colleagues found that 85% would be willing to carry a handheld computer during patient care activities. Characteristics especially valued by family physicians in decision support software included: the ability to update information, a uniform interface, drug information, current treatment recommendations, and the ability to print patient educational materials.[21] Handheld computers

Table 17-2. Web-Based Sources of Evidence-Based Clinical Information

Site and Web Address	Comment
Journal of Family Practice POEMs http://www.infopoems.com	More than 320 critical appraisals of key primary care research literature; updated regularly, with 96 new POEMs added per year
Turning Research Into Practice (TRIP) http://www.gwent.nhs.gov.uk/trip	Excellent Welsh site lets you search more than 12 evidence-based sites at once
Cochrane Database of Systematic Reviews http://www.update-software.com/ccweb/ cochrane/revabstr/abidix.htm	Abstracts only of more than 500 systematic reviews
Bandolier http://www.jr2ox.ac.uk/Bandolier/index.html	Popular British site—includes essays and features a good sense of humor
Primary Care Guideline Repository http://itsa.ucsf.edu/~petsam	Excellent collection of practice guidelines, mostly evidence-based
Agency for Health Care Policy and Research http://www.ahcpr.gov	Access point for the Agency for Health Care Policy and Research's Clinical Practice Guidelines and the U.S. Preventive Services Task Force screening recommendations, among others
National Guidelines Clearinghouse http://www.guidelines.gov	Large collection of guidelines, with detailed descriptions of how they were created

POEMs = *p*atient-*o*riented *e*vidence that *m*atters.

appear to be a promising tool for quickly answering physicians' clinical questions in any location because they are highly portable, turn on and off immediately, and have adequate memory and speed for the task of medical information management and reference.[22] Eventually, these units will provide inexpensive, continuous, wireless connections to the Internet and local area networks.

Many physicians have computers at or near the point of care. Excellent sources of evidence-based information for desktop computers include the Cochrane Library (http://www.update-software.com/ccweb/cochrane/cdsr.htm) from the Cochrane Collaboration and the Best Evidence reference from the American College of Physicians and the British Medical Journal Publishing Group (http://www.acponline.org), both available on CD-ROM. Useful Web sites for answering clinical questions using evidence-based information are shown in Table 17-2.

At Michigan State University, Ebell and colleagues have developed a handheld software program that brings together a variety of evidence-based sources of information.[23] The design goal was to allow physicians to answer clinical questions with evidence-based, relevant, valid information in less than 1 minute. Resources on InfoRetriever include:

1. Abstracts from the Cochrane Database of Systematic Reviews (more than 400: 100 new abstracts added per year)

2. *Journal of Family Practice* POEMs critical appraisals (more than 300: 100 new abstracts added per year)
3. *Evidence-Based Practice* newsletter brief critical appraisals (300: 300 new abstracts added per year)
4. Key evidence-based guidelines
5. Detailed history, physical examination, and diagnostic test information integrated in a calculator for interpreting results
6. Validated clinical prediction rules
7. Drug information

The software originally written for the Newton series of handheld computers (now discontinued) has been ported to the Windows 95, Windows NT, and Windows CE operating systems for desktop and handheld computers (http://www.infopoems.com). Studies to evaluate the impact of InfoRetriever on student learning, physician behavior, and a physician's ability to answer questions are under way.

Certainly, more research is needed on the information needs of primary care physicians. First, we must collect and classify clinical questions in a variety of settings, creating a taxonomy of information needs. Other studies will include comparisons of different types of physicians who might have different needs,[5,7] a focus on the effect of interventions on both patient outcomes and information-seeking behavior,[7] studies that consider physician characteristics and learning styles, and interventional trials of comparing different methods of information delivery. In addition, informatics researchers and software designers must develop systems that help physicians frame an answerable question using the language of clinicians rather than researchers and develop tools that act as servants or even agents of the physician (rather than the other way around!).[5]

How Can I Get Started?

You can immediately take several steps to more effectively answer clinical questions at the point of care. They are as follows:

1. *Reflect on your practice on a regular basis.* As a medical student, resident, and practitioner, you have built an extensive database of clinical experience and medical knowledge. Like any database, however, it can grow outdated. Regularly reflecting on your decisions and practices stimulates clinical questions. Answering these clinical questions using valid, relevant information keeps your database up-to-date. A simple way to do this is to keep an index card in your pocket and to write down questions that you cannot answer immediately. Commit yourself to answer at least one or two of the most compelling questions each week.

2. *Inquire, do not advocate.* Too often, physicians advocate their own plan for a patient or their own belief about a condition rather than inquire into the best possible approach for our patient(s). Advocacy is characterized by statements such as, "I think . . . ," "I believe . . . ," "The facts are . . . ," "Experience says . . . ," and "My colleagues always . . . ." Inquiry, on the other hand, is characterized by statements such as, "What do you think . . . ," "I wonder if there is a better way to . . . ," "Should I keep doing this . . . ," and "Why have I always . . . ." When you find yourself making advocacy statements, ask yourself whether you could instead inquire. Whereas advocacy tends to uphold the status quo, inquiry leads to new knowledge and new insights.

3. *Feel good about not knowing everything.* It is impossible for any physician, especially a primary care physician, to know everything. Ours is a specialty defined in breadth rather than depth.[24] Your reading, therefore, should focus on problems common in or important to your patients. When you find an article about such a problem, make sure it uses outcomes that matter to your patients, such as symptom improvement, mortality reduction, cost, or quality of life. Such an article that is valid and would change your practice is a POEM. Approximately 2% of the medical literature, however, is POEMs,[25] so this approach will help you eliminate the stack of unread journals at your bedside! Because the findings of a POEM have been shown to improve important patient outcomes and because they differ from your current practice, Slawson and Shaughnessy argue that you are ethically obligated to know about POEMs and apply them to your practice.[19] To learn more about

POEMs, visit the *Journal of Family Practice* POEMs Web site at http://www.infopoems.com.

4. *Learn to ask a focused clinical question.* Too often, our clinical questions are couched in terms specific to a particular patient. Asking, "What test should I order for this 28-year-old woman with chest pain?" is appropriate when talking to a human consultant, but not when searching a medical reference. Instead, asking, "What is the best test to rule out myocardial infarction in this person with chest pain and a low likelihood of disease?" is more likely to lead you to the information you need to make a decision. David Sackett and colleagues have written an excellent chapter on this topic in their book *Evidence-Based Medicine: How to Practice and Teach EBM.*[16]

5. *Let someone else do the heavy lifting.* Several excellent sources of what is called *secondary literature* are available. Each has a group of physicians trained in critical appraisal, epidemiology, and research design who identify important articles, critically appraise them for validity, and publish the results in brief synopses. Examples include the *ACP Journal Club, Journal of Family Practice* POEMs feature, *Evidence-Based Practice* newsletter, and *Evidence-Based Medicine* journal. By distilling a mountain of medical literature to the 10 or 20 most important pages every month, secondary literature makes it possible for physicians to remain up-to-date without spending inordinate amounts of time in the library.

6. *Learn to use a computer.* The best evidence-based sources of answers to clinical questions are available on computers, and a growing list of highly useful Web sites is available (see Table 17-2). In addition, you can search the MEDLINE database of the National Library of Medicine for free via the Web (http://www.nlm.nih.gov). Become familiar with excellent evidence-based sources of information such as the Cochrane Library, Best Evidence, and InfoRetriever programs. They should be your first stop for answers to clinical questions. Better yet, consider purchasing a handheld computer. Handheld computers can go where you go and help you answer your clinical questions at the bedside, in your office, in the elevator, at home, or wherever they arise.

Only by being critically reflective practitioners will we improve our practice and the health of our patients. This style of practice is not only good for our patients, it is intellectually stimulating and can help primary care physicians successfully address a wide variety of problems with greater confidence.

> Be patient toward all that is unsolved in your heart and try to love the questions themselves like locked rooms and like books that are written in a very foreign tongue. . . . Live the questions now. Perhaps you will then gradually, without noticing it, live along some distant day into the answer.

> — Rainer Maria Rilke

Acknowledgments

I would like to thank the following individuals for their thoughtful, critical review of this work and many useful suggestions: Drs. David Rovner, Margaret Holmes-Rovner, Henry Barry, David Slawson, Allen Shaughnessy, Charles Given, and Laura Bierema.

Disclosure Statement

The author is programmer of the InfoRetriever software discussed in the article and receives royalty payments from its sale. He is also co-editor of the *Journal of Family Practice* POEMs feature and co-editor of the *Evidence-Based Practice* newsletter, both from Dowden Publishing Company.

References

1. Hersh WR, Lunin LF. Introduction and overview (special issue on medical informatics). J Am Soc Inform Sci 1995;46:726–728.
2. Barrie AR, Ward AM. Questioning behaviour in general practice: a pragmatic study. BMJ 1997;315:1512–1515.
3. Covell DG, Uman GC, Manning PR. Information needs in office practice: are they being met? Ann Intern Med 1985;103:596–599.
4. Smith R. What clinical information do doctors need? BMJ 1996;313:1062–1068.
5. Woolf S. The medical information needs of internists and pediatricians at an academic medical center. Bull Med Libr Assoc 1989;77:372–380.
6. Gorman PN, Ash J, Wykoff L. Can primary care physicians' questions be answered using the medical journal literature? Bull Med Libr Assoc 1994;82:140–146.
7. Gorman PN, Helfand M. Information seeking in primary care: how physicians choose which clinical questions to pursue and which to leave unanswered. Med Decis Making 1995;15:113–119.
8. Osheroff JA, Forsythe DE, Buchanan BG, et al. Physicians' information needs: analysis of questions posed during clinical teaching. Ann Intern Med 1991;114: 576–581.
9. Kaiser PK, with the Corneal Abrasion Patching Study Group. A comparison of pressure patching versus no patching for corneal abrasions due to trauma or foreign body removal. Ophthalmology 1995;102:1936–1942.
10. Kaiser PK, Pineda R. A study of topical non-steroidal anti-inflammatory drops and no pressure patching in the treatment of corneal abrasions. Ophthalmology 1997;104:1353–1359.
11. Davis DA, Thomson MA, Oxman AD, Haynes RB. Changing physician performance. A systematic review of the effect of continuing medical education strategies. JAMA 1995;274:700–705.
12. Evans CE, Haynes RB, Birkett NJ, et al. Does a mailed continuing education program improve physician performance? Results of a randomized trial in antihypertensive care. JAMA 1986;255:501–504.
13. Knowles M. Self-Directed Learning. New York: Association Press, 1975.
14. Mezirow J. Fostering Critical Reflection in Adulthood: A Guide to Transformative and Emancipatory Learning. San Francisco: Jossey-Bass, 1990.
15. Argyris C. Reasoning, Learning, and Action: Individual and Organizational. San Francisco: Jossey-Bass, 1982.
16. Sackett DL, Richardson WS, Rosenberg W, Haynes RB. Evidence-Based Medicine: How to Practice and Teach EBM. New York: Churchill Livingstone, 1997.
17. Fitzgerald PJ, Fortner JG, Watson RC, et al. The value of diagnostic aids in detecting pancreatic cancer. Cancer 1978;41:868–879.
18. Shepherd J, Cobbe SM, Isles CG, et al. Prevention of coronary heart disease with pravastatin in men with hypercholesterolemia. N Engl J Med 1995;333:1301–1307.
19. Shaughnessy AF, Slawson DC, Bennett JH. Becoming an information master: a guidebook to the medical information jungle. J Fam Pract 1994;39:489–499.
20. Oxman AD, Sackett DL, Guyatt GH, and the Evidence-Based Medicine Working Group. Users' guides to the medical literature: How to get started. JAMA 1993;270: 2093–2095.
21. Ebell MH, Gaspar DA, Khurana S. Family physicians' preferences for computerized decision-support hardware and software. J Fam Pract 1997;45:137–141.
22. Ebell MH, Hale W, Buchanon JE, Dake P. Handheld computers for family physicians. J Fam Pract 1995;41: 385–392.
23. Ebell MH, Barry HB. InfoRetriever: Bringing evidence-based information to the point of care. MD Computing 1998;15:289–297.
24. McWhinney IR. A Textbook of Family Medicine (2nd ed). New York: Oxford University Press, 1997.
25. Ebell MH, Barry HC, Slawson DC, Shaughnessy AF. Finding POEMs in the medical literature. J Fam Pract 1999;48:350–355.

Epilogue

John P. Geyman, Richard A. Deyo, and Scott D. Ramsey

Although fueling continued intellectual and political debate in medicine, evidence-based medicine seems to be gaining wider acceptance in the United States. These gains can be explained by increasing recognition of widely divergent patterns of health care, the rise of patient autonomy, demands for care that improves function and longevity rather than surrogate end points, advances in electronic medical records and databases, and the increasing need for accountability and control of escalating costs of health care. Two clinical examples illustrate the extent of the problem for which the implementation of evidence-based medicine is being proposed as a logical approach: (1) How can a fourfold variation still exist in adjusted odds ratios for the likelihood of warfarin use for patients with atrial fibrillation in the South compared with the Midwest?[1] and (2) Why is antenatal corticosteroid therapy for preterm labor still used infrequently despite evidence from multiple randomized trials showing risk reductions of 30% for infant mortality, 50% for neonatal respiratory distress syndrome, and 70% for intracranial hemorrhage?[2]

Despite the ongoing debate about the role of evidence-based medicine, impressive signs of its wider application are already evident. Two journals devoted to the subject—*Evidence-Based Medicine* and *ACP Journal Club*—are in their fourth year of publication. Predigested newsletters that publish evidence-based abstracts are increasingly available and popular among primary care physicians. Electronic databases of best evidence, such as the Cochrane Collaboration database, are now widely available and being used more often by practicing physicians. Medical education is beginning to see new initiatives in the teaching of evidence-based medicine at predoctoral, graduate, and continuing medical education levels. The Agency for Health Care Policy and Research, meanwhile, has established a National Guidelines Clearinghouse and 12 evidence-based practice centers in the United States and Canada.[3] The first topics to be studied are important

to primary care, including management of acute chronic obstructive pulmonary disease, management of unstable angina, management of preterm labor and chronic hypertension during pregnancy, treatment of acne, and management of cancer pain.[4]

Although these gains are definite signs of progress, many barriers to the widespread application of evidence-based medicine need to be addressed if its full potential is to be realized. Perhaps most important, the burden of practice, with its requirements to respond to a growing knowledge base and a changing health care system, continue to limit the physician's time to learn and practice evidence-based medicine. In addition, high quality evidence is lacking for many diagnostic and therapeutic interventions because of time lags between the introduction of therapy and clinical trials supporting its use, or because high quality studies simply are not performed. In teaching settings, inertia and resistance are barriers for educators who have spent their careers teaching the traditional paradigm of medical education based more on "expert opinion" than outcomes research. Many of the concepts of evidence-based medicine are new to most physicians in practice today.

What is the future of economic analysis, particularly for the practicing physician? This question is difficult to answer in the United States because cost-effectiveness analysis is a discipline without official endorsement by government authorities or private health care–related organizations, such as the American Medical Association. As such, cost-effectiveness analysis must rely on its "power of persuasion" to influence medical practice. In an ideal world, health plans and physicians would review data from cost-effectiveness studies and select the most cost-effective therapies for use in practice, given the budget constraints of the health plan and each patient. By reducing spending on inefficient health services—that is, those that offer little health improvement for dollars spent relative to alternative therapies—health dollars could be spent where they would do the most good (including providing care for those who currently lack access to health care). Several barriers are blocking the realization of this ideal.

The first important barrier is what we term an *information problem*. There will never be enough cost-effectiveness studies to address the needs of decision makers. The cost-effectiveness analysis literature has not kept up with the introduction rate of new technologies and has addressed only a small fraction of important questions considering use of existing technologies. The former problem may be less of an issue in the future because cost-effectiveness studies are now routinely introduced into clinical trials sponsored by both private industry and government agencies. Another barrier is the fact that decision makers simply do not have the training and time to review the cost-effectiveness analysis literature on every new and existing medical intervention. Although we hope this book helps with the training issue, the problems of keeping up with the sheer volume of information—something we also face with the clinical medical literature—still remains. Nevertheless, as we have seen for evidence-based medicine applied to the clinical literature, not all studies warrant our attention in the first place. We expect to see more systematic reviews that are devoted to reviewing and selecting the most salient, methodologically sound cost-effectiveness studies.

A more important problem than issues of information, however, is that cost-effectiveness analysis operates under a set of assumptions that do not necessarily match those of the primary decision makers in health care—namely, patients and their physicians. As mentioned in Chapter 11, cost-effectiveness analysis seeks to maximize health from a societal perspective. Individual patients and physicians are not expected to act in the best interests of society. Patients make decisions about what is best for them. Because health insurance drastically reduces the out-of-pocket costs most patients face, they can choose relatively inefficient health services that provide small (but positive) benefits at a high cost to their health plan but a relatively low cost to them. This problem can be compounded if the physician has a financial incentive to provide the inefficient service.

Other nations have addressed the problem of getting individuals to act in the best interests of society by creating regulations that ensure cost-effectiveness analysis is part of the decision making process. Canada and Australia, for example, require that information on cost-effectiveness be submitted alongside clinical data before a new drug or device is considered for their national formularies. The United States is unlikely to adopt this type of regulatory approach, however, in the absence of nationalized health insurance or a consensus regarding the scientific validity and usefulness of cost-effectiveness analysis. At present, the introduction of national health insurance seems even less likely than the formulation of cost-effectiveness analysis guidelines! Cost-effectiveness analysis, therefore, remains without "teeth" for the foreseeable future. Decision makers have to determine ways in which economic data can be used to give their organization relative advantage compared with competitors.

We feel that as costs and competition increase in the health care market, clever organizations will see that cost-effectiveness analysis can be used to help them reduce their use of services that offer little benefit for a high cost. Ultimately, by restricting use of *specific* services, cost-effectiveness analysis may be able to help health insurers expand coverage *in general*, at competitive costs. Ironically, the pressures to use cost-effectiveness analysis will likely come from the major purchasers of insurance (i.e., employers and state and federal governments) rather than directly from physicians and patients.

Where does this leave us for the new millennium? We believe that evidence-based medicine has made a good start and shows promise as an integral part of medical education and clinical practice but that it is still a young and emerging field. Evidence-based medicine is a discipline, not a remedy for our shortcomings as practitioners. As such, it is not a panacea, but its adherents feel it has much to offer for improving patient care. In this book, we have introduced primary care physicians and others interested in a changing health care system to the major concepts and approaches developing in this young field. We can be certain that the profile and applications of evidence-based medicine in another 10 years will be quite different from those today. If this book enables more primary care physicians to gain a broader understanding of the strengths and limitations of evidence-based medicine, it will have been successful.

References

1. Stafford RS, Singer DE. National patterns of warfarin use in atrial fibrillation. Arch Intern Med 1996;156:2537–2541.
2. Bronstein JM, Goldenberg RL. Practice variations in the use of corticosteroids: a comparison of eight datasets. Am J Obstet Gynecol 1995;173:296–298.
3. Marwick C. Proponents gather to discuss practicing evidence-based medicine. JAMA 1997;278:531–532.
4. AHCPR announces new studies for evidence-based practice centers. Am Fam Physician 1999;59:14.

Glossary

Evidence-Based Medicine Glossary*

Linda E. Pinsky, Joyce E. Wipf, and Scott D. Ramsey

Absolute Risk Reduction: Absolute difference in the rate of events between the control and intervention groups. Absolute risk reduction = events in control group − events in interventions group[1]

Bias: A systematic error that leads to results that do not represent the true findings.[2] See *lead-time bias*, *length time bias*, and *publication bias*.

Blinding:
  Double-Blind Study Design: Neither the subjects nor the researchers know whether the subject is in the placebo or treatment group.
  Single-Blind Study Design: The subjects do not know whether they are in the placebo or treatment group.[2]

Case-Control Studies: Retrospective studies beginning with people who have a disease and controls who do not have the disease. The investigator then looks retrospectively to see what proportion in each group was exposed to the same risk factors.[3]

Bad outcome → Exposed (a)
Bad outcome → Not exposed (c)

Good outcome → Exposed (b)
Good outcome → Not exposed (d)

Some Strengths	Some Weaknesses
Useful for study of rare diseases	Participants may have a recall bias
Less expensive	Selection bias possible in choice of controls

Findings expressed as an odds ratio.

Causality: Determination of causality.[2]
  Susceptible host → disease
  1. Suspected cause precedes disease.
  2. Association is strong.
  3. No likely noncausal basis for the association.
  4. Association makes biological sense.
  5. Magnitude of association is strongest when it is predicted to be so.
     a. Increased exposure = increased risk
     b. Increased susceptibility = increased risk

---

*Portions of the glossary originally appearing in a University of Washington Web site on Advanced Physical Diagnosis (http://eduserv.hscer.washington.edu/physdx) are copyrighted by the University of Washington and are reprinted with permission.

Chance Node: Chance nodes identify points where one or more of several possible events that are beyond the control of the decision maker may occur. Chance nodes for the same events should align horizontally in the decision tree.[4]

Charges: The posted prices of provider services. Charge is the amount the hospital, clinic, physician, or pharmacy attempts to recover (or bills) for a good or service.[5]

Cohort Studies: Observational studies—prospective or retrospective—in which groups are assembled according to exposure or lack of exposure, then followed longitudinally to determine outcomes (e.g., fractions who develop a disease).[3]

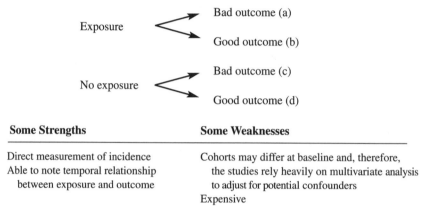

Some Strengths	Some Weaknesses
Direct measurement of incidence	Cohorts may differ at baseline and, therefore,
Able to note temporal relationship	the studies rely heavily on multivariate analysis
between exposure and outcome	to adjust for potential confounders
	Expensive

Findings expressed as relative risk.

Confidence Interval: The imprecision of study sample estimates as population values. The wider the confidence limit, the less precise is the estimate. Confidence intervals of 95% are most commonly presented, meaning that a 95% chance exists that the indicated range includes the true value in the population sampled. Confidence intervals are affected by sample size, variability in the characteristic being measured, and the degree of confidence required.[6]

Confounders: Patient characteristics that may affect the results a study is trying to measure. Because these factors may be unevenly distributed (i.e., nonrandom) between study groups, they can decrease the validity of the study.[2]

Cost-Benefit Analysis: An analytic tool for estimating the net social benefit of a program or intervention as the incremental benefit of the program minus the incremental cost, with all benefits and costs measured in dollars.[6]

Cost-Consequence Analysis: An analytic tool in which the components of incremental costs and consequences of alternative programs are computed and listed without any attempt to aggregate these results.[6]

Cost-Effectiveness Analysis: The efficacy of a program in achieving given intervention outcomes in relation to the program costs. The intervention outcomes are expressed in terms such as years of life saved or cases of cancer detected, rather than in dollars.[7]

Costs: The actual resource expenditure to provide a service, as opposed to the amount charged. Resources can be the value of time or any other input in its highest value use or the benefits lost because the next-best alternative was not selected.[6]

Decision Analysis: An explicit, quantitative, systematic approach to decision making under conditions of uncertainty in which probabilities of each possible event, along with the consequences of those events, are stated explicitly.[6]

Decision Node: Decision nodes identify points at which alternative actions that are under the control of the decision maker exist. In the simplest problem, the decision node describes the problem.[4]

Discounting: A process used to convert future dollars to their present value. For policy making, future dollars are discounted to present terms for two reasons: (1) Money available today has a higher value than the same amount of money that is available in the future, and (2) individuals have a positive time preference—that is, they would rather consume today than delay consumption until some time in the future. Although developed to account for intertemporal decision making regarding money, the method of discounting is also applied to health to express future outcomes in terms of their present value.[8]

Effectiveness: The ability of an intervention to achieve the desired results under usual conditions.[2]

Efficacy: The ability of an intervention to achieve the desired results under ideal conditions.[2]

Incremental Cost-Effectiveness (Ratio): The ratio of the difference in *costs* between two alternatives to the difference in *effectiveness* between the same two alternatives.[6]

Incidence: The number of new cases of disease within a given time.[3]

Kappa Statistic: Kappa is a chance-corrected measure of agreement between pairs of observers. It reflects the degree of agreement for an interpretation, diagnostic finding, or decision. A high level of agreement generally occurs when kappa values are more than 0.5. Agreement is poor when kappa values are less than 0.3.[1]

Lead-Time Bias: Apparent lengthening of survival due to earlier diagnosis in the course of disease but without any actual prolongation of life.[1]

Length Bias: Bias due to the tendency of screening tests to detect a larger number of cases of slowly progressing disease and miss aggressive disease due to its rapid progression.[1]

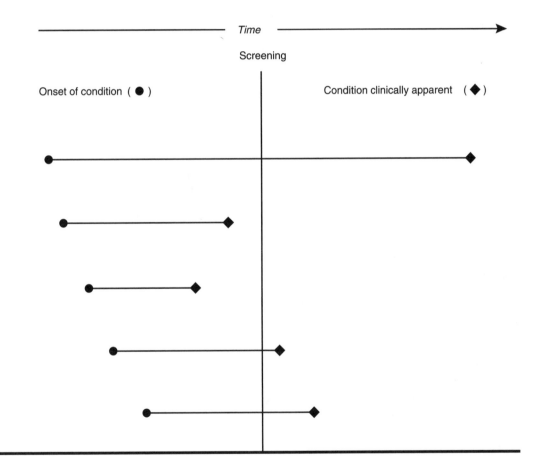

Likelihood Ratios: The odds of disease given a specified test value divided by the odds of disease in the study population.[1] **Negative Likelihood Ratio (LR–):** The ratio of something clinicians do not want (false-negative error rate) divided by something they do want (specificity). It shows how much the odds of disease are decreased if the test result is negative.

$$LR- = \frac{specificity}{1 - sensitivity}$$

How small is a small LR–?

0.0–0.1	Large change from pretest to post-test probability
0.1–0.2	Moderate change
0.2–0.5	Small, but sometimes important changes in probability
0.5–1.0	Rarely important change

Positive Likelihood Ratio (LR+): The ratio of something that clinicians do want in a test (sensitivity) divided by something they do not want (false-positive error rate). It indicates how much the odds of disease is increased if the test result is positive.

$$LR+ = \frac{\text{sensitivity}}{1 - \text{specificity}}$$

How big is a big LR+?

1.0	The test is useless
1.0–2.0	Rarely important change from pretest to post-test probability
2.0–5.0	Small change
5.0–10	Moderate change
>10	Large change

Magnitude Estimation: A technique from psychophysics wherein judges are asked to rate the magnitude of the sensation produced by one stimulus versus another as a ratio (e.g., "2.5 times as much").[6]

Managed Care Organizations: (1) An integrated system of health insurance, financing, and service delivery functions involving risk sharing for the delivery of health services and defined networks of providers.[9] (2) Any system of health payment or delivery arrangements in which the health plan attempts to control or coordinate use of health services by its enrolled members to contain health expenditures, improve quality, or both. Arrangements often involve a defined delivery system of providers with some form of contractual arrangement with the plan.

Multi-Attribute Utility Theory: In measuring preferences or utilities for health states, multiple attributes are often involved: mobility, ambulation, emotional dysfunction, physical activity, and so forth. In multi-attribute utility theory, the evaluation task is broken down into attributes, and single attributes are evaluated using different numeric estimation methods, such as category scaling, standard gamble, or time trade-off. Trade-offs among attributes are then quantified as importance weights or other scaling factors. Finally, formal models are applied to reaggregate the single-attribute evaluations.[8]

Negative Predictive Value: See *Predictive Value.*

Number Needed to Treat (NNT): Number of people needed to treat to prevent one bad outcome.[3]

$$NNT = \frac{1}{\text{Absolute risk reduction}} = \frac{1}{\text{Events}_{\text{in control group}} - \text{Events}_{\text{in intervention group}}}$$

Odds Ratio[3]:

$$\text{Odds ratio} = \frac{\text{Risk of disease in exposed}}{\text{Risk of disease in unexposed}} = \begin{array}{l} a/b \text{ where } a < b, \text{ so } a + b \approx b \\ c/d \text{ where } c < d, \text{ so } c + d \approx d \end{array}$$

To calculate *a, b, c, d*, see the 2 × 2 table.

Opportunity Costs: A term for the costs of not being able to do something because you did something else. It is often used in analyzing the competing costs in medical care when making decisions about allocating resources. For example, if providers spend time with each patient talking about screening for hemachromatosis, they may not have time for discussion of smoking cessation with the patients.[10]

Outcome: The consequence of a medical intervention on a patient.[11]

Outcomes and Effectiveness Research: Sometimes called *outcomes research.* Medical or health services research that attempts to identify the clinical outcomes (including mortality, morbidity, and functional status) of the delivery of health care.[11]

Perspective: The viewpoint from which a cost-effectiveness analysis is conducted. For example, the patient's viewpoint (out-of-pocket costs), the provider's viewpoint, the payer's viewpoint, and society's viewpoint (including medical and social costs) may differ.[1]

Predictive Value[1]:

For both PPV and NPV, use the following table for calculations:

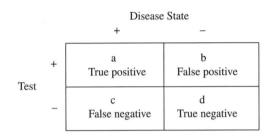

Negative Predictive Value (NPV): Proportion of persons with a negative test result who do not have the condition.

$$ NPV \ = \ \frac{d}{d+c} \quad or \quad \frac{True\ negative}{All\ negative} $$

Positive Predictive Value (PPV): Proportion of persons with a positive test result who have the condition.

$$ PPV \ = \ \frac{a}{a+b} \quad or \quad \frac{True\ positive}{All\ positive} $$

Preferences: Judgements of the desirability of a particular set of outcomes or situations that describe what is labeled "good" or "bad." Connotes the exact meaning of value, desirability, or utility of health states. See also *Utility.*[8]

Prevalence: The number of cases of disease in a population at a given time (frequency).[3]

Probability[1]:

Post-test Probability: The probability of a disease after a given test result. Its value depends on the pretest probability of the disease and the test's sensitivity and specificity.

Pretest Probability: The prevalence of disease in a specified group of subjects. Although the overall prevalence may be known, the disease status for each individual may be unknown before a diagnostic test.

Publication Bias: Bias resulting from the tendency for certain studies, particularly those with positive results or large number of participants, to be published, whereas those with negative results or smaller studies are not.[3]

Quality-Adjusted Life Year (QALY): Quality of life expectancy takes into account not only the length of life but also the quality of life during the period of extended life. It acknowledges that fates worse than death exist.[4] An analysis that uses QALYs seeks to evaluate the trade-off between mortality, morbidity, and the preferences of patients and society to accept a shortening of life to avoid certain morbidities. The concept of the QALY is that people are willing to take a measurable risk of a bad outcome to achieve certain states of health.[4]

Randomized Control Studies: Experimental studies in which people are randomly assigned to an intervention or control group. The randomization refers to allocation among study groups, not to eligibility for the trial.[3]

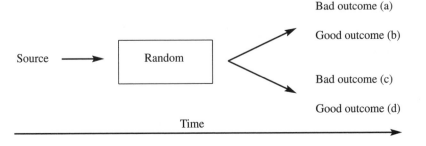

Some Strengths	Some Weaknesses
Randomizing makes group comparable for even unknown factors	May not be appropriate for ethical or practical reasons
Double-blind design minimizes observer	Expensive

Findings expressed as relative risk.

Rating Scale (Category Scaling): Scales comprised of distinct categories. The categories are often numerical, such as 0, 1, 2, . . . 10; the phenomenon being rated must be assigned to only one category. Numeric categories often are treated as equal-interval in analyses. In psychology, sometimes referred to as the *method of equal-appearing intervals*.[6]

Recall Bias: Subjects may inaccurately recall medical history or previous exposures. Such bias is especially a concern in retrospective studies in which the presence of a disease (or a particular outcome) may bias subjects' recall of their exposure to a putative risk factor.[1]

Receiver Operator Curves: A graph plotting the true-positive against the false-positive rate (1 – specificity) over a series of cutoffs for defining a positive test. A diagonal line indicates no ability to distinguish persons with and without the condition. The farther the curve reaches toward the upper left corner of the graph, the better the test is in distinguishing diseased from nondiseased persons.[1]

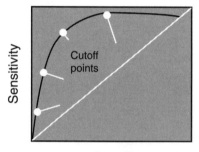

Historical note: Receiver operator curves are derived from British radar operators during World War II. The goal was to find the correct technique to identify all incoming airplanes without giving too many false warnings. By plotting the sensitivity and specificity cutoffs of the more and less successful radar operators, the best combination of sensitivity and specificity could be determined.

Reimbursements: The amount actually paid by the individual or the third-party payer for the good or service.[4]

Relative Risk[6]**:**

$$\text{Relative risk} = \frac{\text{Risk of disease in exposed}}{\text{Risk of disease in unexposed}} = \frac{a/a + b}{c/c + d}$$

To calculate *a, b, c, d*, see the 2 × 2 table.

Reliability: The ability of a test to obtain the same results when repeated under the same conditions.[2]
Risk Aversion: Preference for a certain rather than an uncertain outcome.[8]
Risk Neutral: Indifference to certain and uncertain outcomes.[8]
Risk Seeking: Preference for uncertain rather than certain outcomes.[8]
Sensitivity: Proportion of persons with the condition who test positive for the condition.[2]

$$\text{Sensitivity} = \frac{a}{a + c} \quad \text{or} \quad \frac{\text{True positive test results}}{\text{All patients with disease}}$$

Use the following table to calculate:

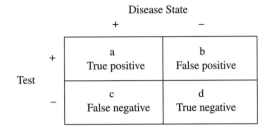

Sensitivity Analysis: A procedure for determining the robustness of an analytic result by systematically varying the values assigned to important variables in the analysis.[8]

Specificity: Proportion of persons without a condition whose test results are negative for the condition.[2]

$$\text{Specificity} \quad = \quad \frac{d}{d + b} \quad \text{or} \quad \frac{\text{True negative test results}}{\text{All patients without disease}}$$

Use the following table to calculate:

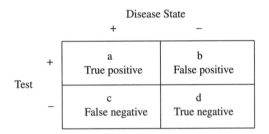

Standard Gamble Technique: In cost-effectiveness analysis, an approach to determining the utility of a particular outcome from a particular perspective. Judges (e.g., patients) must choose between a certain outcome and a gamble—that is, between a "a sure thing" and a gamble in which the probability is P that perfect health is the outcome and $1 - P$ that immediate death is the outcome. The probability P is varied until the preference for the sure thing—the certainty of the particular health state—is equal to the preference for the gamble. The probability P for which the expected utility of the two choices is equal is then a measure of the preference for the health state and satisfies (by construction) the requirements for a von Neumann–Morgenstern utility.[6]

Surrogate Marker: An alternative marker used in studies as a replacement for a true clinical outcome. Recent studies highlight the possible discrepancies between intermediate and end point markers. Encainide and flecainide (anti-arrhythmic medications), for example, were shown to reduce ventricular arrhythmia (surrogate end point) but increase mortality (true clinical outcome).[3]

Table (2 × 2 Table): Epidemiologic investigation into risk factors or test accuracy often uses the 2 × 2 table format.

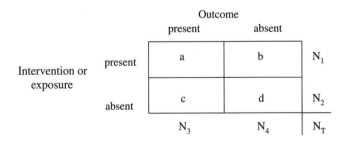

See *Relative Risk*, *Odds Ratio*, *Sensitivity*, and *Specificity* for formulas.

Technology Assessment: A form of policy research that evaluates technology for providing decision makers with information on different policy options. These options may include the allocation of resources to research and development, development of regulations or legislation, and setting standards or guidelines for health planning and health practice.[8]

Terminal Node: An end point in a decision analysis. It usually represents a final, constant state of health or death.[4]

Time Trade-Off Technique: The time trade-off method was developed as an alternative to the standard gamble by Torrance, Thomas, and Sackett.[12] The time trade-off method presents the rater with a choice between two alternatives that both have a certain outcome. The rater must decide how many years of life he or she is willing to give up to be in the healthier state compared with the less healthy one.[4]

Types of Studies: See *Randomized Control Studies, Cohort Studies, Case-Control Studies.*

Utility: A concept in economics, psychology, and decision analysis referring to the preference for, or desirability of, a particular outcome. In the context of health-related quality of life measurement, utility refers to the preference of the rater (usually a patient or a member of the general public) for a particular health outcome or health state. The health state being evaluated may be a state that has been recently experienced by the patient, is being experienced by the patient at the time the instrument is administered, or may be described as a hypothetical health state. It is important to distinguish between utility scores obtained from interviews of patients (especially for states they have experienced or are experiencing) and scores obtained from interviews of members of the general public for whom the health states are generally hypothetical. Scores obtained from members of the general public for hypothetical states are sometimes called *social preference* (or *utility*) scores. If the respondent evaluates the desirability of the health state on behalf of him- or herself, as if he or she were experiencing the health state, then the resulting score is not strictly a social utility. If, on the other hand, the respondent evaluates the desirability of the health state on behalf of members of society in general, then the score may accurately be labeled as a social utility or social preference.[8]

Values: "Standards of the desirable" that influence selective behavior. In this view, "a value is a conception, explicit or implicit, distinctive of an individual or characteristic of a group, of the desirable which influences the selection from available modes, means and ends of action."[8,13]

Variability[3]**:**
   Interobserver Variability: Variation in test results by different observers. This variability is often quantified with the kappa statistic.
   Intraobserver Variability: Variation in test results during repeat testing by the same observer.

Willingness to Pay: A method of valuing health that is based on the amount of money that individuals are willing to pay either to reduce the probability of death due to a given disease or to increase the probability of cure for a given disease. The willingness-to-pay approach is an alternative to the human capital method for expressing health benefits in monetary units.[8]

References

1. Jekel JF, Elmore JG, Katz DL. Epidemiology, Biostatistics, and Preventive Medicine. Philadelphia: Saunders, 1996.
2. Last JM. A Dictionary of Epidemiology (2nd ed). New York: Oxford University Press, 1988.
3. Fletcher RH, Fletcher SW, Wagner EH. Clinical Epidemiology: The Essentials (3rd ed). Baltimore: Williams & Wilkins, 1996.
4. Petitti DB. Meta-Analysis Decision Analysis and Cost-Effectiveness Analysis: Methods for Quantitative Synthesis in Medicine. New York: Oxford University Press, 1994.
5. Medicare Payment Advisory Commission. Report to the Congress: Medicare Payment Policy, March 1998.
6. Gold MR, Siegel JE, Russell LB, Weinstein MC. Cost Effectiveness in Health and Medicine. New York: Oxford University Press, 1996.
7. Rossi PH, Freeman HE. Evaluation: A Systemic Approach. Newbury Park, CA: Sage Publications, 1993.
8. Patrick DL, Erickson P. Health Status and Health Policy: Allocating Resources to Health Care. New York: Oxford University Press, 1993.
9. Washington State Department of Health. Public Health Improvement Plan, A Progress Report. Olympia, WA: Washington State Department of Health, March 1994.
10. Pindyck RS, Rubinfeld DL. Microeconomics (3rd ed). Upper Saddle River, NJ: Prentice Hall, 1995.
11. Physician Payment Review Commission. Annual Report to Congress. Washington, DC: Physician Payment Review Commission, 1996.
12. Torrance GW, Thomas WH, Sackett DL. A utility maximization model for evaluation of health care programs. Health Services Res 1972;7:118–133.
13. Kluckholn CK. Values and Value Orientations in the Theory of Action. In T Parsons, EA Shils (eds), Toward a General Theory of Action. Cambridge, MA: Harvard University Press, 1951.

Index

Note: Page numbers followed by *f* indicate figures; page numbers followed by *t* indicate tables;page numbers followed by *fm* indicate forms.

Other Books from

BUTTERWORTH HEINEMANN

Effective Medical Testifying by William Tsushima and Kenneth Nakano

1998   232pp   pb   0-7506-9986-8

Health Law and Policy by Bryan Liang

1999   352pp   pb   0-7506-71076

Primary Care of the Native American Patient by James Galloway, Bruce Goldberg and Joseph Alpert

1999   416pp   pb   0-7506-9989-2

Neurology in Primary Care by Joseph Friedman

1998   232pp   pb   0-7506-7036-3

Headache by Egilius L.H. Spierings

1998   236pp   pb   0-7506-7128-9

Medical Spanish: The Instant Survival Guide, Third Edition by Cynthia Wilber and Susan Lister

1995   368pp   sb   0-7506-9597-8

Visit our web site at: www.bh.com

These books are available in bookstores or in case of difficulty call:
1-800-366-2665 in the U.S. or +44-1865-310366 in Europe.

JOIN THE BUTTERWORTH-HEINEMANN E-MAIL LIST!!!

An e-mail mailing list giving information on latest releases, special promotions, offers and other news relating to Butterworth-Heinemann titles is available. To subscribe, send an e-mail message to majordomo@world.std.com. Include in message body (not in subject line): subscribe bh-medical